Blood and Sand

THE WEST ASIAN TRAGEDY

Blood and Sand

THE WEST ASIAN TRAGEDY

S. Nihal Singh

CBS Publishers & Distributors

New Delhi • Bangalore

Blood and Sand
The West Asian Tragedy

First Edition : 2003

Copyright © 2003, S. Nihal Singh

All photographs by the author

ISBN : 81-239-0959-4

Production Director : Vinod K. Jain

Published by :
Satish Kumar Jain for CBS Publishers & Distributors,
4596/1-A, 11 Darya Ganj, New Delhi - 110 002 (India)
• E-mail : cbspubs@del3.vsnl.net.in
• Website : http://www.cbspd.com

Branch Office :
Seema House, 2975, 17th Cross, K.R. Road,
Bansankari 2nd Stage, Bangalore - 560070
• Fax : 080-6771680 • E-mail : cbsbng@vsnl.net

Printed at :
Meenakshi Printers, Delhi-110006

Introduction

These are cameos of the tragedy and heartbreaks of the Israeli–Palestinian confrontation, culled from my writings stretching over the past two decades and more. The present selection has been subjected to minimal editing to give a flavour of those times and the hopes and despair that punctuated them. My hope is that this volume will illumine in a measure the ramifications of the Palestinian tragedy as it affects Palestinians, other Arabs, Israelis and the wider world. Oil has not been an unmixed blessing for the states that have this natural resource in great abandon. While oil has brought immense wealth to states, it has attracted the interest of the more powerful nations, in particular the United States, and their desire to gain profit and control access, if not the local governments.

The founding of the Israeli state brought an explosive intrusion into the Arab world, which has been unsuccessfully coping with the ensuing tensions, including wars, ever since. As American power and influence grew after World War II and Britain's contracted, Washington took over London's role with this difference. The absorption of a substantial number of Jewish refugees during and after the war and their wealth and power added an emotional and political edge to American policies, buttressed by American Jews' capacity to influence presidential and congressional elections. Today the American Jewish lobby — lobbies being an accepted part of American political life — pretty much runs the contours of Washington's West Asian policy.

The end of the Cold War and the demise of the Soviet Union brought their own compulsions. Towards the end of his second term, President Bill Clinton unsuccessfully tried to find a basis for a settlement of the Israeli–Palestinian conflict. But the Bush administration has practically given up on such an endeavour, preferring instead to train its guns on Yasser Arafat and give full support to Ariel Sharon while plotting a military invasion of Iraq to take President Saddam Hussein out. American priorities changed after the events of September 11, 2001, the Palestinian suicide bombings merging with the larger American "war on terror" cleverly exploited by Sharon. In any event, the mix of a new American feeling of vulnerability and growing consciousness of its omnipotence has become a deadly combination. The old adage of "if you are not with us, you are against us" has been brought back from the days of the Cold War. The Bush administration's approach is to treat dissenters — individuals and nations — with contempt and there seems little patience or tolerance for the Arab world.

At a time President George W. Bush is planning a new military attack on Iraq, it is interesting to revisit the start of the Second Gulf War through the eyes of one who was in Baghdad. I was witness to the first days of President Saddam Hussein and his government seeking to cope with the American-led attacks to prise Kuwait out of the Iraqi grasp, miraculously leaving him in power after his defeat.

S. Nihal Singh

Contents

5 The Imperial Power   223

6   India and West Asia   299

Epilogue   329

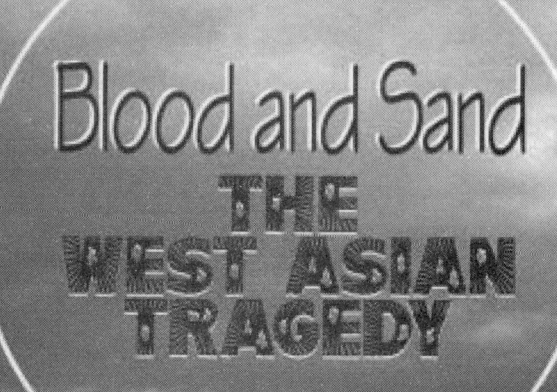

Blood and Sand
THE WEST ASIAN TRAGEDY

What was it like to be in Baghdad as the bombs started falling in the Second Gulf War? Or being cooped up on the floor of the bomb shelter of the Al Rashid hotel while paying for a room that could not be used. These are some nuggets from this selection of the writings of an intrepid foreign correspondent and editor who has roamed far and wide. Painstakingly, over the years and decades, the author has recorded the West Asian tragedy.

The central Israeli–Palestinian confrontation comes in many shapes and sizes but it adds up to the continuing occupation of Palestinian land by Israel, thanks to full-throated American support. The September 11, 2001 events have merely served to enable Israel to wrap up its repressive policies in the new American paradigm of fighting terrorism, with disastrous consequences for Palestinians.

In the popular American mind, there is no distinction between those who took over civilian planes to use them as missiles to demolish the World Trade Centre towers in New York and part of the Pentagon and suicide bombers who answer Israeli F-16s, helicopter gunships and armoured cars with their bodies. If Israelis and their American protectors believe that the scourge of terrorism can be vanquished by depriving Palestinians of their state and nationhood, they are living in a fool's paradise.

If America does go to war against Iraq, its neoconservative rulers would be tempted to reorder the map of West Asia. Along that path would lie more bloodshed, more Palestinian suffering and more terrorism. The injustice being done to Palestinians will continue to fuel terrorism.

Neighbours

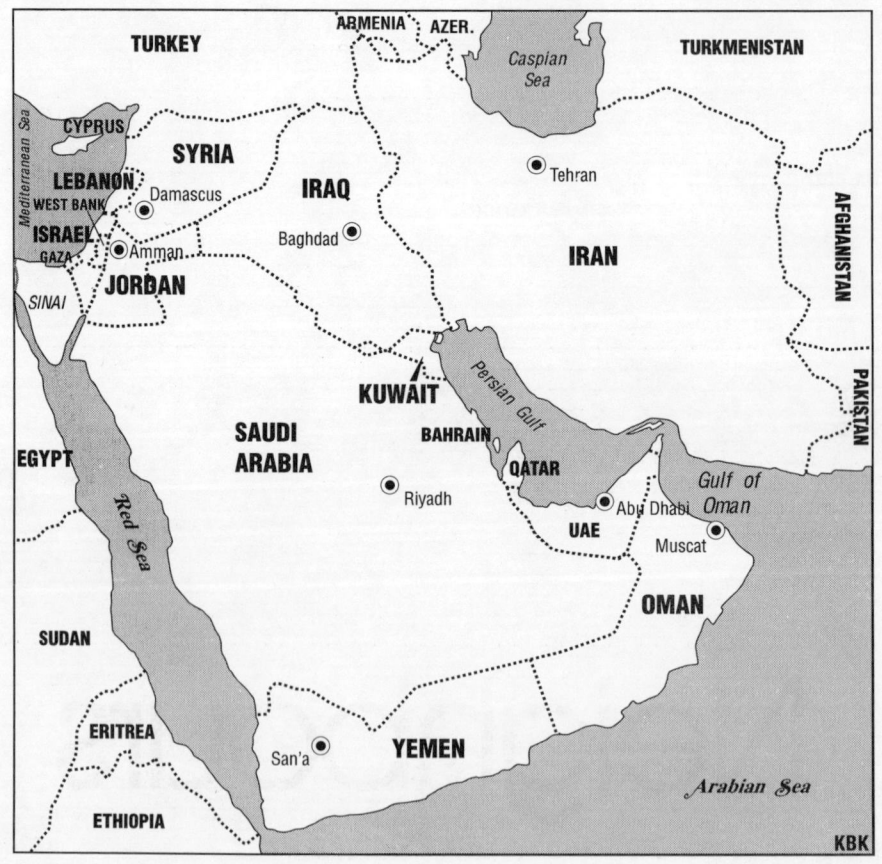

IRAN

The Shah Goes, 1979

The Iranian crisis, the outcome of which was of vital interest to India and the better part of the world, was a classic example of the interaction among domestic circumstances and the instruments of modern power. Shah Raza Pahlavi was an autocrat, an absolute monarch, who suppressed dissent ruthlessly while seeking to take his country to the front rank of industrial and military powers. At the same time, he was able to convince one superpower, the USA, that the American interest lay in giving him more and more weapons of war so that he could be an effective regional policeman to protect Western interests, particularly safeguard the vital routes through the Persian Gulf and the Straits of Hormuz.

The Shah was brought back to the throne with American assistance in 1953 after the overthrow of Mossadeq. He quickly set about buttressing his position and that of the throne and never looked back despite numerous plots. He concentrated all power in his hands; the ministers and the officially sponsored party were his creatures. He kept a watchful eye on the army while pampering it with high salaries and perquisites and the most expensive toys of war. His method of governing was to alternate spells of repression, including torture, with periods of relative relaxation. And his ambitions grew for spreading the glories of the Pahlavi dynasty and his country farther afield.

The Oil Revolution

The Shah's big break came with the oil revolution of 1973 when oil was successfully used as an instrument of power and its price was quadrupled. His dreams grew to seemingly fantastic proportions. He said in October 1975 that his objective was to follow the West German model, implying an increase in the per capita GNP from $1,344 in 1973 to $5,600 in a decade. The targets for the modernisation plan for 1985 were car production passing the million mark, steel production 20 million tons and Teheran as the financial capital of West Asia bridging Zurich and Tokyo.

Together with a wide-ranging industrialisation programme, including the decision to go in for the most ambitious atomic power programme in the region, the Shah set about furiously arming his defence forces with the latest and best in US arsenal. The Americans were, at any rate, grateful to the Shah for not joining the Arab oil boycott of Israel, and the Shah demonstrated his capacity to play the regional policeman's role by sending troops to Oman in support of the Sultan and helping Somalia in its war with Ethiopia, apart from using them to seize three Gulf islands, Abu Musa and the Tunbs, in 1971.

The American involvement with Iran took shape after World War II and grew with the withdrawal of the traditional imperial power, Britain, from the Persian Gulf. US interests were to prevent Russian encroachment (the then USSR shared a 3,000 km long border with Iran), assure the sea lanes and oil supplies for its own profligate style of living as well as for Israel and its allies in Europe, and to have a moderate friendly power to calm Arab passions in the Arab-Israeli conflict. The Shah seemed to fill the bill admirably, and although it became necessary to humour him with more and more arms, paid for in cash, the political price was considered well worth it. Already in 1974 Iran's military budget had jumped to $5,604 million from $961 million in 1970 and in 1976-77 Iran's military expenditure was $9.5 billion, about 45 per cent of its oil revenues. Warnings from such men as Senator Edward Kennedy as early as October 1975 to reconsider

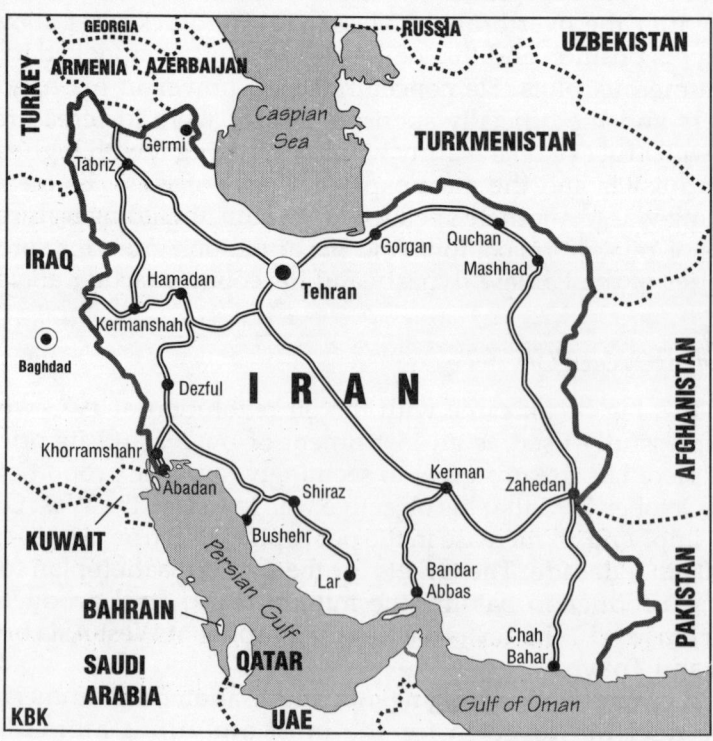

arms sales in the light of their possible repercussions fell on deaf ears in Washington.

The Shah, indeed, proved more than a match for the Americans in diplomacy. First, he convinced everyone that he was synonymous with Iran and ran a successful public relations campaign in the US to soften criticism against his policies of repressing dissent at home, through torture and the nastiness of the SAVAK secret police organisation. His triumph was in befriending President Carter, who had unfurled his human rights programme after assuming office. Despite the Shah's record, Carter paid an official visit to Iran to heap fulsome praise upon his host.

On the other hand, the Shah had not entirely neglected the Soviet Union, the secondary superpower. He came to an agreement with the Russians on exchanging Iranian gas for a steel mill the Russians had agreed to build. Despite his suspicions of the Soviet Union, the Shah was perhaps trying to demonstrate that close as his relations with the US were, he was no American puppet. In any event, his deals with Russia were in tune with his ambitions of what could be described as a West Asian co-prosperity sphere. His dream was to acquire the status of Britain or France in the global hierarchy of powers by 1990.

Like all dictators, the Shah failed to reckon with the strength of dissent in his country. He did not realise that he was building up a revolutionary situation by his own actions. On the one hand, he was sending hundreds of thousands of Iranians for study abroad to help build the infrastructure for a modern Iran, seemingly oblivious of the political and social problems he was creating; on the other hand, he had alienated the religious elements, particularly the *mujtahids*, who traditionally played an important role in the social and moral life of the country. Through curbs on their activities and land reforms and by controlling religious endowments, he created a growing extremist force by the very severity of his regime's repression, the worst phase being the 1971-76 period. Superimposed on these developments was the element of growing corruption at the top which enveloped his own family, and, it is widely believed, the Shah himself.

Tide of Protests

The fuse was lit in 1978 by a relaxation in the repression, and there was no turning back the tide of protest. The religious elements combined with the leftists to force the Shah to take what is euphemistically called a vacation abroad. Ayatollah Khomeini had served as the spiritual mentor of the movement from his perch abroad. Yet the success of the agitation was surely due to the middle class who gave the movement universality. This middle class represented the new elite which was denied its share of the political cake even as it participated in the country's prosperity. It was around 25 per cent of the population, which included merchants and businessmen.

The future of Iran was clouded by the inevitable problems of evolving a new political system out of the debris of the Shah's Iran, with the contradictory pulls of the religious factions and the leftists watched by an army whose officers felt let down by the unceremonious departure of their monarch who looked after them so well.

The events in Iran held lessons not only for the superpowers and countries like India but also, and particularly, for Iran's neighbours of the oil-producing variety. How could primitive feudal countries flushed with funds but with sparse populations, cope with the problem of achieving rapid industrialisation without inviting cataclysmic changes? They did not have a large foreign labour force on a permanent basis, involving as it does in its own problems, and had to build their own infrastructure by training their men and women in modern technology and management. Yet this very action carried the seeds of dissent. People educated in a liberal environment rebel against feudalism and demand a say in governance.

Iran had already overextended itself and was beginning to pare down some of its overambitious plans. The governments of Shapour Baktiar or its successors inevitably needed to take this process further. Iran's oil resources were, in any event, expected to begin declining in the mid-1980s. There were indications that Iran's oil-producing neighbours had been reassessing their plans against the background of the social and political factors involved and many of them planned to further slow down their march into the twentieth century after developments in Iran.

The security and strategic problems thrown up by the Iranian crisis were of greater interest to the superpowers, and also to the rest of the world. For the US, the anti-Shah demonstrations, culminating in the departure of its greatest ally in the Persian Gulf, had been a traumatic experience. There were about 50,000 Americans in Iran in the business, technical, and military fields, and there was total identification of the US Administration with the Shah. This made them the targets of anger. Characteristically, the immediate reaction of Washington was to send a symbolic fire-fighting force to Saudi Arabia to reassure the other staunch ally in the area of continuing American support.

Perhaps Washington had drawn some comfort from the fact that the Iranians were traditionally suspicious of the Russians and did not wish easily to "fall a prey to Soviet blandishments", despite the leftists' sympathies for communism. Besides, whatever the character of the government that was to settle down in office, the Iranians needed to sell their oil to the West and import technology. It was clear that the Baktiar Government or any other successor regime had to be more in tune with Arab sentiment on Israel and the observance of religious codes. If indeed it had been a middle class revolt and this segment asserted itself, Iran might have seen a friendly moderate government in office, instead of an obscurantist one.

A Revolution Gone Awry

Revolutions are seldom gentlemanly affairs, and in as combustible an area as West Asia, it was inevitable that the Iranian revolution did not only claim its own victims but also spread shock waves in the region and around the world. To an extent, Iran had lived up to Ayatollah Khomeini's initial billing; indeed, it had done more by tangling with the Americans and using them as an excuse to explain away its leaders' failures.

The crisis in US–Iranian relations in which the American embassy personnel were innocent pawns was only one facet of a wider canvas of oil, Islam and nationalism. At that moment, the agony of America in watching with dismay the continuing confinement of its men and women overshadowed the other aspects.

There could not be two opinions on the inadequacy of the Iranian religious leaders to tame the revolution and lead it along healthy lines. Iran had to find its own answers to its problems as a long and difficult road lay ahead. If Iran wanted to be a theocratic state, so it was, but its religious leaders should have learned how to administer the country and assure the safety of all its people.

Iran's religious leaders were apparently initially surprised by the students' action in taking the American embassy personnel as hostages, although the students themselves were influenced by Ayatollah Khomeini's sermons. The Iranian leadership was yet to learn that irresponsibility fed on rhetoric and more rhetoric led to more irresponsible acts.

Strangely, Ayatollah Khomeini not only surrendered himself completely to the students' demands in seeking the dying Shah's return for the hostage's freedom but also used the fortuitous Kaaba incident which was condemned by all, calling for a holy war against the US and Israel. This had some tragic consequence in Pakistan and echoes in India.

For Jimmy Carter, the crisis could not have come at a worse moment. Even as he was fighting off a determined challenge to his second-term nomination to the presidency in his own party, he had to combine restraint with some show of force to try to secure the hostages' release. He sought to neutralise the Iranian ban on oil exports to the US by banning its import, froze Iranian currency assets and sent American warships to the Indian Ocean as a flag-waving exercise.

It seemed unlikely that in stirring the cauldron of Islam, oil and nationalism, the Ayatollah was conscious of all the consequences of his actions. The motives of the defilers of Kaaba were unclear, but the act could only cause unease in Saudi royal circles.

The US was not alone in watching the macabre drama being played in Teheran with growing helplessness. In one respect, the US was fortunate in being able to do without oil imports, but much of the rest of the world was hopelessly dependent on West Asian oil and was viewing the symbolic use of oil as a political weapon with trepidation. For the poor countries in particular, it meant further crushing burdens in coping with the astronomical prices even as the oil-rich shed crocodile tears over their plight.

Islam had proved to be a potent force of nationalism, and the fundamentalist streak in the Iranian revolution was apparent from the beginning. But as the people of Pakistan were discovering for themselves, religion could also be employed for giving the people a substitute for freedom and Pakistanis had to find an answer to this question.

India's reaction to the Iranian crisis and the wave of religious revival in parts of the Muslim world had been in an undertone, although the External Affairs Ministry did well in condemning the Kaaba outrage. Any government in power in Delhi has to take into account the Muslim sentiments in the country and India's capacity to act was hamstrung by the caretaker nature of the then government.

The Ayatollah's war against "American imperialism" and zionism had muddied the already turgid waters of the Indian election campaign. Indira Gandhi realised that this particular piece of opportunism was a double-edged weapon and could only serve to arouse religious passions, which were best kept in check, particularly at election time. India could not have been made a party to the Ayatollah's extravagances, and had the Indira Congress persevered in using the Iranian crisis for its own narrow selfish ends, it could only invite retribution from other voters.

Instability Phase

India's problems apart, Iran's was a revolution that had gone awry and although the American hostages, the fulminations against the Shah and the Ayatollah's oratory had diverted the people from their real problems, they could not resolve them. Indeed, with a loose government run by a religious oracle, the semblance of an administration Bazargan tried unsuccessfully to run and growing divisive tendencies as evidenced by the Kurdish revolt, Iran was set for a long period of instability.

The Shah's weakness was that in his inordinate ambition for his country, he set in motion changes at a breakneck speed without taking into account the social and psychological dislocation they could cause or spread political power among the growing technocracy. He not only antagonised the clergy but also the intelligentsia and the middle class by using suppression as an instrument of state policy.

Ayatollah Khomeini's triumphant return to Iran led to the purges and execution of members of the *ancien régime*, and a measure of chaos and confusing centres of command were an inevitable feature of the end of long years of the Shah's inability to bring some order to the country and begin to heal the wounds inflicted by a divisive past.

In his wisdom, Ayatollah Khomeini took the country towards a version of a theocratic state, which could only serve to deepen the divisions in Iranian society. Apart from the problem of minority nationalities, which only patience and generosity could resolve, a turning away from the modern world in social mores and ideology could hardly endear that regime to either the leftists or large sections of the middle class exposed during the Shah's regime to the liberalising influences of the West. It seemed hardly possible that the Ayatollah could succeed in turning the clock back for all time. The Ayatollah, in the meanwhile, could only congratulate himself on humbling a superpower and being a catalyst for change.

The sorry confinement of the American hostages was to bring Iran diminishing returns as the conscience of the world rebelled at this medieval play in which the remaining life-span of a dying deposed monarch was sought to be balanced by the lives of scores of Americans held in captivity against all international norms. Were the play to have a tragic ending, little credence was likely to be placed on Iran's flight against "American imperialism" and zionism.

The Iranian developments were a reminder that changing societies brought in their wake aberrations that distorted ideas, plunging countries in fresh turmoil. It was the hope of all friends of Iran that the distortions that had surfaced in the revolution would yield place to saner policies more in tune with Islam's true meaning and the changing world.

Drinking Poison

In international affairs, as in life, war and peace have a logic of their own. And Iran's acceptance of the United Nations cease-fire resolution in 1988, after nearly eight years of bloody fighting with neighbouring Iraq, flowed from the irrefutable logic of circumstances.

Iraq had recaptured nearly all the territory taken by Iran. The American determination to prevent an Iranian victory by tipping the scales in favour of Iraq was underlined by the tragic and arrogant American mistake in shooting down the Iranian Airbus. And Iran's continuing refusal to accept the year-old UN Security Council resolution as it stood was merely serving to underline its growing isolation in the world. It was only the Soviet refusal to go along with the US that prevented the imposition of a statutory arms embargo.

Signs of a change in Iranian tactics, if not strategy, were multiplying even as the fog of revolutionary rhetoric was kept up. There was the decision to place all the Iranian forces under the Parliament speaker, Ali Akbar Hashemi Rafsanjani. There were the diplomatic approaches made to France, Canada and Britain. There were the secret talks Teheran was holding with the United States through intermediaries. But the decision, when it was finally taken, could not have been an easy one.

The Iranians had charted a course of religious fundamentalism after the revolution to send shock waves throughout the region. And since the Iraqis sought to take advantage of the confusion after the fall of the Shah of Iran to launch a military operation to grab territory, Ayatollah Khomeini and his followers merged the brave new world they were seeking to build with the war against Iraq.

The result had been an estimated million lives lost, and the see-saw battles saw spectacular Iranian advances ultimately to be overtaken by Iraqi counter-attacks and recapture of territory. Iraq also bore the horrendous responsibility of initiating chemical warfare which, to the shame of the superpowers in particular, had still to be outlawed internationally.

It would still be a long process to peace. A cease-fire had first to be enforced, and the various other provisions of Resolution 598 implemented. The UN Secretary-General, Perez de Cuellar, would have his hands full in trying to meet the challenge of implementing the resolution. But the war as it had been waged for nearly eight years was over.

This is something to be thankful for, but the superpowers and the rest of the world were now looking at the consequences of this momentous development. One consequence was obvious. An unstable region prone to fighting its little and big wars was bristling with arms as never before. To the usual mix of arms had now been added chemical weapons and missiles.

American Strategy

Even before the Iranian acceptance of the UN resolution, Henry Kissinger had concluded that America had achieved its basic objectives in the Gulf. These he defined as ensuring freedom of navigation, prevention of Soviet domination of the area and preserving the territorial integrity of "friendly" states and encouraging their progress.

It was, indeed, remarkable that despite the war and the threat America's friends and allies felt they were susceptible to, despite the American hostages held in Lebanon by pro-Iranian groups, Washington had made known its desire to live with Iran, if it is returned to the barest forms of accepted civilised conduct. The Iran-Contra affair was, of course, botched up by grade B amateur strategists operating out of the White House.

The centrality of Iran to America's strategic thinking in the region would now come into greater play. And if the Iranian leaders played their cards well, the pro-Iraqi tilt in American policy would be reversed; the tilt was, in any event, a limited one of denying Iran a victory. Washington believed that Iran needed America to balance its relations with the superpower on its doorstep. Significantly, the first Israeli reaction to the Iranian acceptance of a cease-fire was to express fears about Iraq's expanded fighting machine.

During his tenure as national security adviser and, later, as secretary of state, Kissinger's aim in West Asia was to shut out the Soviet Union from the region. This was an unrealistic goal. It was, for instance, almost universally recognised that in arriving at an eventual settlement of the Palestinian issue, the Soviets would have to be brought in. But given the Soviet Union's domestic agenda, Moscow was not in a mood to take on any new external adventure.

Apart from Israeli fears of a stronger Iraq, the Israeli leadership would come under greater international pressure to tackle the Palestinian issue. It was only the uprising in the occupied territories that jolted the Arab world to try to do something about a problem many would rather forget.

Once the distraction of the Iran–Iraq war was over, the Palestinian question would take the primacy it deserved. In that event, Israeli leaders would no longer be able to stall a solution.

For India and the rest of the Third World, the breakthrough in the Iran–Iraq war held some depressing lessons. The efforts of the non-aligned movement, in addition to those of the Islamic Conference, did nothing in convincing Iran to cry a halt to a senseless war. It was, in the end, the might of one superpower and the distinct lack of sympathy of the other and the situation on the battlefield that forced Iran to accept the year-old UN resolution. And both contestants belonged to the non-aligned movement.

If South–South cooperation had not taken off in the economic sphere, the political field gave one little encouragement to believe that major political disputes could be resolved in future in a South–South setting. This was, of course, not the first instance of its kind, but it was the most dramatic to date. Perhaps the realisation of this failure would help moderate the rhetoric at future gatherings of the developing countries.

Saudi Moves

Apart from Iraq's future role in the region, which Israel fears, Saudi Arabia's moves held much interest. Saudi acquisition of Chinese intermediate-range missiles and the recent major arms deals with Britain were two indications of a desire to cut loose from American apron-strings. Traditionally, the United States was hampered in pursuing its West Asian policy by the kind of strategic relationship it has had with Israel and this dilemma would be compounded by the failure of efforts to resolve the Palestinian problem. The new Saudi assertiveness implied that even the bigger American allies in the Arab world were becoming restive over US compulsions in relation to Israel.

It was no secret that there were doves and hawks in the Iranian leadership, with Rafsanjani being classed as a moderate. Assuming that the Parliament Speaker played an important role in getting the Ayatollah to accept reality in agreeing to the UN resolution, he had an uphill struggle ahead of him in asserting his primacy after the Ayatollah. None of the main contestants dispute—or dare dispute— the fundamentals of the revolution. The disputes concerned personalities, economic policies, and, above all, the promotion of political statecraft.

There could not be two opinions about the need to rebuild the war-ravaged country and get the fighting forces and military equipment in shape. This task would take time and a great measure of flexibility, a quality which had not been much in evidence in Iran. Yet the next phase would necessarily involve a whole set of pragmatic steps not only to get the economy moving but also to deal with the world.

One of the major questions Iran would have to confront was how to deal with the "Great Satan", as the United States has been traditionally called. The division of doves and hawks was likely to show up on this question. The circumstances that led Iran to accept the UN resolution would indicate that the moderates had more than an even chance to set the course for the country for the next few years.

Managing Contradictions, 1993

At Imam Khomeini's shrine outside Teheran, pallbearers carrying a coffin made their way to the tomb shouting slogans to the glory of the revolution. More martyrs were being discovered every day as the debris of the eight-year fruitless Iran–Iraq war was cleared. An odd car in Teheran and in the holy city of Qom carried photographs of other martyrs on its rear window.

But for these reminders of a grim war, Teheran wore a relaxed confident look. The Islamic revolution was in place, with women suitably attired in black chadors, their heads covered. Men were tieless, neckties having been decreed as a symbol of Westernisation which the revolution sought to supplant with the Iranian version of Islam.

Girls were required to wear the headscarf from the age of six, but the younger women of Teheran sought to give some character to the shapeless chador by throwing the end of the scarf over their left shoulders or wearing chadors of lace. The more daring ones, usually Iranians settled abroad, made long fashionable overcoats do duty for the chador, their heads covered with silk scarves.

Women were not allowed to wear make-up, except when attending a wedding. Alcohol was, of course, banned. Apart from those daring to break the law, men were required to drink non-alcoholic beer if they wished to indulge in their fancies. There was no exception to observing the dress or alcohol codes for foreigners, diplomatic missions being unofficially allowed their preference in the latter field.

Satellite dishes were, strictly speaking, illegal but were tolerated, confined as they were to a small number. Iranians talked nostalgically about Indian films, which were not allowed to be screened because of their dance numbers. Thousands of cassettes of these films, however, did the rounds, thanks to the marvel of the video cassette recorder.

There was a Ministry of Culture and Islamic Guidance and no one was left in doubt about the country's pecking order. Imam Khomeini of course remained supreme and his still unfinished shrine continued to draw trickles of men and women outside of Friday or special days. At Qom, where the Imam spent much of his time following the revolution, the mosque renamed after him drew a steady stream.

An arrow marked the spot where he prayed and the pulpit stairs were revered. The faith and devotion of the young and the old who came to pray were impressive. Outside in the teeming bazaar, photographs of the Imam, Ayotollah Khamenei, his successor and the present spiritual leader, and President Hashemi Rafsanjani were spread out on pavements, somewhat incongruously juxtaposed with pictures of cherubic European and American children with inscriptions emphasising love and faith in God.

In representations depicting the three leaders, the Imam and Ayatollah Khomeini were shown on one plane, the lower plane being occupied by President Rafsanjani. The spiritual leader, in fact, commanded the armed forces and had men overseeing the work of each ministry. This inevitably led to different centres of power, another important functionary being the speaker of the Majlis (parliament).

Despite their shapeless forms and scrubbed faces, Iranian women have a personality and good looks. I asked several of them what they thought of their dress code. Some said bluntly they did not like it, others preferred the more diplomatic "not much" answer. The men responded to the question quite differently. They said Islam required women to cover their bodies. One answered, " It's all right by me, but my teenage son doesn't like it."

Women's Dress Code

How long women would be required to cover themselves from head to foot, but for their faces, is anybody's guess. The chief editor of Teheran's largest selling newspaper, *Ettela'at* said half in jest that it wouldn't surprise him if there was an edict 10 years from now that the dress code for women was not necessary. Whether the women would wait that long was another matter. For the present, Iranian women expressed their personalities by the avidity with which they drove cars—there must be more women drivers per square mile in Teheran than anywhere else in the world. At the equivalent of one rupee a litre of petrol, some 40 per cent of Teheran's population owned cars.

At the sprawling radio and television complex in Teheran, the vice-president of external services, Shahidimoddab, told me that he was receiving hundreds of letters from the Indian subcontinent supporting the *fatwa* against Salman Rushdie. Teheran Radio's Bengali service was more popular than BBC's, in Bangladesh in particular, he said.

That was the only reference to Rushdie I heard in Iran during a week's stay although local newspapers featured the winning entry in an international cartoon contest on him. It was on predictable lines.

Iran was still in the process of reconciling its devotion to the cause of the revolution with the dictates of running a nation state at a time of international turbulence. President Rafsanjani had already taken the country some distance in meeting the modern world. Iranian dilemmas were in how far to act as the world's guardian of the Islamic faith, with its repercussions, and in the manner of attaining the welfare of all citizens in a world weighted against the developing countries.

The different power centres in Teheran spoke of the internal problems that arose out of a declared ideological state with a worldwide mission. Clerics of a conservative bent could, and did, act as a brake on President Rafsanjani's pragmatic policies. Besides, it was open to question whether a nation ruled by more than one power centre could function efficiently.

What was praiseworthy was Iran's desire to see the world without blinkers, despite the rhetoric of the mass media and the politicians. The symbol of this approach is the lavishly funded Institute for Political and International Studies, a branch of the Foreign Ministry. Researchers study different segments of the world with unbiased eyes. Unlike many other think tanks, the Institute had a direct input into the making of Iranian foreign policy, and was encouraged by the Foreign Minister, Ali Akbar Velayati.

The coming into being of the Central Asian States as independent entities was a particularly exciting event for Iran because it offered the country an avenue towards its cherished goal of opting out of the West Asian sub-group. Iran shares borders with Azerbaijan and

Turkmenistan and has Kazakhastan, Turkmenistan and Azerbaijan sharing access to the Caspian Sea with it and Russia. To the land-locked nations of Central Asia, Iran offers a route to the Gulf and the Indian Ocean. Iran views itself as the guardian of the Gulf, does not class the Gulf states as Arab and would rather forget the quarrels and contradictions of the Arab world.

President Rafsanjani had tempered the original enthusiasm of the revolution to try to befriend the Gulf states, despite the unwelcome consequences of the American-led war with Iraq. The United States had forged new defence agreements with some of the Gulf states and was pumping arms into Saudi Arabia and Kuwait. And in an ultimate insult to Iran, Washington pointedly left it out of a new defence arrangement between the Gulf Cooperation Council and Syria and Egypt.

President Rafsanjani's suggestion of an India–Iran–China alignment was very much in the nature of exploring all options to meet the new and dangerous world. Iran was also seeking to build good relations with Europe, particularly Germany and Italy, and was not adverse to talking to the US, Washington permitting.

Among the points that remained to be determined was whether the beguiling vision of showing the wayward states of Central Asia the light would lead Iran to ideological excesses. President Rafsanjani's tour of four of the five Central Asian states—Tajikistan was pointedly left out—was part of his policy of an intense cultivation of these states.

But the eight-year war had led to tremendous reconstruction problems and with a galloping population, Iran's considerable oil revenues were insufficient to meet the needs of essential imports and find resources for major new undertakings. Here lay the crunch. The more lustily Iran flew the flag of Islam to claim an international constituency, the greater the hurdles it faced to break out of its relative isolation.

Iraq of course was humbled and defeated for the present. And another rival of Iran is Saudi Arabia, now buttressed by dollops of American arms. They both claimed a share in power and influence in the Gulf. Iran was also acutely aware of the consequence of a drop in oil prices and how they could be manipulated. Teheran was therefore eager to be seen cooperating with the Organisation of Petroleum Exporting Countries because stable and predictable prices of oil remain the country's lifeline.

Indeed, the logic of the situation would suggest a continuation of President Rafsanjani's pragmatic policies, but the ideological centre of the world when the other world ideology, communism, had come a cropper, cannot be underestimated. The obvious dilemma was how to reconcile the role of the world missionary with promoting the country's interests.

Shah on Display

The Shah of Iran's palaces in Teheran are open to the public. Hordes of school girls and ordinary Iranians visit them every day to gawk at the opulent lifestyle of a disgraced and departed monarch. Among the rooms on display was the gambling room complete with billiards and playing card tables and one-armed bandits. Also on display were the glitzy dresses and accessories of the Shah's mother as well as gifts from India, Pakistan, China and European countries.

One palace was devoted to a display of the Shah's collection of works of art. His taste in painting was rather indiscriminate and the only famous names I saw represented were a Picasso and a Miro. The collection reminded me of the acquisitions of Indian maharajas in the old days.

I asked a girl student, her head appropriately covered, what her impressions of the Shah were. "I am too young to know of his time", she answered. Although the authorities presumably hoped that the people would draw the correct lessons from the bad old days, this openness in a strict and missionary Islamic state was surprising. In the carpet museum in Teheran, for instance, among the feast for the eyes was a carpet depicting Omar Khayyam carousing with a lady friend with a jug of wine by their side.

On one plane, it would seem, the Iranian leadership was confident enough of the people's acceptance of the Islamic revolution to let them see the heresies of the past. Gambling, liquor and the display of feminine form were banned. On other plane, there was some concern over the cultural invasion from the West, particularly through satellite programmes and the ubiquitous cassettes.

In the attractive city of Isfahan, I saw a couple, the woman appropriately dressed according to the Iranian Islamic code, holding hands as they walked past me in a street. According to the chief editor of *Ettela'at* in Teheran, there are some immutables in Islam and other precepts that were capable of change. He mentioned the place of women in society in the latter context. Women drove cars and took on jobs in a mixed environment as long as they were suitably clothed, according to the dictates of Islam as decreed by the ayatollahs.

But there was an undercurrent of concern. At the Ministry of Culture and Islamic Guidance, I was asked how India coped with the problem of invasion from the skies. And in the shopping arcades of Isfahan, jewellery shops stood cheek by jowl with shops displaying posters and postcards, most of them of European and American origin. In the tea houses of Iran, customers avidly watched American cartoon films on television, dubbed in Persian, and Bruce Lee was a favourite with Iranian teenagers. There was a plentiful supply of imported consumer goods and American cigarettes had many takers.

Striking Contrast

It is this contrast between openness and a strict Islamic code that was most striking. Iranians are an attractive and hospitable people, but the consequences of a modern-minded population in the cities and towns colliding with a more traditional rural folk and the clerics remain to be determined. In a sense, this conflict is amplified in the different power centres that operate in the country.

The contradictions were apparent in Iran's interest in attracting more tourists. In Isfahan, I saw European tourist groups in the famous Abbasi hotel, notable more for its ambience than comfort, savouring the history and atmosphere of a famed ancient city. The women wore long overcoats and headscarves and they and their men companions had to forgo the pleasures of an appetiser and wine with meals. There were hardy souls who would brave the adventure of a trip to a missionary Islamic state out of curiosity or a desire to see Iran's magnificent past, but tourism has its limits in such an environment.

Iran thus operated at various levels. Given the limitations of a codified Islamic state, the openness of an administration that is attunded to the world and sought to exploit Iranian strengths was remarkable. For instance, the soft-spoken director of the Institute for Political and International studies, Dr Sohrab Shahabi, told me that his organisation gave its opinion on world developments and trends untrammelled by the public exposition of Iranian foreign policy.

Developments in Russia occupied an important place in projecting future patterns. Contrary to the popular view of the Russian crisis, tinged as it was with an anti-Western slant, the Institute believed that President Boris Yeltsin, or men of his ilk, would emerge stronger out of the crisis. Iranians were also guided by the sensitivities of the Central Asian states whose leaders believed that the forces represented by the Alexander Rutskoi faction in Moscow would have meant a more oppressive Russian control over them.

There seemed to be unanimity among the different Iranian power centres about the importance of the Central Asian states for the country's foreign policy options. Teheran tended to emphasise the influence of Iranian civilisation on the region over the ages. Dr Ali Khoram, in charge of strategic studies in the Foreign Ministry, told me that the Central Asian states had been given freedom, rather than winning it.They had therefore to be made aware of the value of freedom.

Apart from interacting with Central Asia, the Institute in Teheran is concentrating on new research topics such as the role of the United Nations and its future, the North Atlantic Treaty Organisation, the Conference on Security and Cooperation in Europe and prospects for European unity. It was also studying what "Islamic human rights" mean.

I asked Dr Khoram to amplify President Rufsanjani's proposal for bringing Iran, India and China together. His answer was to suggest that while Europeans wanted to be European, countries such as India, Japan, China, Iran and South Korea and some others could emphasise their Asianness. "India and Iran have friendly relations", he said, "and we could be more Asian than tilting towards the West or the East. Other friendly countries like Pakistan could come together with India and China."

"India, China and Iran are three major civilisations. We can find common goals," Dr Khoram emphasied. Dr Khoram believed that instability in the Central Asian states could last from five to 15 years and would depend upon stability in Russia. "If Mr Yeltsin remains in power," he suggested, "Central Asia would find its independence sooner than if the Rutskoi faction were in command. This is the analysis of these republics."

Iran emphasised its independent policy in contrast to the pro-West inclination of the Shah regime. Its slogan is "Neither East nor West", but the nuances of the foreign policy go beyond such slogans. Policy-makers hardly mention the United States nor talk about it in derogatory terms.

Iran recognised that American power was a fact of life and although its public posturing was attuned to America-bashing and even more to attacking the perceived stooges in the region, there was little tendency to launch a tirade against Washington in informal discussions. In the short run, Teheran could do little to reverse the defence and strategic linkages the US had built up in the Gulf and in countries such as Saudi Arabia, now reinforced by the consequences of the Second Gulf War.

Rather, the Iranian policy was to try to expand its own options. Hence the devotion to the Central Asian states and the consequences of Russian developments on them, the attempt to use confidence-building measures in improving relations with the Gulf nations and the policy of cooperating with OPEC.

In the long run, there is little doubt that Iran views the present arrangements in the Persian Gulf as highly inequitous and unjust. It had been argued with some justification by Iranian academics that more than half of the Gulf belongs to Iran and that its population and resources made it potentially the undisputed dominant power in the region.

It would seem that the Iranian opposition to the Israeli–Palesitine Liberation Organisation accord on beginning the process of a Palestinian entity through autonomy for the Gaza Strip and the town of Jericho was being used as a lever to emphasise Teheran's importance to the region. It did not suit the United States to acknowledge this fact at this juncture, with Iraq humbled and the Gulf states nervous about their security. But possibilities existed for softening the American posture towards Iran if President Rafsanjani was able to have his way in taking his country towards a better future.

Bottomless Pockets

More than a decade after the Khomeini revolution, Teheran wears a relaxed look and is a more open city than one would expect after the frenzied days of the end of the Shah regime. Indeed, the transition after the death of Ayaytollah Khomeini, referred to as the Imam, had been remarkably smooth, with Ayaytollah Khamanie taking over the spiritual legacy while President Hashemi Rafsanjani ran the presidency.

After one gets used to the ubiquitous black chadors, with women's faces peering out of black headscarves, and men in suits without ties, the pulsating rythm of Teheran with its streets crowded with cars and bustling shoppers is infectious. The chadors are a testimony, multiplied in millions, of the world's vanguard Islamic state.

Iran's largest and oldest newspaper, *Ettela'at*, selling half a million copies a day, supports the revolution as it supported the Shah in former days. It devoted over 30 per cent of its space to foreign news, indicating the limitations of commenting on domestic affairs and Iranians' interest in the wider world. Despite the frozen state of relations with the United States, the paper ran extracts of Ronald Reagan's memoirs and was running Margaret Thatcher's memoirs.

Ettela'at is a publishing empire bringing out a whole range of magazines and journals in the fields of science and technology, economy, literature, youth and sports. It also publishes books one of which on Kashmir is titled "A Wounded Heaven". It was setting its sights on a London edition in 1994 through satellite transmission.

The surprise is not in newspapers dutifully following the revolution's path, but the hunger that exists for information and knowledge, unihhibited by ideological considerations. Nowhere was this more apparent than in the impressive Institute for Political and International Studies. It is a think tank and a training centre rolled into one and boasted a staff of 200 in its plush building. To a foreign office depleted by the exodus or expulsion of the Shah's loyalists and the entry of untrained men, it provides training in addition to longer range policy formulations.

While this quest for knowledge and expertise proceeded apace under the watchful eyes of President Rafsanjani's dedicated team, in particular the urbane foreign minister, Dr Ali Akbar Velayati, Iran faced immense problems. They were of two kinds. There was the problem of reconciling the different centres of power, the two principal ones being President Rafsanjani and the spiritual leader, Ayatollah Khamenie. And even as the country faced the task of reconstruction after the eight-year war with Iraq, it had to get to grips with the changed scenario after the Second Gulf War and the emergence of newly independent Central Asian states.

It was taken for granted that the main decisions on foreign and security policies as on domestic affairs would be approved by Ayatollah Khamenie. The spiritual leader had his own set of advisers and men keeping an eye on the various ministries. The armed forces were answerable to him. The two main centres of power, with subsidiary centres—the majlis speaker was an important functionary— provided clerics with a conservative bent scope for obstructionist tactics.

Economic Tasks

On the economic plane, the task of reconstruction was beset with difficulties of attracting foreign investment in view of Iran's relative isolation—the United States was still not ready to talk to Teheran except on its own terms. Iran's oil income was not sufficient to cover massive reconstruction needs in addition to essential imports. And a frightening population explosion after the revolution was beginning to cast a lengthening shadow. The Iranian leadership has woken up to the dangers represented by the latter and had taken steps to curb extravagant consumer imports but remained resistant to seeking the help of the World Bank or the International Monetary Fund to stabilise its economy.

Iran remained neutral during the Second Gulf War, wining some sympathy from the West, which had aided Iraq during and after the eight-year war. But rather like the consequences of the Soviet invasion of Afghanistan on India, Teheran found that the United States had sewn up bilateral defence agreements with the Gulf states, an area of its primary concern, and encouraged the Gulf Cooperation Council to have Egypt and Syria in a new defence arrangement to the exclusion of Iran, apart from Iraq. Iran had traditionally considered the Gulf states as its area of influence, although it had rivals in Iraq and Saudi Arabia.

President Rafsanjani's approach had been to adopt a pragmatic policy of befriendimg the Gulf states while in an effort to stabilise oil prices and ensure their predictability, he held out an olive branch to Saudi Arabia by cooperating with the Organisation of Petroleum Exporting Countries (OPEC). Iran could do little about the massive amounts of American arms being pumped into Saudi Arabia, except to modernise and expand is own defence forces.

The coming into existence of the Central Asian states as independent entities presented Iran with opportunities as well as dilemmas. It had been more prudent than Turkey in not rushing to recognise them, but Iran had made no secret of its affinity with these countries or its unique geographical position to provide outlets for the new land-locked nations.

Iran's efforts at cultivating the Central Asian states encompassed a range of fields. The Teheran institute ran courses in diplomacy for candidates from Tajikistan, Turkmenistan and Kazakhstan. It opened a department dealing with the region and published a quarterly journal on Central Asia. Iranian radio beamed broadcasts to Tukmenistan, Uzbekistan, Azerbaijan and Tajikistan, in addition to telecasts to Azerbaijan. According to the man in charge, Shahidimoddab, the programmes carried information on Islam and the new nations' history, interspersed with music and poetry, but no display of dancing. "We show Iran as it is", he told me.

Which brings us to Iran's dilemmas. The Islamic revolution had a tremendous impact on the Muslim world. The actions of the Islamic government denoted a missionary zeal in spreading its massage to the *ummah* across national frontiers. The Islamic state was based on an anti-Western foundation in rejecting the concept of the secular state and identifying the new nationalism with indigenous and religious values presented as a complete answer to living and running the affairs of the state. It had also a pronounced anti-monarchical tinge.

Iran's thrust to export its revolution caused a crisis in relations with Saudi Arabia, the case of the Haj incident representing its nadir, the Gulf States took fright and Egypt and Algeria were antagonised. Iran gained a new constituency in many countries somewhat in the manner of the Soviet Union through its creed of communism. The results of the American-led war on Iraq largely worked against Iran's interests although its rival Iraq was humbled and weakened. Saudi Arabia became a bastion of the United States acquiring immense quantities of weapons and Kuwait as well went on an arms buying spree.

Dose of Pragmatism

President Rafsanjani sought to temper his country's ideological zeal by his pragmatic policy of undertaking confidence-building measures with the Gulf states even as he sought to root the ideological Islamic state in Iranian nationalism. The Shah had, in fact, tried to take Iran to its pre-Islamic past to emphasise nationalism. His credo of "Both East and West" was changed by the revolutionaries to "Neither East nor West", but the President sought to build his country on a "negative equilibrium" favoured by the Shah, although in a different version.

Iran could not wish away the existence of nation states and the fact that Muslim countries were ruled by monarchs or an elite that wished to keep Islamic practices within the bounds of their personal or state compulsions. The end of the Cold War, in fact, changed the world scenario with the need to win new friends while exploring openings to Central Asia.

Would the new Central Asian nation states lead to a revival of the old Iranian missioniary zeal? The temptation of showing these states the light was great and the rise of Islamic militancy in many parts of the world was an encouraging sign for Iranian ideologues.

The answer lay partly in President Rafsanjani's ability to continue to promote his policies, partly on the limitations imposed by the United States and circumstances on the autonomy of Iranian action. The people of Iran seemed more concerned with their own welfare. Unlike the press, the people talked frankly about their concerns although popular support for the revolution was not in doubt. An Iranian woman told me, "The Shah's men filled their pockets but when they were full, they sought status. Today the clerics have bottomless pockets".

Khatami Glasnost

There are moments in the history of relations between two countries when a single symbolic act encompasses a new beginning. It was so in the "ping-pong diplomacy" in the case of American relations with the People's Republic of China, and decades later, the interview given by Iran's President Mohammad Khatami in January 1988 to CNN in an address to the "American people" was a pregnant symbolic act that will go down as the beginning of a rapprochement between Teheran and Washington. The interview—for the most part a monologue—was being analysed threadbare in Washington and, thanks to the medium used, it could be watched repeatedly by experts.

The initial reaction was that President Khatami did not go far enough and stopped short of seeking an official dialogue, but it was an unrealistic expectation, and once American policy-makers mulled the interview, they found much food for thought. Indeed, at one level it was a masterful presentation. Given the level of hostility between the two countries, President Khatami made his points clearly and sensibly, giving nothing away while taking a giant step towards a rappro-chement.

Not only was such an interview a 'first' since the Iranian Revolution but for the first time an elected president of the Iranian people praised the basis on which the American state was founded and sought a parallel between the compatibility of religion and liberty in the US and events in Iran with the fall of the Shah of Iran.

In calling for an exchange of intellectuals and journalists with America, he was faithful to his earlier call for a dialogue between civilisations. But calmly and surely he dotted all the i's and crossed all the t's. He berated America's policy of trying to dominate the world and remaining a prisoner of Cold War psychology. He said that on the West Asian peace process, American policy was made in Tel Aviv, not in Washington. Iran would not stand in the way of the peace process but he was convinced it would not work because it was unjust. And he categorically said he was against terrorism and was against the killing of innocent civilians in any circumstances.

But the nuances in President Khatami's address to the American people, as it was billed, were unmistakable. He ascribed the long holding of American hostages in Teheran virtually to the early excesses of the Iranian revolution and acknowledged the hurt it had caused Americans, carefully juxtaposing it with the hurt caused to the Iranian people by several American acts, including the US complicity in the 1953 coup and the humiliations meted out to Iranians during the Shah regime. Anti-Semitism, he suggested, was a Western phenomenon whereas Jews and Arabs had coexisted in the region in the past and, in his view, the "racist terrorist" regime in Israel did not serve American interests or those of the Jews themselves.

Khatami Move

What did this great *tour de force* portend? First, that President Khatami was determined to use his popular mandate to move the country away from its stalemate with the world's sole surviving superpower and was prepared to take risks in the process, given the differences of views among the leadership.

Second, the President was keen to present his country, known more for its radical rhetoric than reasoned argument, in a new light. Third, he was signalling that, after nearly two decades, the Iranian revolution had taken a new turn towards a more rational and liberal dispensation.

That the entire interview with CNN's Christiane Amanpour was rebroadcast on Teheran television was an interesting indication of how President Khatami was cultivating his constituency at home while moulding fence-sitters to his views by exposing them to such heretic sentiments as the greatness of the American people and civilisation.

Such historical inaccuracies as the comparison between the antiquity and greatness of Iranian civilisation and the rather recent American experiment need not surprise us. President Khatami was obviously taking poetic licence in driving his political point home.

Anyone familiar with Iran's recent history would realise that the evolution of President Khatami's *glasnost* will encounter many twists and turns, but he was banking on his intuition that his constituency at home was growing and desperately wanted a change from the straitjacket of the official version of the revolution.

One revealing indication was the disregarding of imposed conventions when Iranian girls joined revellers in the Teheran stadium to celebrate Iran's success in qualifying for the World Cup final.

Intriguingly, President Khatami had tied the liberal trends in his country with the state of relations with the "Great Satan", a new touchstone for the Iranian revolution. Despite the conventional rhetoric, having better relations with the US was popular with a majority of Iranians. For the young, it meant a less restrictive life and for many others a chance to visit and host relations living in the US. There is a large Iranian diaspora.

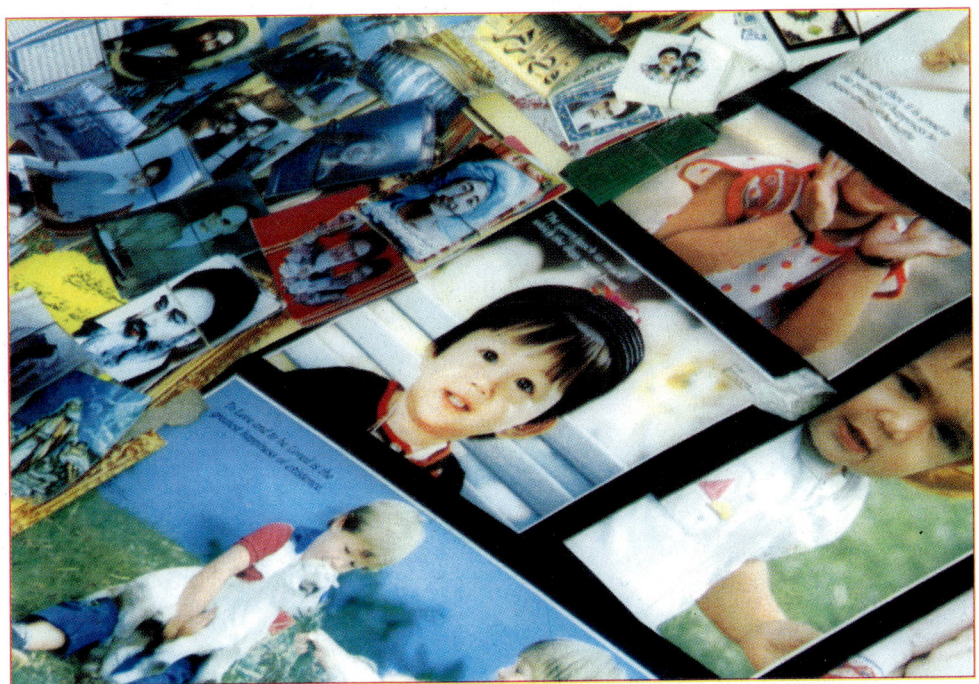

Clerics and cherubic Caucasian children share the pavement in
the Iranian holy city of Qom.

Siesta time in an Iranian mosque.

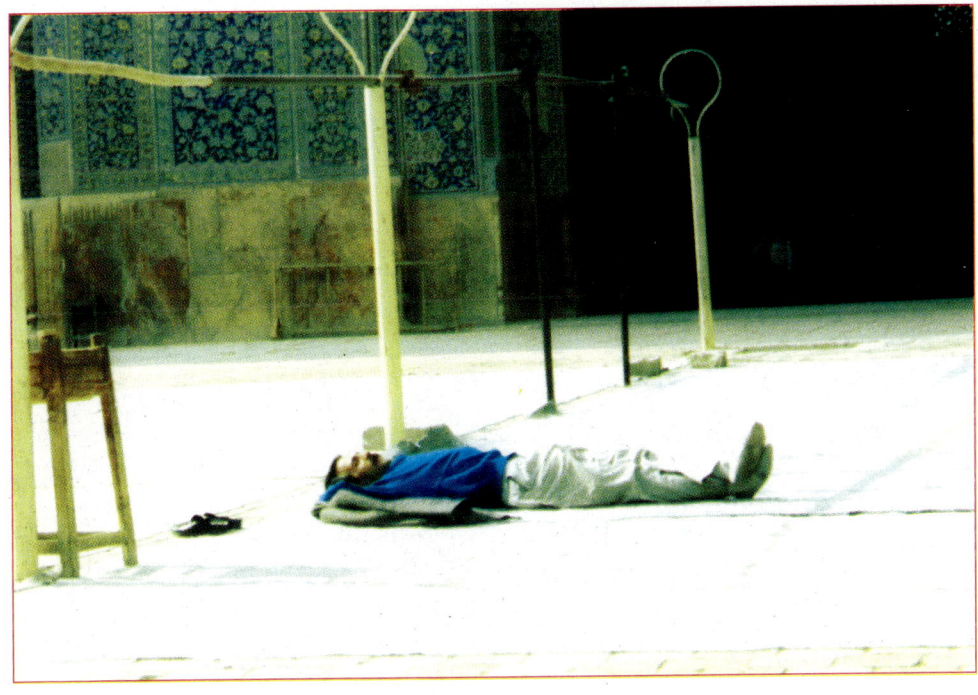

Plate **1**

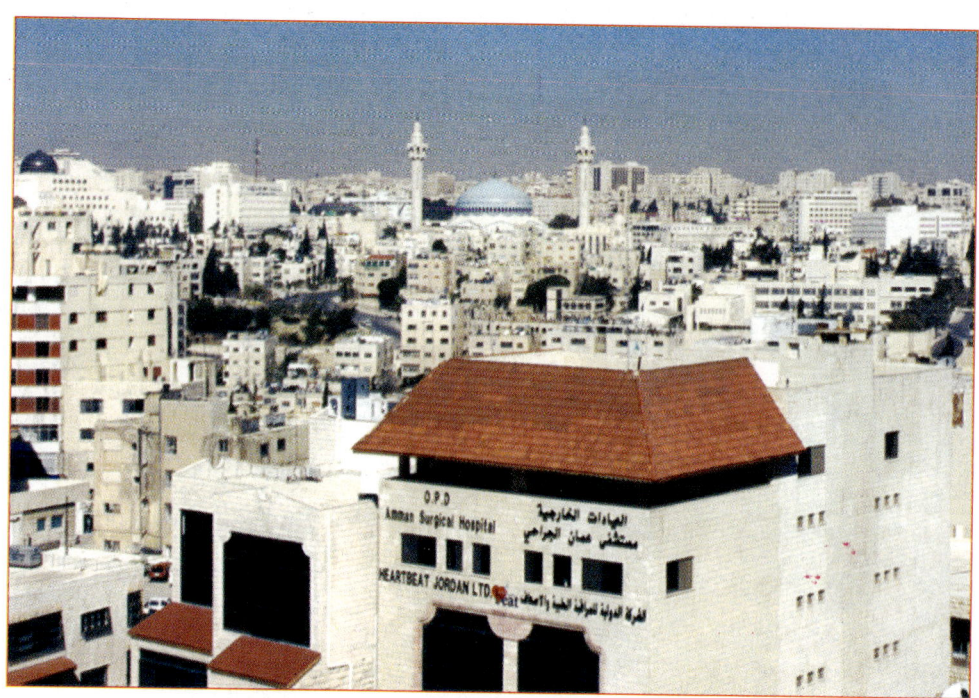

The attractive capital of Jordan, Amman.

The modern face of the Gulf: Dubai, the commercial capital of the UAE.

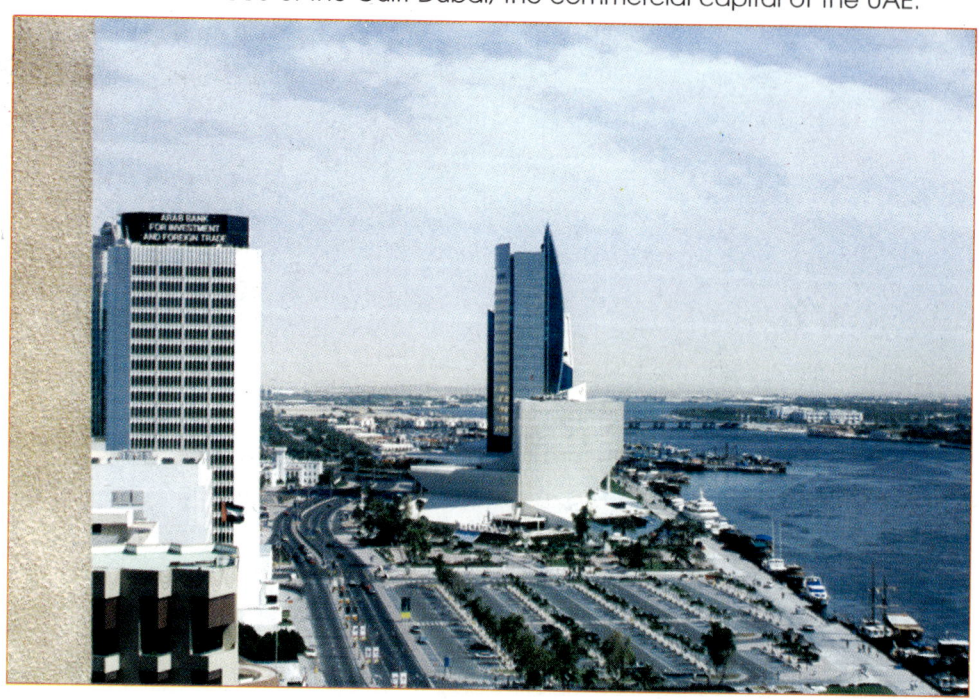

Plate **2**

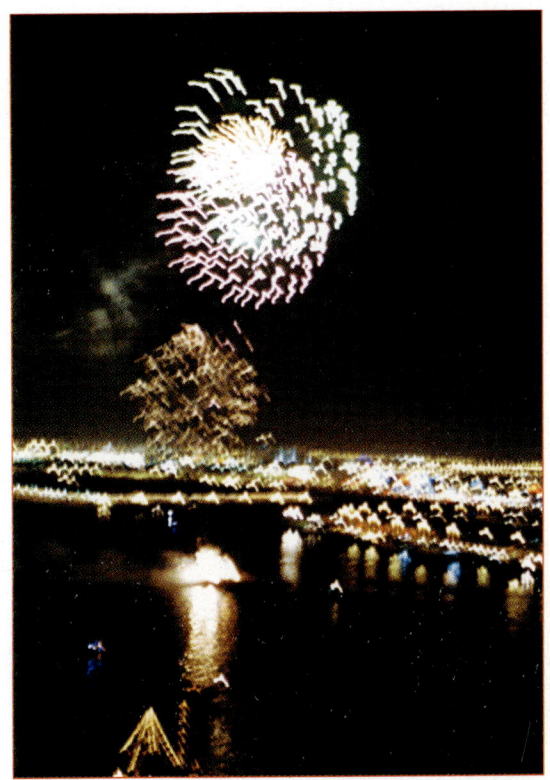

Festivities in Dubai.

'Portrait of a Woman', an exhibit
hanging in Bahrain's art museum.

A young Marrakesh citizen peeps out
of his perch on his mother's back.

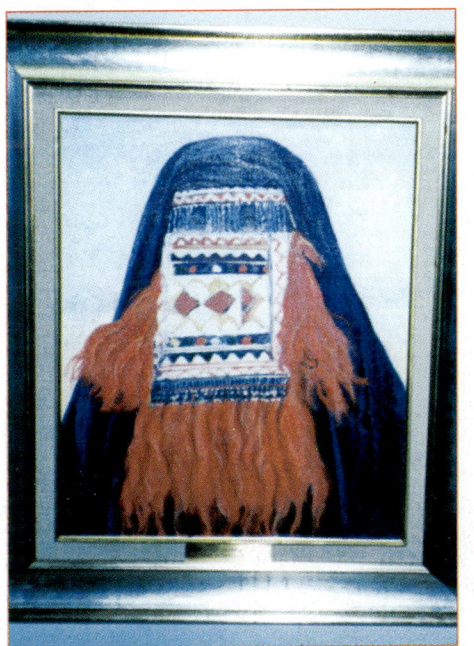

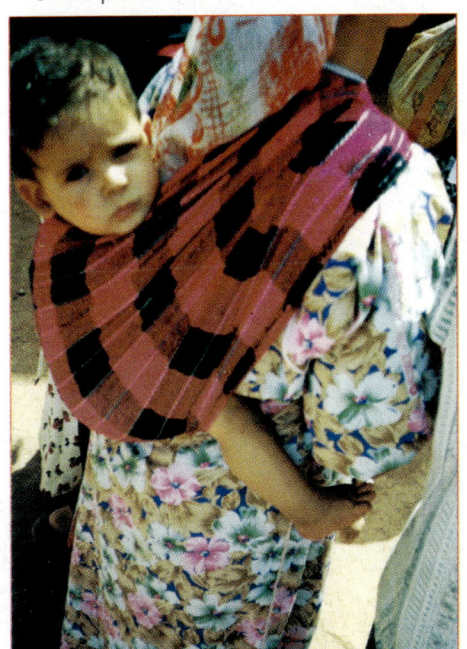

Plate **3**

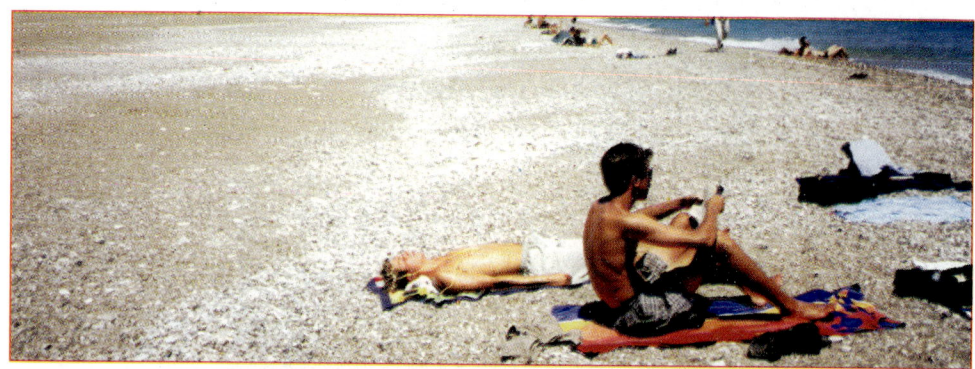

Sun, pebbles and beach: a Turkish rhapsody.

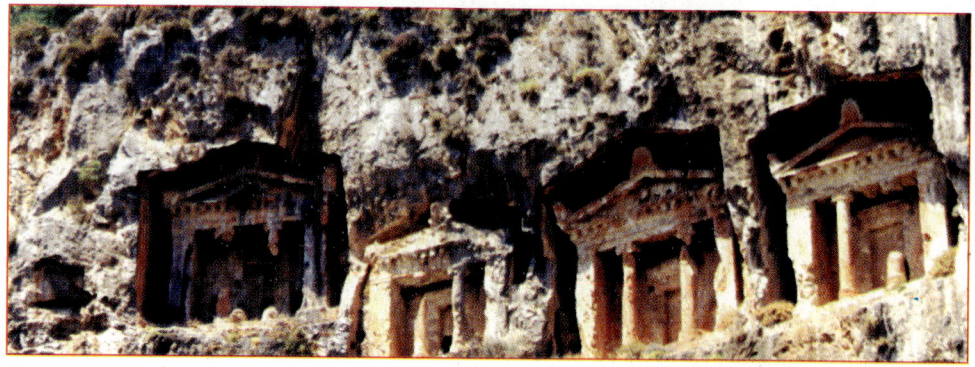

Tombs high in the mountain in Turkey
— to be closer to the gods.

The Sultan's gilded cage in the
palace in Istanbul to keep an
eye on his ministers.

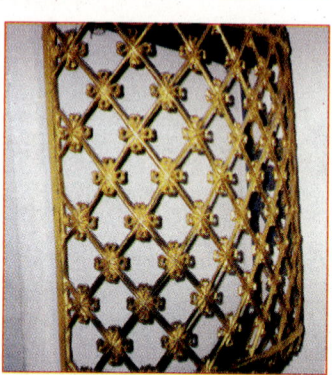

Istanbul stretches from Europe to Asia.

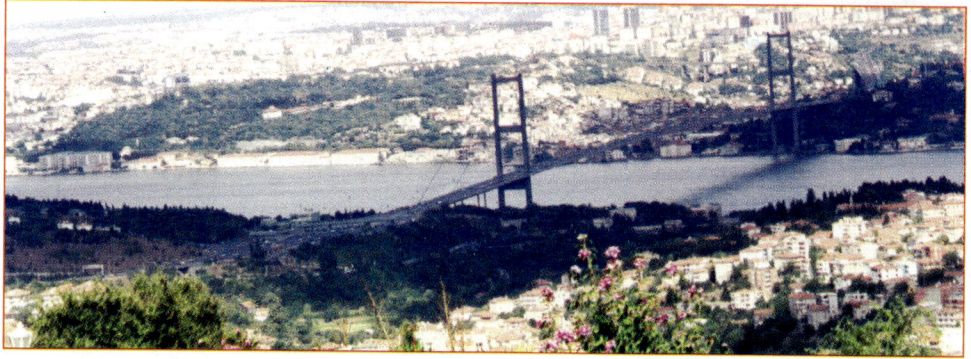

Plate **4**

EGYPT

Living on Hope, 1988

Egypt, the eternal land of the pyramids and the Pharaohs, lives on, and the Nile flows in Cairo, lending a spectacular air to a city of chaotic traffic and an ambience of bonhomie. Israeli tourists took in the sights of Cairo, and *The Jerusalem Post* was available at news stands. Cairo was the Israelis' window on the Arab world even as the rest of it still frowned on the Jewish State.

President Mubarak's Egypt is not Nasser's country. Sadat made peace with Israel under American auspices to regain his territory in the Sinai, to the anger of the rest of the Arab World. Egypt suffered ostracism, and earned a suspension from the Arab League for making a separate peace with Israel.

But the mood in the Arab world was mellower than it was a decade earlier, with one exception, the Palestinians. The uprising in the occupied territories was a rude reminder to the Arab world, as much as to other nations, that it could not sweep the Palestinian problem under the carpet. A people fighting for their homeland and independence demanded to be heard.

For Egypt, the Shultz Plan on West Asia was a life-saver for a variety of reasons. It offered a country alienated from the rest of the Arab world by the Camp David accord a chance to speed up the process of its true return to the Arab fold. It made Egypt's close military and economic relations with the Americans less awkward. Third, it attempted to defuse a dangerous situation in the occupied territories, which had its inevitable repercussions on Egypt.

No responsible Egyptian seriously believed that the Shultz Plan would get very far, but for the record and diplomatically, Egypt had grasped the plan for all it was worth, initiating hectic diplomacy with Tunisians, the Palestine Liberation Organisation and Jordan. It suited Mubarak and his government to talk tall about talks on peace, and since it served the American interest to keep the plan afloat for its own reasons, there was much toing and froing of American and Egyptian envoys among the Arab capitals. In general terms, it suited the Arabs not to present an intransigent front to the world and Egypt, among others, chose to see "positive elements" in the Shultz Plan.

Egyptian ministers made no secret of the fact that they had learnt their lessons from the past and were not too unhappy over seeing Shamir's public recalcitrance, most recently during the Israeli Prime Minister's visit to Washington.

Egyptians said they were in a unique and privileged position in the Arab world, being the only country of the region to have an Israeli embassy in its capital, and with its diplomatic relations restored with much of the Arab world. They were conscious of the traditionally pivotal role of Egypt in West Asia, with a thriving arms export industry, and knew fully well that public Arab postures did not square up with their private diplomacy, as far as Israel was concerned.

The Palestinian uprising in the occupied territories was both a problem and an opportunity for Egypt. It made Cairo's relations with Tel Aviv more difficult, even as Egypt enjoyed the fruits of the Camp David accord with the restoration of the Sinai. At the same time, the prospect of peace—however remote—gave Egypt greater room for diplomatic manoeuvre.

The director of the Israeli section in the foreign office in Cairo, Badr-Hammam, found hopeful trends in Israel, which was divided down the middle by the happenings in the occupied territories. Israeli elections were due in November, but the Egyptian official feared that Shamir might call them early to avoid giving a final answer to the Shultz Plan.

Egyptian Recipe

Egyptians believed that the key to making the plan work lay in Washington, if only it would push Israel hard enough. There was little conviction in Cairo that the US Administration would want to go too far in an election year. But it suited Cairo to pretend that the Shultz Plan had a chance.

The situation on the ground had not changed much. Palestinians continued to demonstrate in the occupied territories, with some getting beaten and others shot. Egyptians said they had advised the PLO not

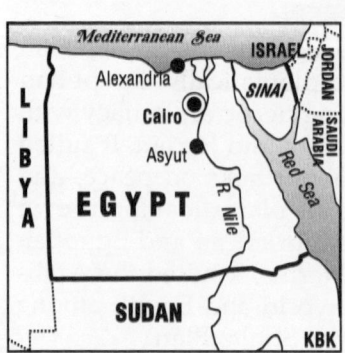

to reject the plan outright, if only because it had not been formally presented to them. Cairo called the bypassing of the PLO in the plan "a big mistake", and suggested that the Palestinian delegates to the talks must inevitably be representative, i.e. approved by the PLO leadership, but did not find the problem insurmountable.

We—a group of foreign journalists—were treated to a unique session between an Israeli, Amos Kenan, and the PLO adviser to Yasser Arafat, Nabeel Shaath, in Cairo. Kenan, unre-presentative as he was of his country because he belonged to the small peace camp, talked in apocalyptical terms. The uprising, and more particularly the recent Palestinian attack in Israel, in his view, had set back the beginning of a very gradual rapprochement between elements in Israel and among the Palestinians. Kenan, who believed that things would get worse before they got better, was for giving back every inch of land—in the Gaza Strip and the occupied territory of the West Bank to the Palestinians who were already an entity.

According to Kenan, the present US Administration could not hope to resolve the Palestinian issue in the remaining six months. In any event, an American-administered peace without Soviet acquiescence would not succeed. "No *Pax Americana* is possible", he said. Nabeel Shaath, on the other hand, declared that the world forgot the Pales-tinians when there was no violence. The Western world, in particular, reacted when there was violence. But he was not optimistic about an early end to the Palestinians' suffering. Firm in his conviction that an independent homeland would come, he agreed with Kenan: "Yes, Israel and Palestinians can be close allies". Kenan confirmed that Israelis were truly divided. Half of Israel, he said, was afraid of war and other half was afraid of peace. But, unfortunately, Israel and Palestinians equally suffered from weak leaderships although they could in future be natural allies in an Arab world which feared both Israeli and Palestinian dynamism. But the future was not the present, and as this somewhat surrealistic debate proceeded apace, there was news of more beatings and more killings in the occupied territories. And the tempo of diplomatic activity in and around Egypt reached a feverish pitch. To what purpose was unclear.

Egypt would like to see a future Palestinian State remain in a federation with Jordan, but protested that it was a question for the Palestinians to decide. It warned all who would care to listen that Israel would have to deal with a more radical leadership in the future if the Palestinian question was not resolved, and the Palestinian undertaking, given in the Cairo Declaration, not to attack Israeli and other targets outside the occupied territories and Israel, would not hold. Egyptians said the Palestinians problem could not wait for the American and Egyptian elections to be completed.

Despair in a Refugee Camp

The uprising in Israel's occupied territories had brought the world's newest divided city to the fore. It is the town of Rafah in Egypt and lies in Sinai, handed back to Egypt in 1982 as part of the Camp David agreement.

The dividing line ran through houses as the bilateral part of the Camp David agreement between Israel and Egypt was implemented to the letter to restore the old international boundary destroyed by Israel in the 1967 war. But Rafah, adjoining the Gaza Strip still under Israeli occupation became known for one thing: the Canada camp of 5,000 Palestinian refugees. The name it acquired after the Canadian forces of the United Nations, which were originally gathered there.

Rafah is a five-hour drive from Cairo across the Suez Canal, and a visit to the camp gave the dimension of the West Asia conflict. Having made a separate peace with Israel, Egypt now faced Israel in Gaza through a high barbed wire fence topped by watch towers on the Israeli side. An ordinary iron gate led a traveller to the Israeli side and vice versa.

This was used by the residents of Camp Canada, the main border crossing lay elsewhere. Less than 100 people used this crossing every day— people working in Israel, or relations visiting their near ones with Israeli permission, given after a month's delay for one visit a year.

It was a windy, cloudy day. Two Egyptian armed police guards sat and smoked in their guard station. Israeli soldiers watched the goings-on from the Israeli side. Nature had retrieved part of the ugliness. Further on, one Palestinian shouted to another across the fence, unable to sit down together.

As refugee camps go, Rafah is far from one's conception of such a tragedy. It had a number of stone houses and its streets were relatively clean, with homes sprouting a sea of antennae, some capped with the defiant Palestinian flag, which fluttered almost next to the Israeli flag across the border. Teenagers and children crowded round visitors, raising their hands in the V sign. They were on the surface like their counterparts elsewhere, but their scars ran deep, and their cause, avowedly espoused by much of the world, remained unfulfilled.

Rafah fell in Egyptian territory through the restoration of the old boundary. Other Palestinian refugee camps lay across the border in the occupied territories. Sara Zaqoot, head teacher of the preparatory class of the only school in Rafah, told us that she heard gunfire from across the border almost every day, saw Israeli planes, and from high ground saw Israeli troops raid a girls' school and beat up pupils.

Palestinian Spirit

The uprising in the occupied territories which had brought the Palestinians situation again to the fore naturally affected the Palestinians most acutely. Every man, woman and child we talked to said that he or she would rather be in Palestine, their home, fighting the Israelis, rather than stay where they were.

There was tension in the town when we visited it because of the deaths of two Palestinians killed in Israel across the border, and riot police sporting shields still stood guard. The elders of the community said that they tried to exercise restraint upon the young who wanted to demonstrate to urge Egypt to do more for their cause.

"People here", explained Mohammed Hasan Al Majjar, the school supervisor, "listen to radio and watch television every hour to find out what is happening to their brothers". There was almost a tinge of despair in his voice as he tried to formulate an answer to the question: When will the independent Palestinian state arrive? "It will not be soon", he finally answered, firm though he was in his conviction that it would come, step by step.

"We tell the young not to do anything to embarrass the Egyptians, who are our friends", Hasan declared. But he made no attempt to hide his feelings. "We feel that we are isolated from our people and our country after Sinai's return to Egypt. We are not better off here. It is better to be home. We are Palestinians".

Even as Rafah represented the hopelessness of 5,000 Palestinian refugees, seemingly left by events in the limbo, Palestinian determination shines through. I asked 12-year-old Abdel Salem how he felt. "I am very happy with what is happening in the occupied territories", he said, "I want to be there to fight". Another student showed me the back of his palm sporting an ink drawing of the Kalashnikov. As if by reflex action, all hands join in the V sign to denote their ultimate faith in Palestinian independence.

The school in Canada Camp had around 1,500 pupils in the three segments: elementary, preparatory, and secondary. What happened to those who graduated from the school? Some went to Egyptian universities, others to other Arab countries for jobs.

Hasan is an intense man whose home was in Ashdod, now in Israel. He came to the camp in 1973 after being uprooted from the original camp by an Israeli road-widening programme to police camps better.

Along the way to Canada Camp from Cairo, a neglected sign painted on a roadside wall proclaimed: "This is Greater Israel". Further on, a check post of the MNFO, the Multinational Force and Observers, set up under the camp David accord, was evidence of the agreement working in one respect.

Egyptian Perestroika, 1990

In a world in flux, Egypt was seeking to carve out for itself a dominant position in the Arab region. There was a high level of emotional satisfaction in Cairo over the Arab world's acceptance of Egypt, despite its separate peace with Israel, represented most recently by Syria's rapprochement. But Egypt's efforts to take centrestage in the Arab world were hampered by fears about the economic outlook, with the country under a crushing foreign debt burden.

Egyptian officials in Cairo spoke about the need for turning attention to economic issues. "Nasser and Sadat involved themselves with major political issues. President Hosni Mubarak believes it is time to tackle the economic problems," said one official. And a political analyst suggested, "There is no way we can repay the $44 billion debt, however much you might squeeze the country."

In many ways, Egypt has come a long way from the days of 10 years ago or more. It had been accepted back in the Arab fold while the Israeli flag flew defiantly in the heart of Cairo (the only Arab country then to have diplomatic relations with Isreal). Inter-Arab traffic met at the crossroads of Cairo once again, and President Mubarak had achieved something of a key position on the Palestinian issue in the Arab world.

Yet events in the wider world were casting shadows on Egyptian optimism. Egyptian analysts were not certain that Mikhail Gorbachev could surmount his problems, with one of them suggesting that the Soviet Union could become a neo-Stalinist state. But all decried the expected mass migration of Soviet Jews to Israel as a factor that could complicate the resolution of the Palestinian issue. And there were worries that the Western world, the US in particular, would focus on East Europe, to the detriment of Egypt and the Arab world.

There were other question marks as Egyptians looked at the future. What impact would East European events have on the Arab world? The communists in particular and the Left in general in Egypt were seeking to explain away the events, not dissimilar to the embarrassment the Indian communists were facing. The liberals, on the other hand, were suggesting that the Arab leaders should heed the warning and move towards democratisation. While some believed that the bulk of the Arab regimes was capable of projecting selective censored information, others said that in the modern age one could not keep a people insulated. "There's the BBC to turn to to know the truth", said one.

Egypt served as the role model in the region and the present political phase in the country was described as "controlled pluralism". The press was, in the Arab context, relatively free and Egyptian intellectuals suggested that their regime was not particularly oppressive. The key question remained the issue of presidential succession, with President Mubarak hesitant in introducing a new constitution. Thinking Egyptians tended to view the President as a sincere man with right instincts but a man of limited vision.

"Perestroika in Egypt started in the mid-seventies," an Egyptian explained. "But it has been a slow process. Sadat had the foresight and he could control the process. Egypt, therefore, avoided the convulsions of Algeria, Morocco and other countries."

Signs of religiosity were apparent in Cairo, as they were elsewhere in the Arab world, with new mosques being built and a large number of women sporting head scarves. But the Muslim Brothers, it was suggested, did not pose an insurmountable problem. They were in the People's Assembly and, according to one analyst, they were middle class people who wished to operate within the system. The influence of the Iranian revolution, many believed, was on the wane.

The liberals in Egypt were encouraged by the signs of change, however symbolic, appearing in the Arab world. In Saudi Arabia, they had elections to the chamber of commerce. Human rights groups were emerging in the Arab world and were being tolerated by some regimes. And the trend, in common with world events, was towards a less ideological view.

Egyptian Opening

"In the sixties and even seventies, our intellectuals argued that democracy was bad and bourgeois and served only vested and capitalist interests," an Egyptian explained. "But nobody is talking that language any more." Egyptians expected a surge of privatisation in the Arab world because of falling oil revenues and the fall from grace of communism.

Egypt was heartened by the growing amity in the Arab world, a precious commodity it was seeking to nurture. Such amity was a prerequisite for Egypt's leadership role and could serve as an instrument to cope with the world of the future. Indeed, senior officials in the Egyptian foreign office were looking at the world's emerging economic contours with some foreboding.

One senior official put it thus: "The economic blocs are being formed. There are the United States and Canada; there's the European Economic Community of 1992 and there are Japan and the rich industrialised East Asian Countries. Hence the feeling among Arabs that we must come together. Economic, rather than political, questions will determine the future."

Egyptians were quite clear that their country could not be the leader of a sub-regional grouping. They talked about the Maghreb Union, the Gulf Cooperation Council and Egypt. The obvious implication was that only the Arab region as a whole, under Egypt's leadership, could play an effective role.

When Sadat signed the Camp David agreement with Israel under American aegis, he did so keeping his country's interests in mind in titling towards the West. He put non-alignment on the back burner. Egyptians were split on the accord although the majority, it would seem, was for it, in view of the benefits it had brought.

Non-alignment remained on the back burner. Egyptians made no secret of their view that the concept had lost its relevance and had been unable to tune in to twenty-first century.

There had been the question of dilution of criteria for membership, which had reduced it to another Group of 77. Second, Egyptians felt that the movement kept repeating the clichés of the past, long after the circumstances which brought it into being had passed into history. Egypt, at any rate, had little time for non-alignment.

Egypt's attention was focussed on the Arab world and Africa—the latter by virtue of President Mubarak's presidency of the Organisation of African Unity. In diplomacy, priority is given to the Palestinian issue. As one Egyptian explained, "We must resolve the Palestinian problem because it is using up so much of the Arab nation's energy."

Egyptians believed that the key impetus to keeping the Palestinian issue alive was provided by the intefada in the Israeli-occupied territories, rather than any of the various plans on the table. They were equally convinced that if the problem was not resolved within a reasonable time-frame, the Arab world would revert to terrorism and violence.

There was hope in Cairo that the Palestinians problem would be resolved during the present decade. It was based on the evolution of the Israeli political process. But Egyptian officials made it clear that despite Israeli prodding, Cairo would remain "a postman". Egypt would continue to play its role as one of bringing the Israelis and Palestinians closer without impinging on the Palestine Liberation Organisation's status as the sole representative of Palestinians.

There was no air of apology in Cairo about Egypt's pre-eminent role in the region by virtue of its population and industrial and military capability. During a visit across the Suez Canal I was shown an old Israeli headquarters in the sandy dunes captured by Egypt in the 1973 war. Some distance away, an Egyptian colonel proudly posed for a photograph in front of a derelict Israeli tank commanded by General Assaf Yagory, now an Egyptian showpiece.

I asked the colonel what thoughts were uppermost in his mind about the country's defence after 18 years of "no war". "We have to be strong to safeguard peace", he answered with unaffected confidence.

JORDAN

Walking the Tight Rope, 1988

Among the Arab states, the resurfacing of the Palestinian question presented the most acute dilemma for the kingdom of Jordan. It is a small state with a small population, which lost the West Bank to the Israelis in the 1967 war. Palestinians constitute a majority in its present borders and Jordan cannot afford to be too far out of step with the Arab world in seeking to resolve the problem.

Jordan has the largest number of Palestinian refugees, most of whom are automatically granted Jordanian citizenship, unlike in Syria which takes pains to maintain the Palestinian identity for its own reasons. Its salvation lies in making a joint approach to the problem with the Palestine Liberation Organisation, but its last attempt to do so failed because Yasser Arafat, the Palestinian leader, has had to contend with differences in his camp. And the abortive Amman Agreement has been replaced by the PLO official credo of an independent Palestinian state, to which all Arabs states pay lip-service.

Like Egypt, Jordan put the best face on the Shultz Plan on West Asia because, at the very least, it kept the pressures created by the uprising in the occupied territories within manageable limits. In common with other Arab capitals, the uprising is top television news every evening even as the Jordanian authorities from King Hussein down, try to temper the Arab rhetoric. King Hussein had proved to be an impressive tight-rope walker during much of his long reign, but the problem he and his country faced was that the uprising had created a new situation, increasing the risks involved for a frontline state like Jordan.

Understandably, it was in Jordanian interest to keep the Shultz Plan afloat·even while undertaking an intensive round of diplomacy through visits to neighbouring capitals. Against the background of the traditional litany of Israeli wrongs, repeated by newspapers and television stations every day, the Jordanian leadership gave the impression of being very clear headed about the dangers of the uprising on the future of West Asia and where Jordanian interest lay.

The official Jordanian stance was to look at the positive aspect of the Shultz Plan, namely, that the United States had chosen to get involved, and, what was contended in Amman, had accepted the principle of self-determination for Palestinians.

But Jordanians at the same time made no secret of their belief that no eventual West Asian settlement would be possible without Soviet cooperation, as opposed to continuing American efforts to keep the Soviets out of West Asia. And the Jordanian leadership looked with horror at some scenarios being painted in the United States on how to limit its international commitments by making Israel an even more important strategic ally of Washington.

Jordanians said that they and the Palestinians were "one people" even as Palestinians' attempts to keep their identity were apparent in the country. The contradiction involved in the claim colliding with reality could be seen in the Palestinian refugee camps. Press visits to camps were conducted under tight control. With officials and secusiry men outnumbering journalists two to one, there was not much chance for the inhabitants to speak their mind. And even as the refugee camps became more permanent in their ambience, the political questions they posed were many and prickly.

Indeed, the relationship between UNRWA, the United Nations Relief and Works Agency for Palestine Refugees in the Near East, which ran 10 camps in the country, and the Jordanian government was a delicate one. White UNRWA ran the camps under the United Nations mandate, the Amman authorities sought to promote their national policies through these camps. Palestinian refugees formed nearly a third of Jordan's total population.

The director of the UNRWA field office in Jordan, E. Saaf of the Netherlands, who took us to the Baqa camp, said that his organisation built the first concrete school in Jordan three years earlier. It had been difficult to make improvements in camps earlier because such undertakings represented a political decision. He felt that there was a greater sense of realism now.

Baqa had some 80,000 inhabitants out of a total registered refugee population of 850,000, but these figures were at best notional because of the movement of the refugees in and out of camps.

Playing Games

The last census of refugees was permitted by the government in 1973. Jordan refused an UNRWA request for a new census citing its inappropriateness "at this delicate time". Saaf admitted that the refugees could play UNRWA against the Jordanian government and also against the PLO factions. According to Saaf, the question why refugee camps remained—some of them were almost 40 years old—was determined by political, social and financial reasons. The refugee camps were a political statement. The refugees lived in their own tribal groups after they lost their homes. Besides, land outside was very expensive and shopowners in the camps did not pay taxes. Some of the refugees living in camps had two homes. By and large, UNRWA did not hand out doles—most people were employed, with the unemployed rate running at 10 per cent. UNRWA provided nine years' schooling and health care, in addition to minimal facilities to other Palestinian refugees living outside camps.

In political terms, the Jordanian stance was to emphasise the need for Israeli withdrawl from the occupied territories. Official spokesman said that they would not force a confederation of the West Bank with Jordan on the Palestinians while suggesting that Israeli and US acceptance of an independent Palestine state was remote. If such a state did emerge, it would be at the end of a long process, Indeed, in realistic terms, Israeli withdrawal from the West Bank and Gaza Strip and a confederation of these territories with Jordan would by itself represent a major diplomatic achievement as and when it came about. It would be so even without contending with the problem of Israeli withdrawal from East Jerusalem and the Syrian Golan Heights, areas formally annexed by Israel.

Less rhetorical though the Jordanians were in Arab terms, they practised various forms of make-believe. A visit to the Royal Committee of Jerusalem Affairs, formed to look after Jerusalem and find out what was going on there, revealed the extent of Jordanian obeisance to the understandable Muslim attachment to the holy city. After welcoming the international media as "soldiers of justice and truth", thanks to their making the world aware of Israeli repression on the West Bank, committee spokesmen relapsed into standard propaganda, laced with half-truths, which carried little conviction.

Nor was the Jordanian effort to have well-schooled village notables meet the press in the Baqa refugee camp very convincing. Resplendent in their traditional robes, the notables' refrain was, "We shall return home when the big powers will do justice to us". The other answers were equally pat: "There is no separation between Jordanians and Palestinians. We have always lived as one people. We are just like a family".

Life swirled on in the Baqa camp outside the conference room, with people buying and selling goods in the bazaars, and impish children followed the press party, only too keen to have themselves photographed. An old woman in the bazaar cried out: "You are like gold. You have helped us". Her reference was to the new perception of the world's, specially Western, media in highlighting Israeli repression in the occupied territories.

At the end of the day, Jordan fell back on the familiar Arab theme: The United States holds the key and can force Israel to do the right thing by withdrawing from the occupied territories. The shrewd Jordanian leadership, meanwhile, was probing and interacting with the Americans, the Soviets and fellow Arabs to try to defuse a very explosive situation.

A Bridge on Jordan River

The King Hussein Bridge (the old Allenby bridge) is a symbol of the Palestinian crisis for two reasons. It is one of the two bridges linking Jordan to the occupied territory of the West Bank, and the tensions created by the uprising were palpable on the Israeli side. Indeed, the bridge was a reflection of the uneasy peace that existed between Israel and the Arab states, best described by the awkward phrase "no war", as diplomatic moves gathered momentum.

I got a taste of the tension during a visit to the bridge, 50 kilometers from Amman. The Israeli soldier on the other side of the bridge, an unimpressive structure some 25 meters long, objected to photographs of the crossing being taken from the Jordanian side. "No pictures", he shouted from his end of the bridge. The warning was disregarded by the cameramen in the press party comprising nine journalists from around the world.

The soldier worked himself into a veritable rage seeing his orders disregarded and paced up and down his side, finally coming to the centre of the bridge to demand that he talk to the amiable Jordanian in charge of bridge security, Captain Mohammed Amin. The captain listened to the soldier's monologue in good humour, reminding the Israeli that pictures had been taken from the Israeli-occupied side a day earlier. "That was one picture", he retorted. "People are taking a thousand pictures". Frustrated, he stalked back to his side of the bridge, throwing an unprintable expletive at us.

The old bridge across the muddy Jordan river was destroyed by the Israelis in the 1967 war and the present King Hussein Bridge was built by the side of its ruins. There were no markers or flags denoting the end of Jordanian control. For Jordan, the West Bank was part of its territory, admittedly under occupation. The Israeli flag fluttered on the Israeli side. Jordan liaised with the Israelis through the mechanism created by the Armistice agreement.

A Lifeline

Apart from the tourists who go across the bridge with Israeli permission, the bridge was a lifeline for a large number of Palestinians who went home or came to visit relations in Jordan. The bridge was under Jordanian police control, and the director of the bridge's security service, Colonel Khaled Shaheen, harped on one theme is his talk with us: the humiliation meted out to the Palestinians who cross the bridge. "We want the world to know the facts", he said, "maybe it will help decrease their humiliation".

According to Col. Shaheed, Arabs crossing the bridge were stripped. Palestinian maps on chains were torn away from the necks of their wearers and cigarette lighters were confiscated. He added, "Later, the Israelis put the lighters in their pockets".

Quotas for the bridge crossing were fixed by the Armistice agreement. In summer, there were about 4,000 bridge crossings a day, tapering off to 2,000 in winter. But the Palestinian uprising had decreased the number by almost one-third. The Israelis charged 35 Jordanian dinars (US$105) for each person, counting every child, crossing the bridge.

We saw trucks laden with fruit, the produce of occupied territories, roll across the bridge; they were surrealistic trucks, with their engines uncovered. Inside, the seat for the driver was bereft of cushion, and the wheels were sealed with wires fixed to the bolts holding them. Colonel Shaheen said the trucks had to pay the equivalent of US$310 for each crossing and were not allowed to carry a spare tyre. The trucks were required to return to the Israeli side the same day.

A million people crossed the bridge every year in normal times. For individual crossings, the bridge was open from 7 am to 3 pm in summer and from 8 am to 1 pm in winter.

Colonel Shaheen ended his talk with a hope. He said: "The international community can force Israel to be realistic. We hope there will be no bridges, no suffering, no such river crossings in the future".

It was a hope.

A Prince Explains

In one of the clearest expositions of Jordan's key role in the evolving Palestinian situation, Crown Prince Hassan told a group of nine journalists from around the world that there was a linkage between the Afghanistan and Palestinian situations. In both cases, he said, "the main concern is to achieve withdrawal. That is the ultimate objective".

The second most important man in the kingdom implied that the Soviet position on West Asia was "realistic". And it was conceivable that, despite denials, the convergence of several regional conflicts— the Arab–Israeli problem, the situation in the Gulf, the Iran–Iraq war and the Lebanon problem—could lead to a superpower trade-off.

The Crown Prince, in his early forties, was clear headed and to the point in an hour-long discourse on a whole range of issues affecting the Palestinian question, lacing his comments with flashes of humour. Wearing a conservative lounge suit, he met us in the complex of the sports city in the attractive Jordanian capital of Amman.

The Crown Prince did not mince his words in frankly acknowledging that Jordan's relationship with the Palestine Liberation Organisation was ambivalent and said it was time for the PLO to clarify its approach to the peace process. He described it as a sad fact that the PLO had different patrons in the Arab world. He declined a high-profile role for Jordan in relation to the occupied West Bank and the Gaza Strip. In his view, first things must come first. "There should be a clear assurance on the final status. Palestinians have to be given their right to determine their future".

In an equally forthright enumeration of Jordan's approach to the Shultz Plan, he said an alternative to the peace process was "an unprecedented wave of terror in the Middle East as a whole". If the Palestinian question was not resolved, the region would be "drowned in a sea of nationalism". The whole fabric of the sovereign state was being torn by sectarian and ethnic conflicts. "The mosaic of Lebanon is quite clear".

The Crown Prince said the scope of an international conference would have to be determined, but it would have "a clear referral role". There was, he added, "a better alignment of the stars" for convening an international peace conference on West Asia.

"This region", the Crown Prince said, "is looked at as one of terrorists or barrels of oil. Put us in human terms. The humanising process is beginning to happen". Ridiculing the concept of Israel being surrounded by "a sea of enemies", he said that each Arab state had its own problems.

"Egypt had signed an agreement with Israel and was working for an international conference. Syria had its own problems because of its involvement in Lebanon and in relation to the Gulf, the Gulf states were for an international conference. The Arab region was a pluralistic world".

Jordan's Problem

Pinpointing Jordan's problem, he said that when it tried to appear reasonable, it had to consider its own constituency, which was the Arab world. It shouldered much of the financial burden in supporting the administration of the occupied territories, but it was suggested in a poll among Palestinians on the West Bank that King Hussein's popularity was three per cent. "I would be very happy if the King's popularity would be zero per cent because it shows our objectivity".

The Crown Prince cast some doubt on the proposed confederation of the West Bank and Jordan by referring to "the concept of confederation if it ever emerges at the end of the day". He suggested that to talk about the confederation now would be putting the cart before the horse.

Crown Prince Hassan said it was encouraging that US diplomacy could accept self-determination for the Palestinians. "Americans have always said that you have to deal with the incumbent". The Shultz initiative, he felt, was "very much to stay in 1988".

But he did not hide his fears about recent American trends. One of Jordan's basic fears was the feeling of American retrenchment which would encourage the "self-image of strategic Israel in this context". The Right in Israel would be bolstered by the feeling that it was the safeguard against Khomeinism in West Asia, and hence could ignore the question of politics in which people mattered.

"Our cards are on the table", the Crown Prince said. "In Jordan's East Bank, the impact of the uprising was that the people were torn between supporting Palestinians in terms of money while at the same time they did not wish to divert attention from what was happening there". This remark was made against the background of official Jordanian discouragement of Palestinian demonstrations in the country.

King Hussein's Surprise

In March 1988, Jordan's Minister for Occupied Territories, Marwan Doudin, told me in Amman that he hoped his ministry would be abolished "one day". He could have scarcely imagined that his wish would be fulfilled in a matter of months, rather than years or decades, in dramatically different circumstances than he had envisaged.

In moves that stunned his officials and the outside world, King Hussein renounced responsibility for the Israeli-occupied West Bank and Gaza, withdrew the development plan for the area, dissolved Jordan's House of Representatives, which had significant Palestinian representatives, and announced the laying off or retirement of 20,000 employees in the territories. In short, the most durable king of the Arab world stood conventional wisdom on its head.

The conventional wisdom was that if the United States mustered the will to pressure Israel, the occupied territories could be given freedom, over time, in a confederation with Jordan. The eight-month-long uprising in the occupied territories forced the Arab world and the United States to look at the problem again.

Despite the lip sympathy they gave the Palestinian cause, most of the Arab states had their own compulsions for according low priority to the issue while the US, Israel's strategic ally and benefactor, was for the better part marking time. Thanks to the uprising, the US Secretary of State, George Shultz, conducted vigorous shuttle diplomacy to sell his plan.

The plan itself was an inadequate answer to the problem. It promised a somewhat symbolic international conference leading to direct talks between the Israelis and the Arabs, including Palestinians, but not the Palestine Liberation Organisation, on an association of the occupied territories with Jordan. But most of the Arab states, to appear to be doing something, encouraged Shultz to persevere, and nobody rejected the plan out of hand, except of course the Likud wing of the Israeli government.

Overnight, the Shultz Plan seemed to have become irrelevant. But King Hussein had posed problems for all the others involved as well: the Palestine Liberation Organisation, Israel, Syria and the other Arab neighbours. All these countries and the PLO were still recovering from the shock waves created by King Hussein's brilliant move.

Two questions arose: what led the King to make the move and what would be its likely consequences? It was clear that there was growing frustration in Jordan over a no-win situation. Yasser Arafat had to repudiate his agreement with King Hussein last year on a joint strategy for tackling the Palestinian issue. Jordan, itself a Palestinian-majority country, was not popular among the Palestinians of the West Bank and Gaza Strip, and yet was carrying most of the burden of supporting the infrastructure and services and giving almost automatic Jordanian nationality to Palestinian refugees.

There were 13 Palestinian refugee camp in Jordan and, according to the Labour Minister, Rasheed Oraykat, 273,000 Palestinians holding Jordanian passport lived in the other countries of the Arab world. An independent Palestinian state, several officials explained in Amman, was an impractical idea. The Information Minister, Hani Khasawna, protested: "The Palestinian dilemma has many dimensions. Palestinians are a disappointed people. West Bank Palestinians' unhappiness with Jordan doesn't matter to us. They don't like the Syrians either. We don't want to impose ourselves on anyone".

Crown Prince Hassan explained it somewhat differently. "There is a misperception of Jordan's role", he said. "We shoulder much of the financial burden of the administration in the occupied territories".

Making a Point

King Hussein had gone as far as he did in dissociating his country from the occupied territories to make the point that it was not merely a tactical exercise. A statement of intent would have led to the obvious interpretation that he wanted the PLO and the other Arab states to come to him to help resolve the Palestinian problem.

Whatever King Hussein's motives, one consequence of his moves was that they helped to unfreeze a situation that was becoming more desperate each day. Until now, the vicious circle had remained unbroken. The Likud Prime Minister of Israel was simply refusing to give up any territory, the Americans had gone as far as they could go in an election year, the deaths in the occupied territories kept mounting as the Israelis used various forms of repressive measures to try to contain the uprising and the PLO, of course, stuck to its guns in demanding an independent Palestinian state.

The challenge King Hussein had presented was, first of all, to Yasser Arafat and his organisation. The King had earlier accepted the common Arab position of the PLO being the sole legitimate representative of the Palestinians and had now stated that he would immediately recognise a PLO-initiated government in exile. It was easy enough to form such a government, but could a revolutionary movement such as the PLO help run the administration of the occupied territories even in providing the necessary financial support? The Arab states had not been particularly generous to the PLO. A new twist had been added by Libya's offer to make good the money Jordan paid for the salaries and infrastructure in the occupied territories, estimated at one million dollars a month.

One factor that would weigh in the possible formation of a government in exile was the containment of the Syrian-supported dissident PLO factions. Besides, whatever the mechanics, money would need to be sent to all the thousands in the occupied territories now denied of their sustenance. The mood in these territories seemed confused.

For Israel, its problem had been compounded. The right-wing demand for the annexation of the territories had been rejected by the government. The dilemmas of the Labour Party were greater because the Jordanian option no longer seemed to exist. It was also Israel's election year, but the sooner the Israelis realised that the costs of occupation would go on mounting, the better it would be for the country's welfare and peace in the region.

The American administration was stymied by the compulsions of the Presidential election. But President Reagan would have to take some tentative decisions to cope with the new situation. To suggest, as American spokesmen had thus far, that the Shultz Plan stood was to beg the question of recognising the PLO.

For the other states as well, King Hussein's moves posed difficult problems. If Yasser Arafat boldly seized the initiative, it would imply that the Syrian-supported PLO dissidents would be at a greater disadvantage. Syria, it would seem, could not go beyond a point in trying to dethrone Arafat in order to coopt the PLO for its larger purposes in the region.

Although the credo of an independent Palestinian state was unanimously accepted by the Arab countries, there were differences among them, ranging from lack of enthusiasm to fears about the dynamism of the Palestinians. Egypt, as the only country to have made a separate peace with Israel, had to tread particularly warily.

Abdul Jawad Saleh, a deposed mayor from the occupied territories, told me in Amman in March: "We are asking the Arab states to leave us alone, and we'll take care of ourselves. We need a little help". King Hussein seemed to have answered his prayers.

At the very least, King Hussein had added a healthy dose of realism to the resolution of a vital problem in which many of the principal players were living in a make-believe world. The uprising forced the Arab states to take note of the Palestinian problem, and now the King's dramatic moves might bring Palestinians nearer the goal of independence.

A King Departs

K ing Hussein's extraordinary rule of 47 years encompassed the history of nearly half a century of West Asia's tempestuous politics and it was remarkable that for a monarch living in as troubled and divided a neighborhood as he did, he was receiving encomiums from both sides of the political divide. And it spoke volumes for his survival instincts, not merely in the physical sense of escaping coups and assassination attempts, that he was able to carve out a special role for himself and his country.

Ascending the throne in his teens, King Hussein had to learn on the job at a time the world he lived in was convulsed by wars and Israel's formation. Staying afloat in such a world was an achievement; to become a key player in the politics of war and peace for the ruler of a small, largely resource-scarce country burdened with refugees created by a state carved out by the Western powers showed political astuteness of a high order.

Living an events-filled life, the King made mistakes. He reportedly acknowledged the 1967 war one such mistake. Whether his decision to sign a peace treaty with Israel following the Oslo accords was a mistake depends upon the perspective of the person pronouncing the verdict. But King Hussein rode two horses with agility and kept Jordan as a nation knitting its tribal and Bedouin-origin population with the Palestinians who sought refuge and settled down. His deepening relationship with the United States stemmed from his country's needs and the compulsions of maintaining good relations with the sole surviving superpower, his more controversial connections with US agencies aside.

The King left a difficult legacy to his son and successor, Prince Abdullah, because the process of reconciling the Israelis with Palestinians had met great boulders, put in place by Israel's Benjamin Netanyahu among others, and Palestinians were being denied the crumbs they were offered by the flawed Oslo accords. The King's passing would mean that it would be that much more difficult to implement an agreement that was being eroded every day.

It was clear that Prince Abdullah's principal tasks would primarily be to attend to domestic affairs first. Although long in the making, the transfer of succession from the King's brother Prince Hassan, who served as the Crown Prince for nearly 34 years, to his oldest son came as a surprise. And this was followed by the equally surprising return of the King to his American hospital bed and his sad return home on a stretcher. Events had followed in too quick a succession for Jordanians to absorb them fully.

Neighbours' Welcome

Prince Abdullah had the support of Jordan's army—he was a senior officer in it—and this should stand him in good stead. Several of Jordan's neighbours were quick to endorse and welcome him as the Crown Prince, again a good augury because the country would need all the help it could get in moving the economy and tackling high levels of unemployment. The UAE's gesture in announcing its intention to transfer money to Jordan to shore up its economy would be particularly welcome to Amman.

It would obviously be more important for Prince Abdullah to set his own house in order than to cut a dashing figure on the regional or world stage. He was untested politically although no one who had lived in the King's proximity could remain ignorant of some of the wheels within wheels that exist in West Asian politics. But King Hussein had built his web of ties in the region and the world even as he balanced political forces at home and no successor could easily acquire these qualities.

Starting early, King Hussein had known and dealt with an amazing number of world leaders who had come and gone and had survived the upheavals of the region and his own involvement in some of them. He lost the West Bank and East Jerusalem in the 1967 war with Israel although he continued to retain an oversight role on Al Aqsa and the Dome on the Rock; he went against many of his Arab friends in tilting towards Saddam Hussein following Iraq's invasion and annexation of Kuwait; and the Palestinians remember only too vividly the Black September of 1970 when the Army fought the Palestine Liberation Organisation to expel its fighters.

In a sense, King Hussein converted the vulnerability of his country into an asset and with his decision to sign the peace treaty with Israel in 1994 he made peace and moderation his watchwords. That Israel made his task as difficult as it became was not his fault nor was the unravelling of a process that became a mockery of peace. Even the Wye River Memorandum he got up from his sick bed to help save remained unimplemented, despite all those hours and prestige President Bill Clinton put into it. The American compulsion vis-à-vis Israel is another story.

As King Abdullah tried to pick up the threads of his father's illustrious legacy, he would primarily seek the help of his Arab friends in the first instance. It was a tough act to follow, but as a perceptive observer suggested, the teenager Hussein had fewer assets and advisers to bank on at a worse time when he ascended the throne.

LEBANON

A Nation Bleeds

The tragedy of Lebanon, a fractured country which was bleeding to death, illumined the tragedy of how a local crisis had got enmeshed in the larger Arab-Israeli conflict, and there was no end to the larger crisis in sight.

As far as Lebanon is concerned, the imperative need for a new constitution to take the political and demographic realities into account had brought in many outside powers. Syrian troops went in under an Arab League mandate and stayed there to underline their leader's concept of his sphere of influence. Iraq, after its stalemated victory over Iran, was flexing its military muscles by supporting the Maronite Christians against Syria.

The Iranian revolution spilled over into Lebanon to harry the United States and to underline the new power of Khomeini's Islam. The Israeli invasion of Lebanon and subsequent retreat while retaining a border strip under their control added a new complication. And the Palestine Liberation Organisation, often routed in Lebanon, had retained its supporters.

Of the two superpowers, it was the aim of American policy during the long Kissinger reign to try to keep the Soviet Union out of the region after Egypt's turnaround. And the United States had not regained its composure in Lebanon after the spectacular murders of US marines and had relapsed into reactive diplomacy.

At a congressional hearing, frustrated senators grilled a senior Bush administration official on Lebanon for hours. The thrust of the senators' questions was whether the United States had a policy on Lebanon, apart from waiting on the Arab League. The answers were not convincing.

The Soviet Union had built a rather spectacular bridge with the post-Khomeini Iran, in addition to the arms-giving relationship it enjoyed with Syria and Iraq. It had counselled realism and moderation to the PLO even as it sent similar signals to Israel. While the Soviet Union was prepared to play a greater role in the region, it was understandably wary of rushing in where angels feared to tread.

Arab efforts at securing a solution in Lebanon had been frustrated by intra-Arab rivalries, the Iranian dimension and the fact that there was no sign of a resolution of the Arab-Israeli conflict. The three-member committee appointed by the League got nowhere.

Meanwhile, Lebanon continued to bleed, week after week, month after month, year after year. In a sense, it is a chicken and egg argument. What comes first—the resolution of the intra-Lebanon fight or the beginning of a solution to the Arab-Israel conflict? If the former, who would impose a solution on the bitter murderous quarrels of the Lebanese rivals—the Syrians, the Iraqis, the Iranians, the Israelis?

New French diplomatic efforts to try to bring a measure of peace to a country for which they bear a historical responsibility had not led very far. The killings continued day after day, cease-fires by the hundred were declared and broken. As the United Nations is the conscience of the world, its secretary-general was stung by the horrendous tragedy to invoke a rarely used power to summon a meeting of the UN Security Council.

It was clear that the UN could not wave a magic wand to bring peace to Lebanon overnight, but the Security Council meeting could be the beginning of a serious search for a step by step de-escalation of a situation in which two "governments" in the country, allied with groups and outside powers, were fighting one another to the last Lebanese.

It was equally clear that the two superpowers should act in concert to try to douse the flames of war. But the United States' moves could only be tentative because it was hamstrung by a number of constraints. Foremost among them was the symbiotic relationship with Israel, which went beyond a military and strategic relationship.

Ironically, the Bush administration started rather well, with the new secretary of state, James Baker, giving hints of new thinking on West Asia. It also agreed to build on the parting Reagan legacy of a dialogue with the PLO. But the administration's momentum on West Asia soon flagged as the traditional factors again came into play.

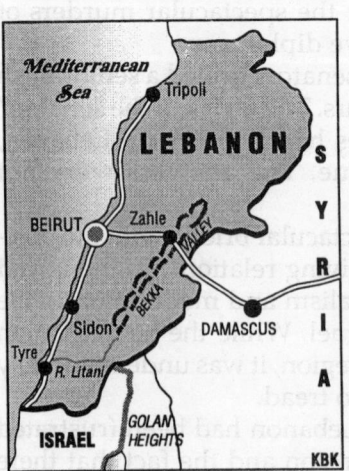

A Sham Plan

The US continued to embrace the Shamir peace plan, which the latter rescued from the clutches of his Likud party. The plan itself was an Israeli diplomatic offensive to counter the world's opprobrium on Israeli killings of Palestinians in the occupied territories in the long and continuing intefada. It offered little hope of a solution but remained an American talking point in talking about peace. The

PLO, which had now accepted Israeli's existence, continued to nag Americans to action, with little immediate result.

The Israeli leadership had given no indication that it was of a stature that could play a statesmanlike role in beginning to break out of the stalemate. Hanging on to the occupied territories in perpetuity offered no solution, and the painful process of rebuilding links and friendship with Arabs should begun. But Israeli leaders remained obdurate because they rightly assumed that they would continue to enjoy full US support.

A further American constraint in Lebanon and West Asia was the question of American hostages. Israel's abduction of a Shia cleric and the hostage-takers' apparent response in killing one of the American hostages created a major problem for President Bush in seeking to adopt diplomacy in resolving an issue that struck at the American jugular nerve.

The United States was continuing to sift the Iranian tea leaves in sending signals to the new executive president, Hashemi Rafsanjani, that Washington, for its part, was prepared to turn over a new leaf. The immediate price demanded was Iranian help in the release of the hostages. The signals from Iran, on the other hand, remained mixed, signifying divisions in the post-Khomeini leadership on dealing with "the Satan".

The initial results of the Security Council's call for a cease-fire were hardly encouraging. Efforts to arrive at a limited, but enforcable disengagement in Lebanon should be the first step in the long road to eventual peace in Lebanon. The strands of the larger Arab–Israeli conflict should be disentangled from the intra-Lebanese fighting. The Security Council's support to the Arab League for continuing its barren efforts would not take the world very far.

A new essential step would be called for. Israelis should be made to withdraw from their self-proclaimed security belt in Lebanon. Syria would not agree to withdraw its troops but they should be placed in a new, more limited framework under the supervision of the United Nations. Once peace returned to Lebanon after its seemingly never-ending nightmare, the United Nations should convene a conference of all Lebanese parties to evolve a new constitution, which would inevitably be less weighted in favour of Maronite Christians.

Merely to pose these possible solutions is to state the Herculean efforts that would be required. The alternative was to kill what remained of Lebanon and further exacerbate the consequences of the Arab-Israeli conflict, for the region and the world. The ballooning nature of the Lebanon crisis carried the warning that time was running out.

The Arab League, riven by divisions, proved incapable of bringing peace to Lebanon. Before we pass too harsh a judgement on it, we should remember that the League was trying to tackle problems left over by history and compounded by outside powers' strategic and political interests. Members of the League, it is no secret, were themselves attached to particular, often antagonistic, outside powers.

The onus was on the two superpowers to agree on a set of measures on Lebanon. A prerequisite was American acknowledgement of an equal role for the Soviet Union in the region. The United Nations and its secretary-general could merely highlight and dramatise the Lebanese tragedy, but there could be no workable solution unless the Big Two were willing to lend a hand in unscrambling what was perhaps the greatest post-war tragedy in the world.

Lebanon was a country that was literally moving towards extinction by the daily decimation of its people. For the Lebanese, it was a fate worse than a foreign invasion. If the daily carnage proceeded apace, there would be no Lebanon left.

Come One, Come All

Everybody was betting on peace in Lebanon—or almost everybody in July 1999—as hoteliers refurbished their hostelries and tourism officials sang the praises of nature's bounty, mountains and beaches and archaeological and historical sites that would keep any history buff contented. Being the only primarily service-oriented country in West Asia, any blip in the peace process registered immediately and tourists from the West and even the Arab world made themselves scarce.

The Israelis hit Lebanon hard on June 24, destroying the power station in Beirut and frightening away the lifeline of Lebanon, the tourists. But they came right back, and Lebanon was now preening itself as the cultural capital of the Arab world and a country of relaxation. Despite a look of disorganisation, things were moving in Lebanon and the hotelier who talked only in superlatives told me that he was betting on peace within a year.

Lebanon was at the crossroads in many ways. The Rafik Hariri era that brought much vitality and the amazing Beirut Central Distinct project had given way to a new regime that was pausing to take a look at the ballooning budget deficit. The assumption of office of Ehud Barak in Israel and his moves towards peace were music to Lebanese ears, in particular his recognition of Syria's central role in a Madrid process gone awry. Hotels were planning to expand and investors were being wooed assiduously.

Despite the interregnum, there was vitality in Beirut. The central district, the legacy of Hariri, who remained a major shareholder in the Solidere company building it, was taking shape although the preceding year was overshadowed by the worldwide economic recession and domestic factional politics. Spread over 120 hectares—50 hectares were being reclaimed from the sea—the new city centre, with marinas and promenades, was an impressive development project that would vie with the best in the world when completed.

Hariri took to newspaper columns to lecture his successors on their new austerity programme. The way to future prosperity, he said, was to expand, rather than contract, and as he showed during his eventful tenure, risk-taking was a central aspect of his vision, with multilateral funding and foreign capital scarce. Hariri might have been discarded politically for a time, but he was remembered by the Lebanese with much affection. They spoke of his charisma and his dynamism, in spite of the mistakes he made, among them surrounding himself with greedy men who had sticky fingers.

Beirut built a brand new airport which could handle six million passengers a year. There was a turnover of three million passengers before the civil war and the figure had reached barely 1.5 million. International airlines using Beirut were reduced to three climbing to 33, including all the major European carriers. A senior Middle East Airlines official told me that the civil war of nearly two decades meant that Lebanon regressed while the rest of the world progressed. Beirut lost its place as the banking and pleasure capital of West Asia. "We have lost not merely to Dubai," he said, "but to other places such as Larnaca and Cairo".

A New World

The airlines industry knew that it had to restructure to survive and Hariri was telling his countrymen that it was now a new world and a new ball game, the information age and the almost universal acceptance of the virtues of the free market. It was his hope as well as the hope of others in Lebanon that the Lebanese ambiance of a free environment culture and the capacity to enjoy life would bring back hundreds of thousands of Arab and other visitors to a country richly endowed by nature. Hariri's admonition was that what he describes as confessional politics—the cause of the civil war—should be kept in check.

There were 640,000 tourists visiting Lebanon in 1998 and the estimated tourist influx a year later was 800,000. The President of the National Council of Tourism, Fouad Fawaz, told me that visitors from the fellow Arab world had never deserted Lebanon, even during the civil war. The effort was to cast the net wider, to Europe and the United States. Germans and French in particular had a strong presence while Americans remained shy. Tourism officials complained that Westerners tended not to distinguish between the security problems in South Lebanon and the peace that prevailed in the rest of the country.

The Gulf Arabs were prominent in such watering holes as the mountain resort of Broumana, a mere half-hour drive from Beirut.

Saudis and Kuwaitis formed the largest contingents, with the UAE behind them. They maintained homes to escape from the summer heat of their home countries among the pines and moderate temperature. Pierre Askhar, the affable president of the Hotel Owners' Syndicate and owner of Printania hotel in Broumana, was planning a spa resort and was scouting for property for India's Taj hotel group in Beirut.

It is in the field of culture that Lebanon is truly amazing. Summer is the time of a rash of festivals featuring such world-renowned artists as Luciano Pavarotti and Placido Domingo as well as the singing heartthrobs of the Arab world. The festivals run for weeks among several centres. I asked the tourism minister, Arthur Nazarian, who filled the seats at these events. About 80 per cent, he said, were Lebanese although there were visitors from the neighbouring countries and further afield. There were planeloads of enthusiasts who came for the Pavarotti concert. How about attracting "war tourism?" I enquired, pointing to the many telltale signs of the infamous civil war. "We want to forget about the war", he countered.

I asked the information minister, Anwar Alkhalil, what the country's biggest problem was. He said that apart from the security aspect, it was the budget deficit, leading to a five-year austerity programme Hariri scoffed at. Perhaps the most abiding impression of Lebanon was of the people's capacity for enjoying life. The Broumana cafés and night clubs were full of Lebanese as well as visitors singing the night away. The *joie de vivre* is infectious. Such dalliance had its critics, the painter Ghada Saghieh for one; she casts a caustic eye on the nocturnal habits of her countrymen and women.

The Bristol hotel in Beirut, now run by Starwood as its "Luxury Collection", was undertaking a refurbishing programme, and its Italian general manager, Franseco Borrello, was dusting the history of the 50-year-old hostelry with reminders of the famous men and women who had stayed in Le Bristol—the legendary Umm Kahltoum and France's President Jacques Chirac among others. The hotel was not damaged in the war.

UAE

A Successful Experiment

In the turbulent world of West Asia, the United Arab Emirates was trying the experiment of building a modern welfare state on the basis of a tolerant version of Islam. The route it had chosen was not through a multi-party democracy but by harking back to the Bedouin virtues of consultation and conciliation to form an appointed Federal National Council. The Supreme Council of Rulers remained the top policy-making body.

Much of the success of the experiment thus far was due to the leadership of the ruler of Abu Dhabi and the long-standing President of the federation of seven emirates that came into being in 1971, Sheikh Zayed bin Sultan al Nahyan. He was the country's friend, philosopher and guide and spent two months in the year travelling to the far concerns to listen to the people's grievances and finding solutions.

The first oil well was drilled in 1950 but it was only in the late fifties that the first oil export shipment was made, catapulting what became the UAE into the twentieth century. Since then history was being continuously telescoped, with the UAE unabashedly set to reach the material standards of the world's most advanced countries. Thanks to its great oil worth—it is the region's third largest producer after Saudi Arabia and Iran—the Emirates' achievement was striking.

The UAE's per capita income was the equivalent of more than $15,000 a year. The literacy level of its indigenous population was 80 per cent. Infant mortality was 11.7 per thousand, life expectancy 73 for women and 70 for men. Education was given more than 15 per cent of the federal budget, the highest after defence. And under a new "special marriage fund", young UAE men who wish to marry were given a grant of the equivalent of more than $19,000 to persuade them not to seek foreign brides to circumvent the crippling traditional marriage expenses. The state entirely funded the education of 2,000 students abroad and education in the country, as its health services, was virtually free.

Which brings us to some of the unique characteristics of the Emirates. The population of the country of some 600,000 inhabitants was boosted by an expatriate population to a total of over 2 million, the bulk of them from the Indian subcontinent. According to a landmark court rulling in 1989, non-Muslims were not governed by the Sharia courts and a temple and mosque stand in juxtaposition in Dubai.

More than 90 per cent of the UAE's revenues came from oil, but in an effort to diversify, the Emirates had succeeded in bringing oil to below 40 per cent of the gross domestic product (GDP). The diversification was in cement, aluminium and light industry. The UAE had invested heavily in infrastructure to make the country an inviting place for foreign investment.

Schools are segregated along sex lines in the UAE, but in trying to marry Islamic tradition to the demands of the modern age, women were encouraged to study and there is equal pay for equal work. The federation had produced its first home-qualified women doctors, a women's contingent had graduated from the military academy and women occupied positions of some influence in the government and the public sector. The country's only university at the oasis town of Al Ain in the Abu Dhabi emirate had nearly 12,000 graduates, with women outnumbering men and outperforming them in studies.

These developments had to be set against the backdrop of the UAE's surroundings. The Second Gulf War after Iraq's invasion of Kuwait was a shock and marred the Emirates' economic performance. Expatriates took their money out only to return it after the war and the UAE bounced back. But the experience of the war left a scar, what Foreign Minister Rashid Abdulla described as a "blow to Arab unity from within."

The UAE tried to ensure its security in concentric circles in the Gulf Cooperation Council (and its foreign protector, the United States), the larger Arab world, principally the Damascus Declaration allies, Egypt and Syria, and, in a symbolic sense, the United Nations.

Big Brothers

The UAE remained wary of its two "big brothers", Iran and Iraq. Officials in Abu Dhabi emphasised the theme of reconciliation but suggested,

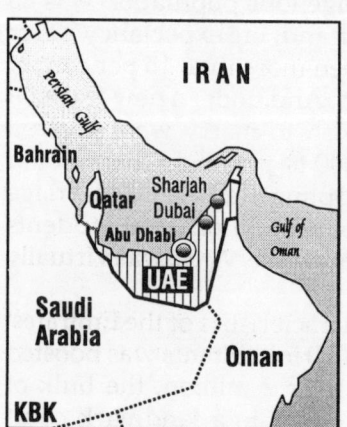

with some regret, that Iraq had not taken initiatives that would encourage its return to the mainstream. With Iran, the UAE had the problem of Iranian occupation of the islands of Abu Musa and the Greater and Lesser Tunb the Emirates claim. Officials declared that they were considering taking the dispute to the World Court at The Hague.

The UAE welcomed the Israeli-Palestine Liberation Organisation agreement on limited autonomy for the Gaza Strip and Jericho, with Sheikh Zayed asserting, "Whatever pleases the

Palestinians pleases us". The Emirates were distressed by the PLO's attitude to the war as also by Yemen's support for Iraq but officials stressed that their theme was forgiveness and reconciliation.

The UAE Foreign Minister would rather not pronounce on who the aggressor in the eight-year Iran–Iraq war was. And on Iran, he pointedly left open the question to Teheran's policy option of respecting neighbours and practising peaceful coexistence and being against the export of revolution and interference in other countries' affairs by threat of force. Officially, the UAE described the Gulf as Arabian, rather than Persian, and spoke about the islands occupied by Iran as Arabian.

Traditionally, Sheikh Zayed had spoken in a forthright manner against extremism in the Muslim world and had often struck the theme of tolerance as being the assence of Islam. At the same time, officials in the UAE were conscious of the West's need for painting Islam as the new enemy after the demise of communism.

It is understandable for a country wedded to moderation and striving to reach out for the twenty-first century that it should seek the path of reconciliation in the Arab world. But "the soil", the Foreign Minister warned, "must be ready" for such a reconciliation. Iraq's stance would seem to rule out a reconciliation for the present, as far as Abu Dhabi was concerned.

As in many other oil-rich countries, oil was at the centre of the Emirates' concern. Iraq had traditionally blocked an increase in the UAE's quota, but with the war the country's production had spurted to 4.5 million barrels per day (mbd). Its production came down to 2.16 mbd, and the Petroleum Minister, Yousuf bin Omeir bin Yousuf, said he was satisfied with the present production level but wanted higher prices.

While the Emirates' oil resources were expected to last another 100 years, the stress in Abu Dhabi was on branching out into other fields. Singapore remained an example to emulate. And in this respect, Dubai's role as an entrepôt centre and the expansion of the Jebel Ali free trade zone near it assumed importance. With Lebanon's demise as the traditional re-export centre following the disastrous civil war, Dubai had set its sights on its position as the undisputed commercial centre in the region. Around 70 per cent of the UAE's imports were routed through the Dubai emirate.

About 90 per cent of the UAE's crude production was exported, with Japan occupying a pre-eminent position, taking as much as one million barrels per day. Japan again was a primary export market for liquefied gas taking most of it. Some 40 per cent of the UAE's oil exports went to Japan.

If Israel had made the desert bloom, the UAE was equally proud of transforming a largely arid and desert land into towns and cities of gardens. The country had pumped in about $3 billion into afforestation programmes and 20,000 new date trees were planted every year. The oasis town of Al Ain, the seat of the country's university, is a veritable garden city and the federal capital, Abu Dhabi, boasts of vistas of green-fringed avenues and gardens.

How the unique UAE experiment in controlled democracy would develop in the future is of interest beyond the country's borders. Imported printed material was censored, largely to protect the nation's cultural values, officials asserted, while the skies were free. The government oversaw the press while running the sole news agency, WAM, and controled the electronic media. The Information Minister, Khalifan al Roumi, asserted that the press was free although it should strengthen federal institutions and moral values flowing from the attributes of a Muslim Arab country and "should not harm others".

The future seemed secure for the UAE, regional turbulence permitting, as long as Sheikh Zayed's fatherly presence was there to guide the country. The Emirates was seeking to ensure the future by investing in human resources, a laudable and somewhat rare goal in a developing country.

A Tough Neighbourhood

How does a small rich country with a population of under 2 million live in the predatory world of West Asia? The federation of the seven old Trucial states, the United Arab Emirates, is young as a nation. The federation came into being in 1971 after the withdrawal of the British and the ruler of Abu Dhabi and the federation's President, Sheikh Zayed bin Sultan Al Nahyan, followed a two-track approach.

Sheikh Zayed was seeking an activist role for his country by trying to energise the Gulf Cooperation Council and was breathing some life into the somewhat still-born Damascus agreement linking the Council with Egypt and Syria. At the same time, the education-oriented budget of the UAE aimed at giving the federation's citizens the capacity to stand on their own in the foreseeable future. Side by side, a Herculean effort was on to try to piece together the fragmentary history of a region dominated by Bedouins and known in the pre-oil wealth era for pearl fishing and sand dunes.

A third unstated instrument to seek security in a dangerous part of the world was provided by the thriving city of Dubai and the flourishing nearby free trade zone. If Dubai and the Jebel Ali free zone were enmeshed with the trade and commerce of the region, the Indian subcontinent, Europe and the United States, they built up a web of relationships that could help the Emirates because the world would have some stake in the UAE and its future.

The shock waves of the Iraqi invasion and annexation of Kuwait and the war that followed were still reverberating in the area. The stark question these events posed was how secure can small states be, particularly those with a mountain of wealth which tempted the greedy and the powerful? The answer lay in having a powerful protector and to strengthen the regional underpinning provided by whatever mechanism that existed.

In the wake of the Iraqi invasion of Kuwait, it was Sheikh Zayed who overrode Saudi Arabian hesitation to try to activate the Gulf Cooperation Council. But the GCC proved hopelessly inadequate in meeting President Saddam Hussein's brutal challenge. And post-war efforts to stiffen the organisation with Egyptian and Syrian sinews of power were psychologically nullified by Kuwait's preference for a straight pact with the United States.

Racing Against Time

There was a palpable feeling in the corridors of power in the Emirates that it was racing against time. The federation itself is a loose arrangement and the father figure of Sheikh Zayed provided the cohesion and stability the country so desperately needed to become a nation state in the true sense of the word. Democracy did not have the ring it had in Kuwait because Sheikh Zayed could communicate directly with his people and, in an interesting experiment, the UAE was emphasising its proud traditions of hunting with falcons even as it was reaching out for the twenty-first century.

Indeed, the UAE had produced some notable technocrats as familiar with the gadgets of the information age as any of their Western counterparts. Equipped with cellular telephones and pagers in their pockets, some of them ran veritable industrial empires. One such was Sultan bin Sulayem, chairman of the Jabel Ali Free Zone and Dubai Ports, a 36-years-old man who ran a tight ship, was as artulate in English as he was in Arabic.

I asked Sultan why Jebel Ali was flourishing while so many free trade zones around the world were languishing. His answer was crisp and to the point. "Thee are two reasons", he said. "First, we have the flourishing port and entrepôt centre of Dubai. Second, the free trade zone idea can only work in an environment of free markets. Closed economic societies think they have given great incentives to entrepreneurs but they are relating these to their own systems and that does not work".

Nor was Sultan fazed by my other question. I asked him about the dominant British presence in the federation and how long it would continue. The whole purpose of the federation's accent on education, he countered, was that citizens would replace the expatriate administrator by the turn of the century.

Sultan's aim seemed overambitious but the administration was proceeding along the right path in resolving the dilemmas inherent in leap-frogging generations and centuries into the modern age.

While Dubai and the bustling port area emphasised one facet of the UAE, a perhaps more basic block of nation-building was provided by the oasis city of Al Ain. This is the original home of Sheikh Zayed, and the veritable garden city that has emerged in testimony to the loving care with which the authorities tended trees and gardens and encouraged agriculture.

Sheikh Saeed bin Thanoon is the son of the governor of Al Ain. He is 25, articulate and a member of the federation's Executive Council. At an encounter in the city's guest house one early afternoon, he outlined his work and play priorities.

The irony of it did not elude him when he suggested that one of his major problems was to find markets for his region's agricultural produce. Another was to provide for the future water needs of the area's population. He supported a decision announced by Sheikh Zayed to create a "marriage fund" to tempt more young citizens to marry, an occasion that still involves an extensive series of rituals of feasts and entertainment which make young men chary of wedlock.

Sheikh Saeed remained wedded to hunting for bustards with falcons, but he went for hunts in his own country and in Pakistan after India imposed a ban. In pursuit of this national sport, bustards are bred in Abu Dhabi. "The UAE and Israel are the only two countries where bustards have been successfully bred", he said. There was, of course, no form of collaboration between the two countries on achieving this distinction.

Beyond the garden city of Al Ain, the falconry of Sheikh and the bustling centre of Dubai, conversation often tended to veer round the federation's future. And every such conversation reverted to the role of Sheikh Zayed. Sheikh Zayed had been the ruler of Abu Dhabi for more than a quarter century and the President of the federation since its founding in 1971.

Although the presidency should rotate among the principalities, Sheikh Zayed was always renominated head every five years. The number two slot of Vice-President and Prime Minister was with Dubai's ruler, Sheikh Maktoum bin Rashid Al Makhoum. Not only was Sheikh Zayed universally popular, but he was also generous with his purse and funded a large slice of the federation's activities.

In reality, Abu Dhabi and Dubai practically ran the federation between them. The loose nature of the federation did not worry the rulers much in view of the universal acceptance of Sheikh Zayed. But the inevitable question posed was how bumpy the transition would be to a post-Zayed world. No one had Sheikh Zayed's acceptance, his personal chemistry with the people and the kind of deference from the other rulers he enjoyed.

Would cries of democracy become more insistent in the future? Would the institution of Sheikh become more controversial? These were two of the host of questions Sheikhs Zayed's future successors would face. But the federation was providing for the future as well as human ingenuity and abundant oil wealth could make it.

Education and health care enjoyed enviable priorities, all the more remarkable for the very conservative nature of Bedouin society. Women were traditionally behind the veil, but, as a lady from Bahrain living in Abu Dhabi put it, "Here the authorities are encouraging women to come out while in Saudi Arabia they impose the veil on women from above".

In the end, in social mores as in planning for the future, it all boils down to a question of time. Would the Emirates have the time to evolve into a modern nation state before the next gusts of turmoil appear?

A National Day in 1991

In December 1990, the United Arab Emirates did not celebrate its National Day. President Saddam Hussein had marched into Kuwait to annex it in August 1990 and the mood in the country was hardly celebratory. So it was with a special zest that this federation of seven trucial states of colonial times celebrated its National Day on December 2,1991 complete with a military parade.

The UAE comprises Abu Dhabi, Dubai, Sharjah, Ajman, Umm Al Quaiwain, Ras Al Khaimah and Fujairah. It is a somewhat loose federation composed for the most part of two states that loom large, Abu Dhabi and Dubai.

It is difficult not to be impressed by the UAE. Abu Dhabi was little more than sand dunes while Dubai relied on pearl-fishing. Life was hard because the elements were harsh. The Bedouin attuned himself to his environment. In some two decades, oil wealth and a wise ruler had catapulted the UAE almost into the twenty-first century.

The Second Gulf War was a traumatic experience for the UAE, as it was for the other countries in the region. The UAE made its own modest contribution to the United States and its allies in the Gulf war and never bought President Saddam's argument of equating the annexation of Kuwait with Israel's continued occupation of the occupied territories.

Progress in the UAE had been so dramatic that it was difficult to imagine that Abu Dhabi was less than two decades or so ago a country without roads, infrastructure or a university. The roads were now better than in any Indian city and telecommunication facilities functioned. Admittedly, the oil wealth had given the necessary wherewithal for the country's progress and the small population—the entire federation is under two million spread over an area of 300 square miles—helped spread the benefits.

Sheikh Zayed has been the dominating presence. Abu Dhabi is dotted with modern buildings, including the one housing the Bank of

Credit and Commerce International, crisscrossed by carpet roads. Although the National Day parade, enhanced by the presence of Princess Anne, underlined the military capacity of the federation appropriate to its modest size, it is in other fields that its priorities were striking.

A Moonscape

In some respects, Abu Dhabi reminded a visitor of a hypothetical moonscape on which a resourceful leadership has built an entire new city. Oldtimers reminded newcomers of how they had charted their paths in jeeps over the sand dunes and the people of Abu Dhabi are more proud of the greening of their capital than of almost anything else. Agriculture takes a major slice of the annual budget and the assiduousness with which the administration had gone about cultivating grass and flowers was as amazing as it was touching. Who could conceive of Abu Dhabi exporting strawberries?

The federation had its problems and tensions, with Dubai, the other major presence, having successfully diversified into industry and entrepôt trade, but despite the recurrence of strains and irritants, it had held. UAE officials said that given the setbacks to other federal projects tried in the Arab world and elsewhere, this was an achievement.

Sheikh Zayed is a popular ruler and the personality cult of the leader was not as pronounced in Abu Dhabi as it is in many other Arab lands. It is perhaps because of the small population and the ruler's ability to communicate with different parts of his own principality that, combined with his social consciousness, had helped the federation to be something of a rarity in the region—a haven of peace and quiet. But Sheikh Zayed is far from being an introvert. He wished to play his rightful role in the region and in the United Nations. The queue of foreign dignitaries visiting Abu Dhabi and his own travels in the region bespoke of an activist philosophy.

The federation's rather newly developed oil wealth had given it a per capita income that perhaps rivalled Kuwait's. But Abu Dhabians remained modest and pleasant people, and some of them suggested that if the oil money ran out, they would go back to being Bedouins. This was an expression of their outlook, rather than a scenario for the future.

Shrewd Sheikh

Much in the federation revolved round Sheikh Zayed who proved to be a shrewd and cautious leader. Apparently, he did not believe that the model of the Westminster style of government was applicable to his country. The Sheikh was grooming his sons and the President's National Day address was read by one of a score of them.

Whether Sheikh Zayed can pass on his charisma and cautious shrewdness to his sons remained to be seen, but in the federation and in Abu Dhabi in particular the President had carved out a special niche for himself. It was in ordering priorities for his country that his reign has been most remarkable. In addition to emphasising education and health care, Abu Dhabi was building its own traditions on the basis of the past. A government funded documentation centre located in a refurbished old fort in Abu Dhabi is an indication of the time and effort being devoted to piecing together a somewhat fragmentary history of a region known more for its pearl and fishing pursuits and sand dunes than anything else.

Twelve Europeans and a host of expatriate Arabs were piecing together the archives of the old metropolitan powers to collate material from the European capitals and the seat of the Ottoman empire on the history of what the British called the Trucial States. Portuguese, French, German, Dutch, American and Turkish documents were being translated and indexed to give scholars an opportunity to deleanate the history of an area which is at best patchy and at worst distorted.

The UAE federation is, indeed, a unique example of a country and people proud of their Bedouin past even as they were anxious to reach out to the future. In the modern age, the Emirates started on an almost clean state, with no roads, little schooling and sand dunes for company. Then the accent was placed on computers, modern science and medicine and the compulsions of living in a dangerous world.

Inevitably, the older citizens worried about how the young and very young would brace up to the future. They have not had the experience of living in a harsh environment with little wealth and few resources. And the consumer culture, with the enticing gadgets of modern living, are very much within their reach. Local papers, for instance, reported the rape of a housemaid—an expatriate as they invariably are—in which a gang of teenagers called their friends for the gang rape over mobile telephones.

Such incidents might be rare in the UAE, but they were indicative of the different mores of the younger generation and the sleepless nights they give the old. But the UAE remains a brave experiment in modern statecraft.

THE REGION

An Islamic Wind

From Tunis to Damascus, from Cairo to Amman, the signs were unmistakable. The Arab states, whatever their professed ideology, were returning to the more conservative mores of Islam. In the Palestinian refugee camps girls wore white head scarves with their uniforms, and religious classes were held in schools run by UNRWA, the United Nation Relief and Work Agency. In the streets of the Arab capitals, a growing number of young women walked and even drove cars with their heads covered.

The response of the regimes of the four Arab states I visited in 1988—Tunisia, Egypt, Jordan and Syria—varied in proportion to the danger they perceived from Islamic fundamentalism. But all of them had made gestures to religious sentiments even as they still fought the political dangers represented by the wave of fundamentalism.

The call to prayer was broadcast over the public address system of Cairo's international airport, and in Amman, the modern attractive capital of Jordan, the proliferating mosques were evidence of the regime's concern to appear to do the right thing. In Tunis, even as jean-clad women sat and smoked in cafés, any number of women walked the streets covered from head to toe. In the streets of Damascus, women covered in full black veils were not a rarity. This was so in the Damascus suburb of Yarmouk where 170,000 Palestinian refugees lived.

The Arab regimes' gestures apart, Egypt took the threat of fundamentalism seriously. According to the information minister, "We are the most religious people in the world". But the minister made it clear that his government was against the violent expression of such belief and Egypt did not accept any religious political party although members of the Muslim Brotherhood sat in the assembly. But he confessed that there was a linkage between extremism and socio-economic problems.

The symbol of the religious challenge in Egypt was represented by 54-year-old Ahmad el-Banna, son of the founder of the Muslim Brotherhood. A three-piece suit sat incongruously with his religious beard as his told me in his office in the heart of Cairo city that he had spent five years in prison. His mission, he said, was to train the people to change their habits.

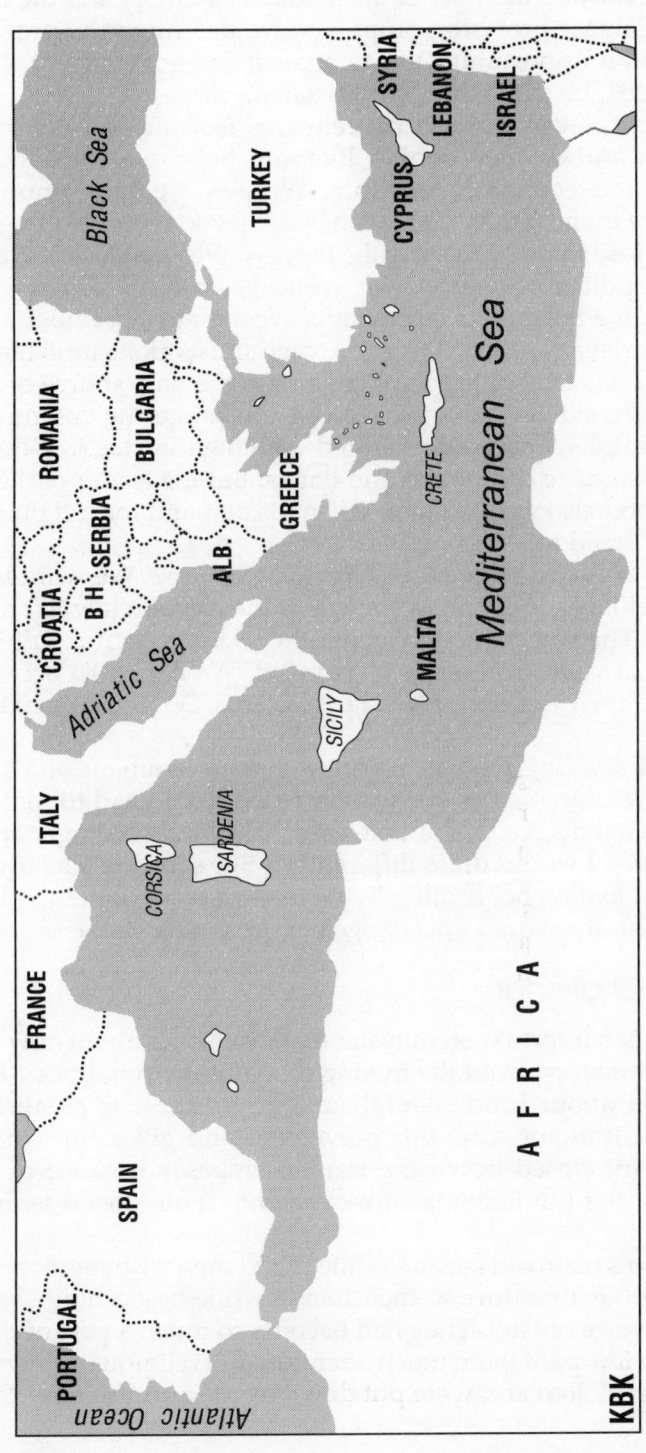

El-Banna was a member of the national assembly and the extension of a martial law provision on preventive detention the previous day gave him an opportunity to rail against the government. "It was a great battle", he said with obvious satisfaction.

El-Banna cleverly mixed his religious fervour and his concept of how men and women should live and behave with demands for political and economic freedom. Women, he said, should build confidence in the family. "This can be achieved by controlling women. They will lose some freedom in the process. We want Islam. We espouse a foreign policy of justice with truth. We are not against Western countries; we need their technology. We are against imperialism. We respect Christian nations. We leave communists alone until they learn".

The Sharia, according to el-Banna, was the only source of law, and although President Sadat was forced to change the common law, it was not implemented. He wanted a change in the work ethic and Islamic insurance companies and banks. But the leader of the Muslim Brotherhood also waxed eloquent on his demand for full political and economic freedom.

"There is no true freedom in Egypt since 1952. We want to change and cancel laws. We want a change in the election law to ensure free elections. The elections are rigged; the 99.9 per cent result is a joke. The normal voter turn-out is 20 per cent. We'll gain 80 per cent from elections if there are guaranteed fair elections. Our movement is gaining strength".

I asked a young woman working in a government office in Cairo why she was dressed as she was, covered from head to foot. "This is what my God decreed", she answered. "He would be angry and would punish me if I would dress differently". She said she was toying with the idea of joining her brother living in the United States to pursue her studies. No, she would not change her dress code in the United States.

A New Challenge

The Egyptian information minister made no bones about how seriously his government viewed the mixing of region with politics. "Everyone is worried about fundamentalism", he said. "It is creating a new challenge. Iran supports this movement and gives fundamentalism hope. Egypt closed down the Iranian embassy because of its inter-ference in the fundamentalist movement. Their slogan is: Islam is a solution".

In Cairo's main old bazaar, white robed men with regulation beards held religious literature in their hands while beseeching shoppers to heed the voice of God. They had become so much a part of the bazaar scene that few paid them much attention. But religious demonstrations could turn violent and were put down by the authorities with a heavy hand.

In Tunis, the civilised pushing out of the secular but increasingly senile Habib Bourguiba was utilised by the successor regime to make gestures to religious sentiment. Several thousand prisoners held on charges of religious-oriented political activism were released. The information minister, Abdul-Wahab Abdullah, said that fundamentalists used Islam for a political purpose and must separate their religious work from politics.

The new Tunisian regime had promised to protect the Muslim character of the country although the information minister said that there was no question of changing the law banning polygamy. He confessed that there had been evidence of Iranian influence in the past although Tunisia was a totally Sunni country, but there was no danger to the government.

The Tunisian foreign minister, Mahmoud el-Mistiri, was candid in suggesting that with the success of the Iranian revolution, the fundamentalists had felt encouraged. Fundamentalists in Tunisia, he said, were very active, but were a minority. They could not have a political party but could run associations. "We have to deal with fundamentalism in a democratic manner".

In Damascus, the minister of state for foreign affairs said fundamentalism was "a worry for all kinds". It was like terrorism, but adhering to rights was sometimes called extremism. "Fundamentalism and terrorism should be condemned, but we should distinguish between fundamentalism and its expanded meaning. Fundamentalism means not using the mind properly".

Jordan's minister for labour, Rasheed Oraykat, opened his meeting with the press in Amman with the invocation, "In the name of God, the Merciful, the Compassionate". Most of the women working in government offices in Amman conformed to the religious dress code.

The chairman of the Palestine National Council, 81-year-old Abdul Hameed Al Sayeh, denied that there was any bloc in the council, which served as the Palestine Liberation Organisation's parliament, based on religion. But he admitted that there were some persons in the council representing religious tendencies in an unofficial way.

Sayeh, who resided in Jordan, was the head of the Supreme Islamic Court in Jerusalem in 1967. He was deported by the Israelis and became Minister of Islamic Affairs in Jordan. I asked him whether he considered himself a revolutionary or a religious leader. "I am both a revolutionary and a Muslim", he answered. The PNC has 425 members and, in addition, had a secret list of members in the occupied territories.

Is the return to old and conservative religious ways a specifically Arab and Muslim phenomenon? No, said many in West Asia, it was a world phenomenon, some pointing to such movements as Moral Majority in the United States. According to Abdul Jawad Saleh, the mayor deported from the occupied territories by Israel, "The whole world is advancing towards a religious trend. It is not only an Arab or Middle East phenomenon."

Apart from the problems the adoption of old religious ways present to women and there role in society, most Arab regimes were willing to propitiate the religious lobby as long as it did not represent a threat to them. Some, like Crown Prince Hassan of Jordan, worried that the United States might be tempted to give Israel an even greater role in the region as a bulwark against Khomeinism. The Arabs had their own reasons to guard against the winds blowing from Iran.

Algeria's Grief

The dramatic happenings in Algeria, which were tantamount to a constitutional coup d'état to forestall the assumption of power of the fundamentalist party, the FIS, sent alarm bells ringing in the area and many parts of the world. But it is essential to separate the alarmist conclusions that were being drawn from the core of the problem.

Islamic fundamentalism is a shorthand term used to connote the use of Islam for political ends. But its capacity to influence events varied from country to country and region to region. In essence, Islam served as a medium not merely of reorienting society, as is the desire of some, but as a vehicle of dissent against traditional rule in a scheme of things that was perceived to be disadvantageous to the underprivileged.

The combustible nature of the appeal of Islam was heightened by the flux the world found itself in, with the virtual demise of communism and the new separateness of the former Soviet Central Asian republics. It was further enhanced by the messianic nature of the Shi'ite revolution in Iran even as it was sought to be tempered by the pragmatism of the dominant strand of the new leadership in Teheran.

In Algeria, it was a simple question of the traditional ruling party, the FLN, having exhausted its political capital, and when economic difficulties began to bite and the people were given the opportunity to express themselves freely, they chose the vehicle of the Islamic party in the face of a divided opposition to voice their dissent. It was a question of the (Western) God that failed.

The consequences of the Algerian developments struck a chord in a number of countries in the region because they were facing their own problems. Despite the winds of change that were gently wafting over Egypt, the establishment there had kept a lid on the Muslim Brotherhood, and it was hardly a surprise that the Egyptian minister of the interior, Abdelhalim Mussa, should administer a warning to the fundamentalists that his government would take all measures to forestall attempts to destablise the country.

Iran as a beacon of Islamic revolution had lost its initial gloss, quite apart from the needs of the government in Teheran to subdue its zeal in order to win friends and influence people in the non-Islamic world, particularly in the West. But countries in the region were keeping a wary eye on Iran's experiment in coopting the Sudan to spread its message through words and trained emissaries.

Egypt, in common with countries such as Tunisia, faced the problem of coping with dissent expressed through religion or a religious-oriented party seeking to challenge the establishment. That most countries in the region were not true democracies in the accepted sense of the term lent substance to their fears that not only were fundamentalists choosing to destabilise the established regimes but sought to turn them away from modern development.

The Poor

Here we should make a distinction between the non-oil producing relatively poor countries of West Asia and the oil-rich states. The Gulf countries had the cushion of the prosperity bulge to dampen dissent. If most of the indigenous people had a vested interest in their prosperity, the appeal of dissenting forces, whatever guise they took, was feeble. In other states, beset with the twin dangers of a one-party rule and economic difficulties, a religious-oriented party inevitably exercised greater appeal.

Iraq, which held aloft the secular banner, was consumed by the bravado and folly of President Saddam Hussein to rule itself out as a major regional player for some time. Syria, whose ruler President Hafez al-Assad was astute enough to bend with the prevailing winds, had won a reprieve but was susceptible to the appeal of Islam in the future.

To jump from this appeal Islam, or an Islamic-oriented party, exercises to suggest that an arc of fundamentalistic countries stretching to the nations of Soviet Central Asia and Pakistan would hold sway is unwarranted. A different set of circumstances was operating in Central Asia even as the newly independent states sought to find a place in the sun outside the orbit of a strong central authority in Moscow.

It is natural that the predominantly Muslim states of Central Asia should want to emphasise their separateness and independence of Moscow by an accent on Islam. It is equally natural that countries such as Iran, Pakistan and Turkey should exploit this factor to forge closer ties. But Turkey out of this trio had stolen a march over the others by its promptness in recognising the independence of these states and the historic nature of Turkish influence in most of them by virtue of the languages they speak and the reach of the old Ottoman empire. Besides, Turkey offered an attractive option because it was both Islamic and oriented towards Europe.

Despite Iranian efforts and the ethnic background of Azerbaijan, there were limits to the spread of Iranian influence in Central Asia by the smaller reach of the Shi'ite sect. And Iran as well as Saudi Arabia, the latter with its Wahabi creed, represented a form of religious zeal which sat ill with the prevailing norms in the Central Asian republics. It is one thing to emphasise Islam to proclaim a new–found independence, quite another to forget the legacy of half a century of Soviet rule in terms of the role of women in society and concepts of social equity, however flawed their practice under communist rule.

The divisions in the world of Islam were as striking as the unity provided by religion. Khomeini succeeded in bringing in a Shi'ite revolution because Iran under the Shah of Iran was ripe for change by the all-consuming corruption in the ruling establishment and the alienation of an increasingly Westernised elite which was kept out of power. The system of one-man rule against the setting of increasing economic difficulties remains a powerful mix to propel a religious-oriented party to bid for power.

There are no short answers to this problem in West Asia. For one thing, accepted notions of democracy do not apply and when an effort is made to apply them, as in Algeria, we arrive at the absurd situation of an army-inspired move to change the rules on the ground that a party on a verge of power would destroy the nascent democracy that was being sought to be introduced. The show of strength by the secular forces in Algeria after the first round of voting was impressive, but there can be no grainsaying the fact that a party all set to achieve victory in the first reasonably democratic elections was denied its chance through an anti-democratic mechanism.

While these contradictions in West Asia would need time to work themselves out through convulsions and changes, it is well to recognise the power of religion or a religious-oriented party to act as a nucleus of dissent against the established order. The very nature of traditional rule, either through monarchies or through the imposition of one-man rule, makes the establishment vulnerable at a time of economic crisis. Islam thus to a large extent coopted the role of the opposition in a number of countries in West Asia, particularly when the creed of communism had been discredited.

The republics of Central Asia have a different set of problems, conditioned by their former incorporation into the Soviet system and their need to find new bearings. They needed to balance their need for interaction through the Commonwealth of Independent States or a substitute with the necessity to strike out on a new path. But a purely religious-oriented appeal was likely to prove counter-productive because they were primarily beset with bread and butter questions.

The scenario of an Islamic green running across West Asia through Central Asia to Pakistan is fanciful because of the divisions in Islam, the contradictory pulls of Islamic states for reasons of national interest and the fact of Western power which should militate against the coalescence of Islamic states to the disadvantage of the developed world.

The only conclusion one could draw is that West Asia and, to a lesser extent, Central Asia would remain a powder keg as the evolution of their societies went through convulsions and hiccups. In the longer term, only the wisdom of the ruling elites in these countries would determine the nature of these changes. To apply copy-book precepts of Western democracy is to beg the question.

Turkey Reaches a Fork

Turkey, the modern nation state, faced its third fork after it was born on the ashes of the Ottoman empire. The first, of course, was the creation of the Ataturk republic which represented a radical reorientation in ordering the affairs of state and religion. The second was the brief and troubled rise of the Islamists who had to bow out in the face of the armed forces' fiat, asserting as they were their self-declared role as the guardians of the secular state.

The third fork was the capture of the Kurdish leader Abdullah Ocalan, triumphantly brought home bound and blindfolded. For the destiny of Turkey would, in a measure, depend upon how it treated this triumph and the European future it had charted for itself. How Ocalan was interrogated and tried would be important; early indications were not encouraging. A bigger, linked question was how Turkey would treat its Kurdish minority of 12 million people.

Prime Minister Bulent Ecevit was right in taunting the Europeans on refusing to have Ocalan. With Italy holding the hot patato and Germany refusing to press charges against the guerrilla leader, Rome finally set him free, only to have him orbit European cities vainly seeking asylum—until he found refuge in the Greek embassy in Nairobi from where he was abducted by Kenyans who handed him to Turkish commandos.

According to the *New York Times*, the Americans helped Turkey track down Ocalan and had been on his trail for four months and were warning European countries not to harbour Ocalan. It spoke volumes for West Europeans' timidity and loss of self-confidence after World War II, stemming from the power of Uncle Sam and their own prosperity spread, that they were only too pleased to deny refuge to the Kurdish leader. Whatever other role Israeli intelligence might have played in the apprehension of Ocalan, the *New York Times* report confirmed that it had tipped off Ankara about Ocalan's departure from Damascus for Russia after Israel had presented an ultimatum to Syria.

Helping Turkey

The Americans had several reasons to help Turkey, a Nato ally, whose Incirlik air base was being used by US and British planes for policing the Iraqi northern 'no-fly' zone and, lately, clobbering Iraqi targets almost every day. Incirlik was also used for electronic surveillance on Iraq. And Turkey was that rare commodity in West Asia, a friend of Israel cooperating with Tel Aviv in the military sphere.

Ocalan presented dilemmas as well as opportunities for Turkey. There are about 12 million Kurds in Turkey out of 25 million spread over Iraq, Iran and Syria. The struggle of the PKK (Kurdistan Workers' Party) against the Turkish authorities, initially for independence pruned to autonomy and cultural and linguistic rights, had claimed an estimated 30,000 lives since 1984, mostly of PKK fighters, and led to a 500,000 strong Kurdish diaspora in Europe as Kurds fled their homeland.

None of the four cities with significant Kurdish populations wished to give its Kurds the status of a nation state. Ironically, the United States had come nearest to giving the Iraqi Kurds something approaching autonomy for its own selfish reasons. The Iraqi tanks that rumbled into northern Iraq at the invitation of the one of the two Iraqi Kurdish factions had meant the destruction of the American-led and funded apparatus to subvert Saddam Hussein. The northern 'no-fly' zone unilaterally imposed by America since the Second Gulf War in 1991 had meant that Iraqi Kurdish factions were free to fight each other or sign a truce as they watched Turkish troops march into and out of Iraq at will to pursue PKK guerrillas.

Since the days of Ataturk, the military role in the governance of Turkey has been legitimised. Apart from periodic coups that punctuated the country's politics and the more recent finger-wagging at the Islamists, Ankara's reaction to the Kurdish problem had been shaped by the armed forces' perception. Understandably, the stick, rather than the carrot, had been the preferred instrument in dealing with the Kurd-inhabited relatively poor and deprived south-east after the PKK raised the banner of revolt.

It was Ataturk who refused to accept the terms of the Treaty of Sèvres which gave the Kurds a state, and the attitude of the Turkish authorities had since then been suspicious of Kurdish aspirations. This explains the fact that the cultural and linguistic rights demanded by Kurds were denied. The pro-Kurdish People's Democratic Party (Hadep) was being investigated. Turkish economic experts believed that it was the combination of poverty—the gap between the south-east and the prosperous west of the country had widened dramatically—and ethnic problems that had fuelled insurgency. The use of force to suppress the revolt inevitably fed further resentment and bred more guerrillas.

Prime Minister Ecevit had made some gestures in promising a measure of amnesty and economic incentives to guerrillas willing to lay down arms. But they were faint and could not hold much attraction for dissident Kurds against the Turkish triumphalism that was daily on display on television as pictures of a captured and subdued Ocalan were flashed on screens. Ecevit, of course, knew his limitations. He was an interim prime minister and he also knew that the military attitude towards the PKK and the Kurdish question left a civilian politician little room for manoeuvre.

Yet Ecevit had the historic opportunity to determine which fork the country would take because, in the end, neither Israelis nor Americans could lead Turkey to salvation. Ankara was very conscious of the risks of the American enterprise with Iraqi Kurds but was insufficiently conscious of Arab sensitivities in teaming up with Israel in the military sphere. Policy questions aside, it was in Turkey's own vital interest to make peace with the Kurds and the only way it could do so was to give them cultural and linguistic rights in an autonomous south-east. That would complete the process Ataturk started in building a modern nation state on the ruins of the Ottoman empire.

Turkish Delight

Few cities in the world have such romantic and historical associations as Istanbul, and the romance comes with more than a whiff of intrigue and mystery. The Golden Horn, the Bosphorus Bridge spanning Europe and Asia, the Topkapi Palace, the Blue Mosque and the 2,000-old mosques dotted across Istanbul are a kaleidoscope of history and the city's unique place in the world. It was the capital of three successive empires—Roman, Byzantine and Ottoman. And in the Basilica of St. Sophia, now the Ayasofya Museum, two civilisations were made to co-exist after its violent capture; the church was not destroyed but converted into a mosque with appropriate symbols.

Istanbul is the tourist's delight, the place to admire and wonder about, the city that took in its stride centuries of history as the Romans, the Greeks and the Ottomans partook of it to leave the modern-day visitor a feast. History competes with shopping as the world of the covered bazaar—a city in itself—displays its wares ranging from the ubiquitous charm against the evil eye to a profusion of products bearing famous brand names, obviously copies.

What I liked about the shopkeepers was that they made no pretence of selling the copies as anything but copies; watches that would cost $ 10,000 in the original sell for $ 25 to make fun presents, and there are the traditional wares, in silk, cotton, copper and the Turkish carpets in all their resplendent glory.

I was returning to Istanbul after about a quarter century. Suleyman Demirel was then prime minister, graduating in the meantime to the presidency. The Topkapi palace complex remains the home of wonder and mystery, with immense halls and cabinet rooms, with a gilded cage-like grill above affording the ruler the opportunity to keep an eye on his ministers. There are the treasures of the past, signifying the opulence and reach of the most recent historical rulers, the Ottomans— the presents and tributes they received, now displayed in the immense kitchens and attached quarters for cooking meals for 10,000 at a time. We have an admonition from Abdulhak Sinasi, "Do not dismiss the dish saying that it is just, simply food. The blessed thing is an entire civilisation in itself".

Turkish Cuisine

Turkish cuisine, which deserves to be better known around the world, bears an imperial stamp in the delicacy, range and varieties of the dishes. The commanders of the Ottoman military elite, the Janissaries, were called Soupmen. What the Turks can do with the aubergine is unbelievable and delicious; one version is called Her Majesty's Favourite, a reference to Empress Eugeine, wife of Napoleon lll, who is reputed to have fallen in love with it during a visit to Sultan Abdulaziz. The varieties of kebabs, for instance, are amazing, each with its own flavour and often its own sauce. Next to the Topkapi is the restaurant that boasts of hosting a fair number of the world's politicians and statesmen, each penning his or her autograph on a photograph for the picture gallery. The restaurant overlooks a vista of water and mosques and palaces.

Turkish coffee, of course, needs no advertisement. According to legend, sacks of coffee abandoned at the gates of Vienna by the retreating Ottoman army in the sixteenth century introduced the brew to the West and made the cafés of Vienna famous.

Istanbul was a fitting beginning to a week of discovery. We took a flight direct to Antalya on the Mediterranean, a centre of attraction for those who like the sun and the beach. There are miles and miles of uninterrupted beaches dotted with tourist hotels. The German accent is predominant as the dresses get skimpier and the pigment of the skin darker. Some covered heads of the local Turkish women were a reminder of more conservative traditions and tastes.

The old city is a labyrinth of lanes, with some old noble houses restored and converted into hotels, complete with Turkish musicians playing to dinner guests around the oriental pool in a languorous atmosphere. A naughty cinema showing exposed behinds of teenagers was, we were told, only for those below 16. *Pensions* abound and charge very reasonable rates for the young wishing to go native.

Getting used to Turkish money was another matter. An ice cream cone was 100,000 Turkish lira. I told the hotel cashier in Antalya that it was the first time in my life that I was a millionaire. "Come again", he answered. The zeros were a legacy of inflation averaging between 60 and 85 per cent a year (in 1994 it touched 120 per cent). One US dollar is around 27,500 TL, but Turks said they have no problem in taking the astronomical amounts in their stride.

The coastal roads are good in Turkey and as we drove up from Antalya hugging the coast, there was an endless vista of the shimmering beautiful sea interspersed with the green of the land. Kemar, Phaselis, Olympos, Kas and then Fathiye, our destination for the night. Along the way we stopped for lunch at a restaurant that must rank as one of the most charming in the world. It is fashioned in tiers along a flowing mountain stream, with tables at the lowest tier reaching out to the ice-cold water, which also serves as a natural refrigerator for cooling mineral water and soft drinks. Its effect on a warm sunny day can well be imagined, with some of my companions jumping into the stream under the spell of nature's bounty.

Marmaris, further north, is a resort of marinas and shops. You take a boat out for a day's trip and then a small boat through tall grass to historical ruins. Our guide had a sense of humour and talked about the tombs of the kings and nobles carved high to be close to the sun, and about a damsel who died in unrequited love. It was hot and our boat ran out of mineral water, but for those with an urge to swim, there was a stop to get cool in the sea.

Parmukkale, another diversion on the way to Istanbul, is where the thermal springs are, some of the many dotted along the coast. A natural wonder are the white rocks. Underground springs have been spouting hot mineral-rich water that has coloured the cliffs white. Parmukkale is literally Cotton Castle. And nearby stand the ruins of the ancient city of Hierapolis, founded in 190 BC by Eumenes II, King of Pergamon, with its copious amphitheatre.

History Galore

Prodded by a tight schedule, we journeyed to Izmir, the reputed residence of Homer in what was Smyrna. Modern-day Izmir is a bustling city whose symbol is the Clock Tower in the Konark Square, built in 1901. Outside Izmir, one rubs shoulders with history again, the theatre in Efes among other ruins and the last resting place of Virgin Mary with its wishing wall outside. And further up, as we go to Bursa, a favourite with visitors from the Arabian Gulf together with Yelova, we savour its most famous speciality, the Kebab Iskander. Bursa fell to Osman Bey in 1326 to become the first capital of the Ottoman empire.

A Turkish friend had warned me before I set out on the week's trip that all I was going to get was an aperitif. That indeed was true, but a good aperitif teases the palate and tempts the diner to await the main dishes with anticipation. In few other countries does one get such a feeling of history, of empires having waxed and waned, leaving their varied legacies in palaces or ruins or in the continuing mouth-watering delicacies perfected over successive generations.

Modern Turks are a very friendly people, ever willing to help the stranger. They are also a proud, nationalistic people. In few other nations does the national flag play such a central role in religious and social gatherings. In Antalya, for instance, the Turkish flag was held aloft in an open-top car carrying young boys to a circumcision ceremony, horns blaring.

The legacy of Kemal Ataturk is jostling with more traditional thoughts, but Turks live with a sense of history and are very conscious of their historical past and greatness. No wonder that Turkey, still a sizable country in its diminished state, attracts more and more tourists who come not only for the sun and the beaches but also for "cultural tourism", associated with Japanese visitors for Turks. In 1996, Turkey received 8.6 million international travellers earning more than $6 billion. But competition is growing and a dip of 8,000 tourists in the first five months of 1998 was making tourist officials sit up. Both Spain and Greece had reduced their value-added tax rates.

Not many Western visitors would know that tulip bulbs taken to Vienna from Istanbul in the 1500s started a tulip craze in England and the Netherlands. In 1634, Holland was in the grip of "tulipomania", which led to the modern-day association of the country with tulips. Seventeenth century Turkey, dubbed the age of elegance and amusement, was called the Tulip Age.

A Choppy Sea

They were inhospitable times for the concept of a Mediterranean identity and hopes to build closer cooperation between the North and the South on the basis of a shared sea. Tunisians made a valiant effort to project the Mediterranean as a logical link between Europe and the Arabs, but in the end there were more questions than answers.

A two-day high-level seminar in Tunis early in November 1992 started with a question posed by the sponsors of "The Mediterranean: What future?" And the questions multiplied as experts and dignitaries, including a panoply of Tunisian ministers, the Belgium minister for external commerce and the Turkish vice prime minister, wrestled with the theme.

Three problems cast their long shadow: the flow of emigrants from the South to the North, Islamic fundamentalism and the South's economic problems. These were compounded by the pessimism engendered by the unresolved crises swirling around the sea—those relating to the Palestinian issue, the Cyprus imbroglio, the tragedy of Bosnia-Herzegovina and Morocco's simmering problem with Spain.

Experts honed in on the urgency of protecting the Mediterranean from pollution. It was like a big lake, they said, subject to great pressures. There had been a spectacular increase in the wastes thrown into it. More than 5,000 ships used the sea each day and millions of tons of oil were transported through it. It was high traffic for a small sea.

The logic of the situation demanded cooperation, but there were few meeting points between the North and the South, except on the need to resolve problems. There was a measure of soul-searching by representatives of the South ranging from Morocco and Libya to Egypt, but their concerns were countered by the concerns of the North. The chasm was both revealing and sad.

It is true that the five countries of the Maghreb are more concerned with the Mediterranean than other Arabs, as pointed out by the Egyptian representative. But Maghrebian integration was "a stop-go" process, as suggested by the Tunisian foreign minister, Habib Ben Yahya, thanks to the crisis posed by Islamic groups in Algeria, and Libya's problems with the West. On the practical plane, Maghreb has closer cooperation with the five European Mediterranean powers and more problems than the rest of the Arab world. Ben Yahya, for instance, complained of "the distorting prism of culture and media" through which Europe viewed the South.

Is there a Mediterranean identity and a common culture? as the Tunisians implied. The answer from Andrea Amato, an expert of the European Economic Community, was frank. "The Mediterranean identity no longer exists," he said. "And a Mediterranean culture has not existed since the Renaissance." And the Maltese foreign minister, Guido Di Marco, confessed that it was difficult to speak of a Mediterranean identity. The Libyan representative felt that the Mediterranean concept "requires us to give up religious, cultural and racial extremism".

The North's point was represented by the Belgian minister, Robert Urbain, among others. He talked of the doubling of Maghreb's population in the next 25 years. And the former French minister, Michele Alliot Marie, spoke of the need for qualitative, rather than quantitative, curbs on African emigration to Europe.

The European Economic Community's representative was somewhat comforting in talking about a Euro-Mediterranean space. He talked of the community's many interests in West Asia, specially North Africa, but said the EEC's responsibility because of its economic weight could only be on the basis of the South assuming its responsibility.

Malta's Di Marco was most positive in suggesting a solution, the creation of a Council of Mediterranean on the lines of the Council of Europe. But there were no takers. Tunisians spoke of the inadequacy of financial instruments alone for Europe's dialogue with the Mediterranean South; it should encompass the whole gamut of relations.

A Nostalgia Trip

Perhaps the most revealing part of the seminar was the spectrum of reflections of the South on the Mediterranean. There was a bit of nostalgia in the Lebanese representative harking back to the time when the Arabs were the masters of the Mediterranean sea from seventh to thirteenth centuries. But he also made the interesting point that without democracy, Arabs would remain embroiled in endless civil wars.

The Moroccan representative talked frankly about Europe's "isolationism" and "racist trends". He said curbs on migration would be dangerous because "Europe needs to know us better" and "we alone cannot solve the problems of fundamentalism and population growth".

The Mediterranean South seemed to have come to the conclusion that the Europe of Maastricht was too preoccupied with its own affairs and with East and Central Europe to engage it purposefully. The North's answer, that the South enjoyed advantages in the North by virtue of sharing the Mediterranean, failed to satisfy the majority.

Indeed, a tone of pessimism pervaded the interventions of representatives from the South. They spoke of the increasingly hostile environment in which migrants lived, with their remittances continuously falling, to be reminded by a Belgian representative: "We are a very small country." A Tunisian representative went on the offensive.

"Terrorism and extremism disturb the concept of a shared Mediterranean destiny," he conceded. "But they are not the monopoly of the South. There is left extremism in Germany, there is the mafia in Italy, terrorism in the former Yugoslavia. It is, however, true that Islamic terrorism has poisoned the atmosphere in the Mediterranean between the North and South."

Perhaps the most philosophical intervention was by Malta's Di Marco. He spoke of the strong "seeds" of Maghrebian unity in a shared language, culture and religion. But he warned that the world was living in an age in search of roots, a journey that could lead to a sectarian and parochial society. Egypt, he reminded his listeners, had the largest population in the southern Mediterranean, and he pointed to the Turkish role.

Di Marco said that Turkey linked not merely Europe and the Arabs but also Europe and the former Soviet Central Asian republics. The last, with their tenuous democratic structures, represented a threat to Europe and the Mediterranean. European security was closely linked to the Mediterranean.

A European Community expert said a strategic Euro-Mediterranean zone should be constituted in the global context. "Let's have an intimate dinner between the EEC and the Mediterranean South." The problem, of course, was that the South remained far from impressed by the dinner invitation.

It was largely left to the Tunisian representatives to try to squeeze out practical initiatives from the seminar sponsored by their ruling Democratic Constitutional Rally. The Turkish vice prime minister, Erdal Inonu, on the other hand, took pains to emphasise his country's empathy for the sufferings of Muslims in Bosnia-Herzegovina.

The European Community and the Maghreb, Tunisians urged, had to find a way of cooperation; the EEC was going East and the Mediterranean was going its own way. And they pinpointed African emigration as the main stumbling block. There was also the debt question, and they asked, "Why not a European-Maghreb bank?" Europeans, castigated the Tunisians, lacked the political will to engage in a real dialogue with the Mediterranean South. For all their kind words for Tunisian efforts to highlight the problems of and need for North–South cooperation, European representatives seemed preoccupied with their agenda. Insofar as it concerned the Mediterranean South, the exploding population loomed large. African emigration to Europe was the starting point for the North's engagement with the South in the Mediterranean.

Over intimate dinners or otherwise, the Mediterranean South had no option but to accept the North's agenda. It remained to be seen whether it would be a convivial dinner or one providing a setting for further recriminations.

A Tunisian Experiment

Tunisia's experiment in attuning Islam to the modern welfare state was of more than passing interest to the world in 1992 because it took a route directly opposed to the Iranian precept. Living as the country does in a volatile area, with Algeria already burnt by an extreme interpretation of Islam and Libya led by an unpredictable leader, the Tunisian endeavour presented a striking contrast.

Five years after the grand old man of the independence movement, Habib Bourguiba, was deposed in a bloodless coup by his prime minister and the present president, Zine el-Abedine Ben Ali, the two continued to exchange civilities and messages. Bourguiba's portrait hung in the presidential palace while he lived a life of retirement in the salubrious seaside town of Monastir, his birthplace.

In these five years of the new era or "the change", as it is called, Ben Ali had consolidated his position. He seemed genuinely popular and although his portrait hung in shops and hotels and newspapers highlighted his decision to make a speech in bold headlines, the personality cult remained subdued by Arab standards. He was often portrayed as a person who cared for the poor and the deprived.

A Tolerant People

Tunisians say they are tolerant people. In a series of spectacular tableaux tracing 3,000 years of history, presented on the eve of the November 7 celebrations marking five years of "the change", one saw a variety of invasions and interactions as the civilisations of Carthage battled with Romans, Byzantines, Shi'ites, Spaniards, Turks and the French. Independence came in 1956.

Perhaps the secret of Tunisians' basic tolerance lay in the high literacy rate, the highest in North Africa, of 57.6 per cent for adults. The state spent 3.3 per cent of the gross national product on education.

The personal status code of 1956, strengthened in 1987, banned polygamy and the status of Tunisian women was apparent from their freedom from the veil and the Western dresses they wore in Tunis. Tunisia boasted of being the only country in the Arab world to have authorised the establishment of an Amnesty International chapter.

A law on political parties adopted one year after "the change" banned any party based on religion. All parties had to respect the "Arab Islamic identity" of the country, however. Mosques were prohibited from indulging in political propaganda. Ben Ali's stated rationale was that a democratic system based on mere numbers was not conductive to effective pluralism in the early stages of the democratisation process. He was for a consensual approach.

The Tunisian state remained very conscious of religious dangers. It was, for instance, officially pointed out: "If it is politicised, any religion whatsoever becomes a formidable tool for brain-washing and incitement to crime in the name of martyrdom and an apology for limitless intellectual and material terrorism. A politicised religion is not a religion any more. Islam is a stranger to these movements which hide behind it. How marvellous Islam would be if it could be snatched away from the clutches of these individuals".

There are reasons for this sensitivity to the abuse of religion. The reaction to the Second Gulf War demonstrated that even in as tolerant a climate as prevailed in Tunisia, feelings ran high on Western "double standards" and the authorities penalised the offending press.

The nucleus of a religious revivalist movement existed, as was clear from the trial of soldiers on charges of seeking to incite people for religious purposes. It was not long ago that the state had to neutralise extremist religious propaganda from Tunisians who had sought refuge abroad. The new era Tunisian state therefore tilted to a benign authoritarianism even as critics asserted that it was overreacting in using a sledgehammer to swat a fly. The official position was explained thus: "In nascent democracies, the state needs, specially in the early stages, to be strong and effectively in control until the new values and norms of behaviour are deeply rooted. Then society is able to defend itself against its enemies, eliminate extremism and fend off reactionary trends by marginalising and absorbing them. The rule of law is important in all societies but is even more important in nascent democracies. Somewhere a 'red line' has to be drawn so that the state is respected and the rule of law prevails."

The surprise was not in the paternalistic trends in the Tunisian version of statehood. It was in the president instituting a commission in 1991 to inquire into charges of abuse of human rights. In its report, the commission said 55 officers found guilty of misdemeanours were sentenced. The report on the implementation of recommendations of the inquiry commission had been published.

Tunisian Concerns

The concerns of Tunisia were reflected in its foreign policy. It was an advocate of the Maghreb Union, which had failed to take off, given the problems of such partners as Algeria and Libya. It was seeking to engage Europe by emphasising the links between the North and South represented by the Mediterranean and as host to the Palestine Liberation Organisation of Yasser Arafat, it was an advocate of the West Asian peace process.

Tunisians were under no illusion that they could by themselves bring about a dramatic change in the animosities that existed. Having invested their modest wealth in educational and socio-economic objectives, they were in no position to flex their muscles. Rather, their attempt was to be a voice of moderation in the conflicts swirling around them while seeking to strengthen their statehood.

Tunisia was in the midst of an economic reform process, a familiar international phenomenon. Liberalisation and privatisation were going hand in hand with an effort to increase direct foreign investment. Tunisians were also instituting a free zone area whose attraction is its proximity to the rich European market, a stone's throw away.

Tunis is but an hour's plane ride from Rome, and its preponderant trade with Europe cannot but he affected by the recession there. Although Tunisians had been allowed a transition period for the preferential treatment they received in the European Community, they were acutely conscious of the effect of European economic union on their future trade relations.

The picture had been clouded further by the strains of intolerance developing in Europe towards migrant communities. France continued to occupy a dominant position in trade and a familiar argument Tunisians offered was that the best means of preventing the outflow of Tunisians seeking a better economic future in Europe was to help the country provide greater employment opportunities to its people. The unemployment rate was running at 15 per cent.

In a sense, Tunisia was fighting two battles at the same time, the two interacting on each other. One was the fight against religious revivalism of a kind that would represent a setback to the tolerant values most Tunisians held dear. The other was an increasingly inward looking Europe preoccupied with its own affairs and with the former communist countries of East and Central Europe to pay more than passing attention to the plight of the countries of the southern Mediterranean.

Tunisia, in common with other countries of the Maghreb, was seeking to engage Europe more directly in its affairs by emphasising the Mediterranean link and suggesting that the countries on the northern shore of the sea could not prosper at the expense of the southern Mediterranean states. Thus far, the debate had hardly been joined by the northern rim.

At the African regional preparatory meeting for the world conference on human rights held in Tunis is early November, the warning of the president, Ben Ali, to the north was clear, "given the fact that Africa remains particularly subject to poverty, disease and hunger, and that our societies still harbour the seeds of religious and racial intolerance that give way to deep divisions."

Ben Ali added: "Herein lies the danger, for in the process of democratic change, these phenomena may find the conditions on which they thrive, and if unchecked, may become the greatest threat to the very democratic environment that has permitted them to emerge in the first place."

Tunisia remained as acutely aware of its vanguard role in the region as it was of the threat from religious revivalism. Rather self-consciously the authorities asserted: "Tunisia was the first country to offer a democratic model in an environment that was unfamiliar, if not outright hostile, to it. It was the first to emphasise the dangers of Islamic extremism in the Arab Islamic region. This alerted many regimes in the area, which initiated their own democratic processes and took steps to consolidate their civil societies in the face of the fundamentalist threat."

Ironically, Ben Ali was an electronics engineer before he went to elite military schools in France and the United States to return home as a young officer of military security in the high command staff. His rise to power began in 1977. He was catapulted to the prime minister's post at 51, a position he used to end Bourguiba's rule, which had outlived its usefulness.

Tunisia represented the moderate face of Islam even as it gave battle to forces of religious revivalism and sought to build a welfare state. A young Tunisian, a businessman, threw up his hands in horror on learning that I was a political commentator. "Give me my card back," he said, "I have nothing to do with politics."

A Failure

After delegates to Mena, the Middle East and North Africa economic conference, had packed their bags and left the Qatari capital Doha, the central impression that remained for those who attended the three-day meeting in November 1997 was that, despite the brave efforts of the Americans and their hosts, politics could not be separated from economics. Arguments why this was not so where trotted out by the president of the World Economic Forum and the senior US representative: the European example of the European Union's humble beginnings in the steel and coal community and the Americans even claimed that economics had won over politics.

Businessman made deals, it was true, and a compendium of business deals between Qatar and American companies was made to arrive at the impressive total of $4.1 billion. Understandably, Qatar was trying to put its best foot forward to present itself as the new boom state in West Asia, with very generous gas supplies becoming the engine of an unprecedented growth rate and a projected per capita income of $50,000. There was appreciation for how well Qatar had managed the conference, with the undoubted help of the WEF and the United States, given its slender experience in the field. And the paucity of hotel rooms in the capital was made good by commissioning three cruise ships as hotels, mostly for the media.

The central Palestinian–Israeli confrontation hung over the conference as a pall of gloom. Even as the various sessions proceeded along their predictable course, the underlying tension was palpable. And outside the conference rooms, reporters plied the protagonists with questions. The Qatari–Egyptian rift was a reminder of disunity in Arab ranks, if further proof were needed after the major economies in the Arabian Gulf had boycotted the meeting. But the central contradictions of Mena were plain for all to see. At one stage, Americans sought to present the concept as a pan-Arab economic gathering. Why then include Israel before the peace process, now nearly in the grave, was restored to health if possible? And if the rule of universality was to be applied, why exclude Iraq and Iran?

There were no convincing answers in Doha because, after what had happened to a process begun in Madrid, Mena was somewhat like putting the cart before the horse. Economic compulsions could help to bring about a historical reconciliation, as between Germany and France, if there was acceptance of reality by both sides. If the Israeli objective was to reduce Palestinians to serfdom and give them municipal powers in bits of territory left them, no deals could bridge the gap or bring about peace. Genuine friendship and reconciliation could come about only through equal partners. Window-dressing was no substitute for the Israeli desire to colonise a whole people in this day and age.

A Great Draw

The Israeli Labour Party leader and former prime minister, Shimon Peres, was a great draw at Mena, and the objective of the organisers was perhaps to soften the feelings Arabs reserved for Prime Minister Benjamin Netanyahu's Israel. Peres was, indeed, an impressive man and knew how to tug at people's heartstrings although the remarkable foreign minister of Qatar, Shaikh Hamad bin Khalifa Al Thani, paid him the left-handed compliment of possessing a romantic view. But for those who were not seduced by the Labour leader's capacity for painting an attractive vision of peace and prosperity, his words brought little comfort. Without saying it in so many words, he was suggesting that the land-for-peace formula, the bedrock of the Madrid process, was inadequate for bringing about peace.

The new slogan of Peres was freedom with peace because land, he suggested, was tangible and was sought to be exchanged for peace, which was a promise. In other words, it was an unequal bargain. Had the giving up of land in Gaza brought peace? he asked. Peres had never publicly spoken in these terms before and the Arab world's attitude to the most famous of the remaining Israeli Labour party leaders could change as the realisation of his new thinking sank in.

It was no surprise that at a gathering of large numbers of businessman, business was discussed and deals were made. But the rationale of Mena surely was that the deals would bridge the Arab–Israeli divide and there were few signs of such activity, with the project under which Qatari gas supplies would go to Israel through the American Enron company still to be publicly revived. And it was a telling reminder of the reality of West Asia that for the first time a Mena conference could not publicly announce the host of its next meeting. The declaration of the senior US official Stuart Eisenstat, who was holding the fort for Madeleine Albright who spent a few hours in Doha, that economics 'bucked' politics had a hollow ring to it, given the prominent reference to the land-for-peace formula in the final declaration, despite Israeli objections.

And the official statements from several delegations, including the Qatari hosts, must have weighed heavily on Israeli minds. The Doha Declaration talked sharply of the plight of the Palestinian economy, thanks to the arbitrary closures of the so-called autonomous territories. Shaikh Hamad bin Khalifa Al Thani, the Amir, made his political point against Israel at the opening while Mrs Albright, in a speech that surprised friend and foe alike, made an attack on Iraq at a meeting the Americans were promoting as an economic gathering. In a sense, Americans never recovered from the gap between their formal stance and Washington's political agenda and fell between two stools.

What then did Mena achieve? It proved that the Israeli factor would continue to bedevil progress as long as the Israelis believed that they could continue to colonise Palestinians. Second, if a pan-Arab dimension to Mena could serve as a catalytic agent, Arab businessmen would take it. Third, globalisation that was one of the major themes of the Mena meeting could never equally embrace Israel and the Arab world until the dissonance caused by Israel's rejection of Palestinian statehood in the genuine sense was recognised.

Peres said at his press conference in Doha that the Arabs had started wars against Israel and the Israelis had won land in the wars, saying at the same time that they should be given up, without defining the extent. Arabs would respond that if Israel wanted to retain its war booty, despite a string of UN resolutions and its own commitments, there would be no peace in the region.

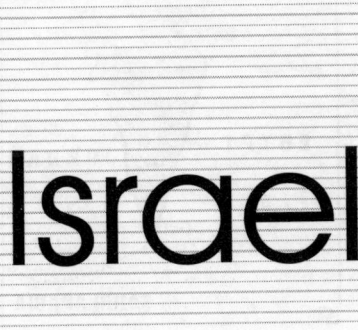

Israel

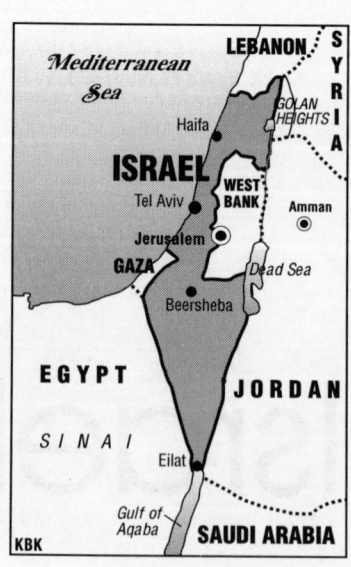

A Soft Landing

The growing number of Soviet Jews migrating to Israel became another flashpoint in the continuing Arab-Israel conflict in West Asia. The Israeli Prime Minister, Yitzak Shamir, publicly declared that some of them would be settled in the occupied territories of the West Bank and the Gaza Strip. This led to strong Arab condemnation. The Arabs feared that the Israelis were seeking to change the demography of the occupied territories. The Israelis imposed censorship on the absoption and placing of Soviet Jews. In January 1990, they expected up to 300,000 Soviet Jews to migrate to Israel in the next three years. I went to an absorption centre near Jerusalem to find out more about it.

Mevasereth on the outskirts of Jerusalem could be just another conglomeration of lower middle class houses. A light drizzle was falling even as clothes hung limp on clothes-lines in gardens. An odd black woman and child on the street were a manifestation of the varied mix of Israel.

Perhaps it was the weather, but the atmosphere in Mevasereth seemed cheerless. As we approached the administrative section, there were few people' around. But soon I was in the capable hands of Zipporah Liben of the immigration and absorption department of the Jewish Agency. She look me to the assembly hall with walls festooned with posters whose central purpose seemed to be to bring home to the new arrivals the unifying force of Zionism.

Liben, who migrated from the United States a few years earlier, had the answers pat. The Mevasereth Centre was set up in 1969-70 for Soviet Jews to begin with. There are 40 absorption centres in the country, each taking in 70 to 100 families at a time. More centres were planned.

In Liben's words, the absorption centre's function was to provide a "soft landing", it was not a rescue operation. There were total immersion courses in Hebrew five days a week, five hours a day, subsidised by the Jewish Agency.

Adoption Rules

"We would like them to stay six months", Liben said. "After six months, they must pay a nominal rent: Each family receives 700 to 800 shekels a month. About 950 people are housed in this centre".

There was the new method of direct absorption, with municipalities in charge. A family of three receives 22,000 shekels in a lump sum in the direct absorption scheme.

"What are the new Soviet arrivals like?" I asked.

"Typically, we get young couples with two children and an aged parent. There are a lot of professionals, with a high skill level. Physicians would have to be retrained".

"How would you rate the Ethiopian Jews?" I enquired.

"Oh, they are from another century", Liben answered.

I was taken to a nursery school in the centre, the most cheerful spot in the whole complex. A varied lot of children, white and black, sat in a circle against a backdrop of the symbols of the Jewish faith. The boys were already sporting yarmulkas. At the teacher's bidding, each child introduced himself and herself. They were from diverse parts of the world—from the Soviet Union, France, Romania, Ethiopia. The whole world seemed represented.

The teacher was teaching them songs, one of which was to welcome the visitor from India. Herself of Iranian origin, she told me that she had gone to India in order to migrate to Israel.

It was a happy group of children I left to brave the drizzle outside. The elders were immersed in their Hebrew lessons, but a break in class enabled me to accost a Soviet Jew. He had a serious mien and not much appetite for conversation. My knowledge of Russian, however, came in handy.

He was a recent arrival and kept puffing away at his cigarette. How did he like it here? I asked.

"I have only been here two or three months", he answered. "Let me see. I shall know later whether I like it or not".

An Indian at Home

The home of 48-year-old Nechmya Tifereth from Paravoor, south of Cochin, in Yuval cooperative near Israel's border with Lebanon had all the attributes of a bourgeois home with a florid taste. A window air-conditioner was mocking the cold winter afternoon in January. A stereo set was mute and a guitar stood on the floor near the dining table.

The pungent aroma of Kerala curry floated in from the open plan kitchen as Tifereth's wife was tidying the dishes. She was in jeans while Nechmya sat in jeans and a windcheater to tell me about himself and his life in Israel.

Yuval had 88 families, originally all of them from Cochin, but as the young married other Israelis, they brought in their non-Cochin brides. Yuval originally was the home of Jews from Kurdistan, but their efforts did not succeed and the land was given to the first batch of Cochin Jews in 1952. Tifereth belonged to the second group of Cochin Jews who came to Yuval in 1955.

Tifereth was a 13-year-old boy when he first came to Israel with a group of 53 other children and after learning Hebrew for three months, he went to the Segera youth centre to study agriculture for four years. Segera, he proudly recalled, was the camp Ben Gurion went to as a daily labourer.

Nechmya's father followed him to Israel a year and a half later. He had a poultry business before he took over as the housekeeper of the synagogue in Cochin. It was tough going for the father, unused as he was to hard labour clearing virgin land.

Nechmya was reticent about his father's experiences, but he said it was a hard life. The climate was difficult. It was cold and there were then no services available in the cooperative. The family first lived in huts. A little part of the present living and sitting room had to house his parents and three children.

Veg to Fruit

Nechmya first planted cucumber and the first five years he devoted to growing vegetables before graduating to fruit trees. Gradually, he built on his modest accommodation to complete the handsome two-storey house. He had five children. Two of them were in the army and two in school. The third boy, 23, helped the father on the farm after his release from the compulsory three-year military service.

Each farm in Yuval was of 28 dunams (1 dunam is a quarter acre). The Tifereth family grew plums and pears and was trying its hand at red grapefruit. But the cooperative experiment at Yuval "moshav" did not quite work out and the members decided to privatise each plot, with the result that Tifereth has to pay off 70,000 shekels (1 shekel was about 50 US cents) over the next 15 years.

Tifereth spoke Malayalam and Hebrew at home but knew little English. Our conversation had therefore to be conducted through an interpreter. He struck me as an intense man wrapped up in his world.

"Are you happy here?" I asked him.

"This was my dream", he answered. "What more can one want? I had dreamt of being a farmer and raising a family on it".

How much money did he make? I asked.

His answer was indirect. "One needs 4,000 shekels a month to be comfortable. I earn only half as much".

It was a subject near to his heart. "We tell the authorities we are living near the border and must be given a remission in repayments, particularly because the committee that managed affairs in the cooperative days was extravagant, and we should not have to pay for their extravagance. We have had demonstrations. We are fighting the authorities".

Had he revisited his original home? I asked.

Nechmya was defensive. "No, I have not revisited Cochin. I don't have the time even for a vacation. How can I go to India?"

Nechmya was wrapped up in his new world and the greatest event of his life, which he recalled in minute detail, occurred on June 15, 1975. It was as if it had happened yesterday.

Four militants attacked the village at night and killed the Mordechai family, man and wife and his brother-in-law. Nechmya was in charge of security and deployed the ten armed men under his command to corner the militants until Israeli security forces arrived. Nechmya had a framed certificate from the authorities praising his courage.

The wife refused to be photographed with him against the backdrop of their home. So Nechmya brought a daughter out of a bedroom to pose for photographs. But his thoughts were far away. They were entwined with that night in 1975 the militants came.

The Diamond Man

The three-tower diamond exchange complex at Ramat-Gan in Tel Aviv is not everybody's cup of tea. It bristled with armed guards and a visitor could enter the building only after surrendering his passport and had to pass through electronically controlled turnstiles which responded to magnetic cards.

The lift operator sported a revolver in his holster as he took me to my floor.

The Israel Diamond Exchange had 2,400 members in 1990, and anything up to $ 5 billion in locked offices which were opened after scrutinising the visitor.

Diamonds and Jews have traditionally gone together for a variety of reasons—among them the fact that many professions were forbidden to them in Europe and elsewhere over the centuries. Israel had the world's largest combined production-export centre for the polished diamond trade. Its overseas sales in 1989 yielded $ 2.7 billion, one-third of Israel's foreign trade earnings.

What took me to Ramat-Gan was to meet the doyen of Indian diamond merchants in Israel, the head of one of the 22 Gujarati diamond merchant families settled there. Ramat-Gan represented a unique meeting of Jewish expertise in diamonds and Gujarati entrepreneurship.

Kirtilal Mehta was on the telephone when I was shown in. Actually, he was talking alternately on two telephones. The result of the two-minute conversation was a $ 2-million deal. He turned out to be a genial soul, and surprisingly sprightly for his 82 years.

Kirtilal had lived in Israel for 25 years. He found Belgium (Antwerp is another world centre in diamond trade) too cold and Bombay was too hot. He liked the Israel climate and spent eight months in Tel Aviv and the remaining four months in India. "The people are nice and friendly here", he said.

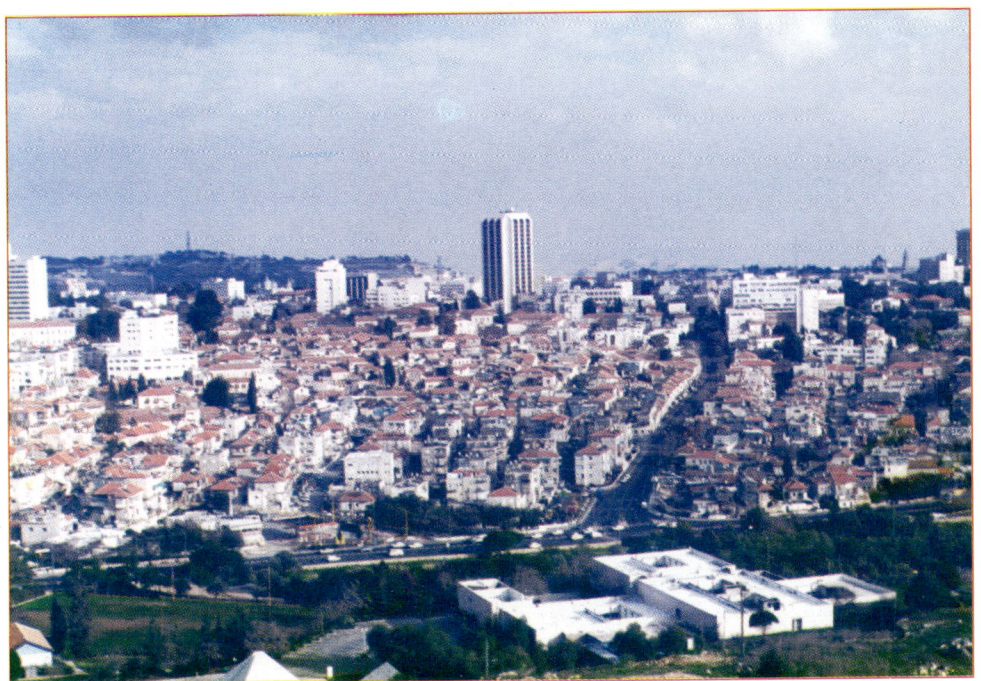

The eternal city of Jerusalem: a bird's eye view of the western district.

Indians in Israel: Nechmiya Tifereth from Paravoor, south of Cochin, proudly poses for a photograph with his daughter outside his house in Yuval cooperative near Israel's border with Lebanon.

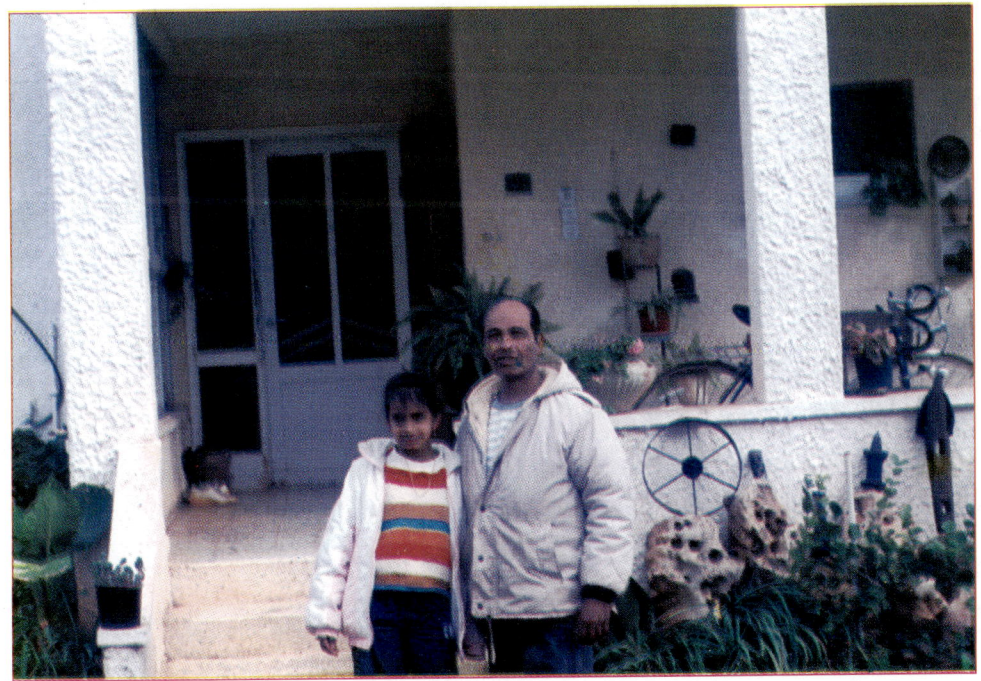

Plate **5**

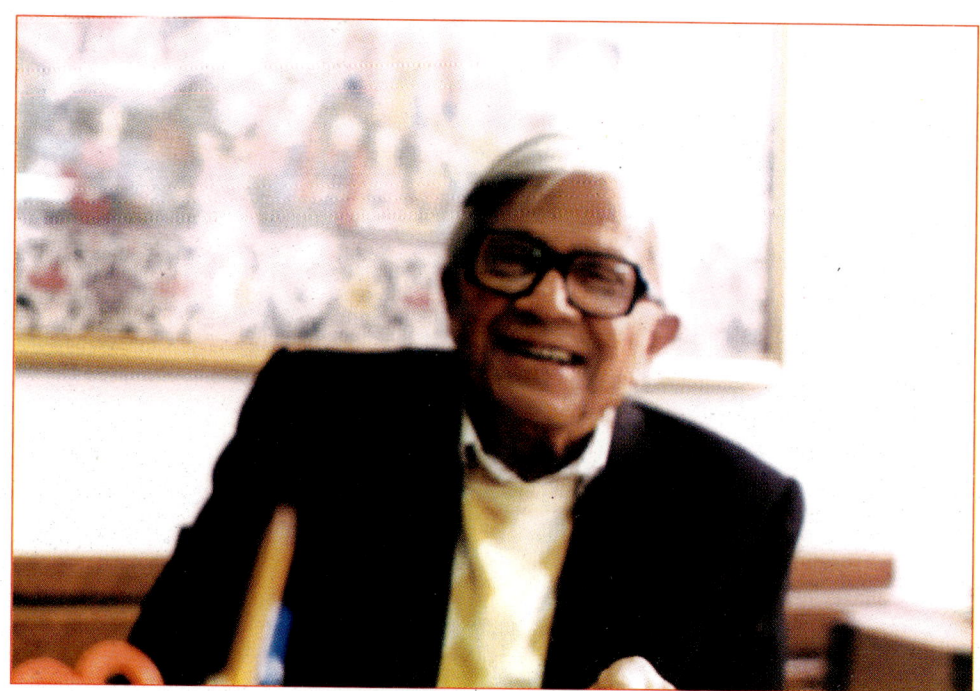

Kirtilal Mehta, the diamond man, poses for a photograph in his office in
Tel Aviv in January 1990.

Children in a school absorption centre for new migrants in Havasereth
on the outskirts of Jerusalem.

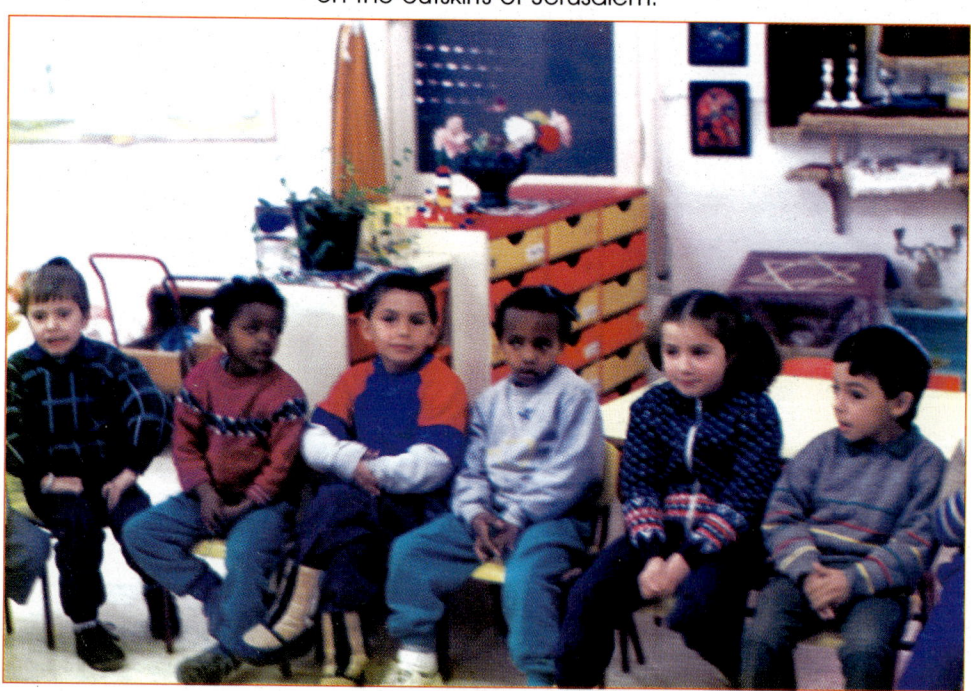

Plate **6**

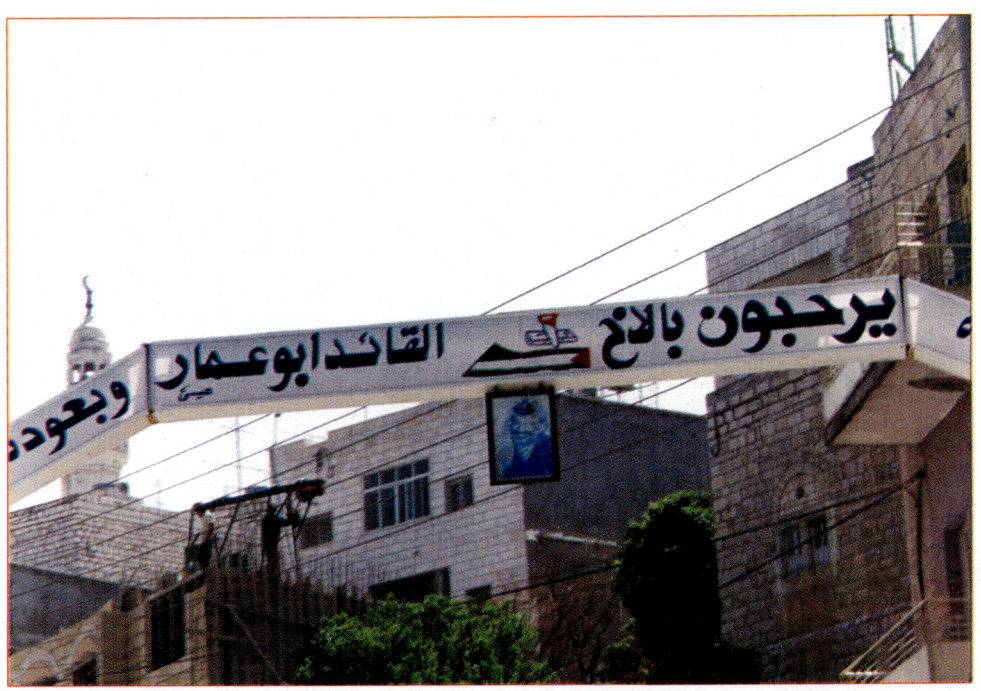

In Bethlehem, the symbol of Palestine, Yasser Arafat, derided and humiliated by Israel's Ariel Sharon.

A traffic ticket for a motorist in Bethlehem before Israel's reoccupation.

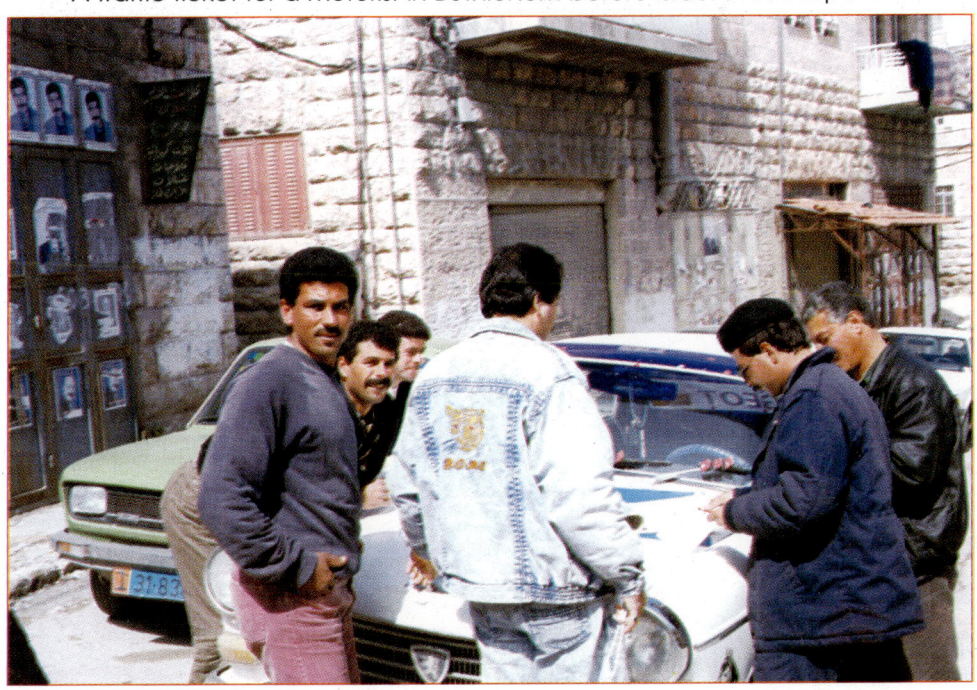

Plate **7**

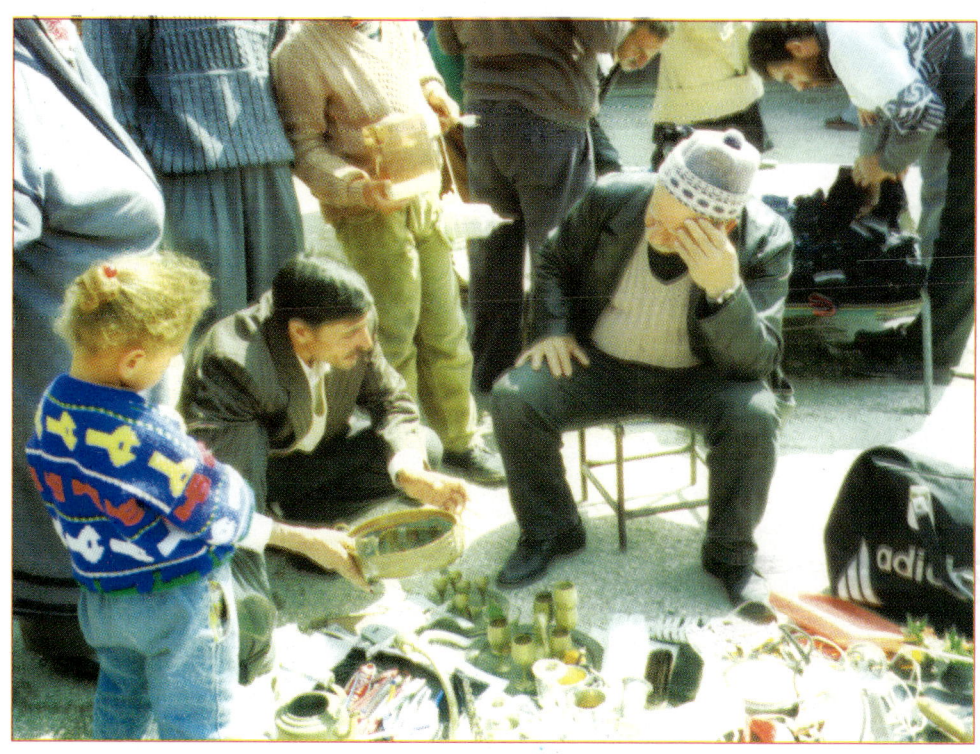

A Palestinian bazaar in Bethlehem (both above and below).

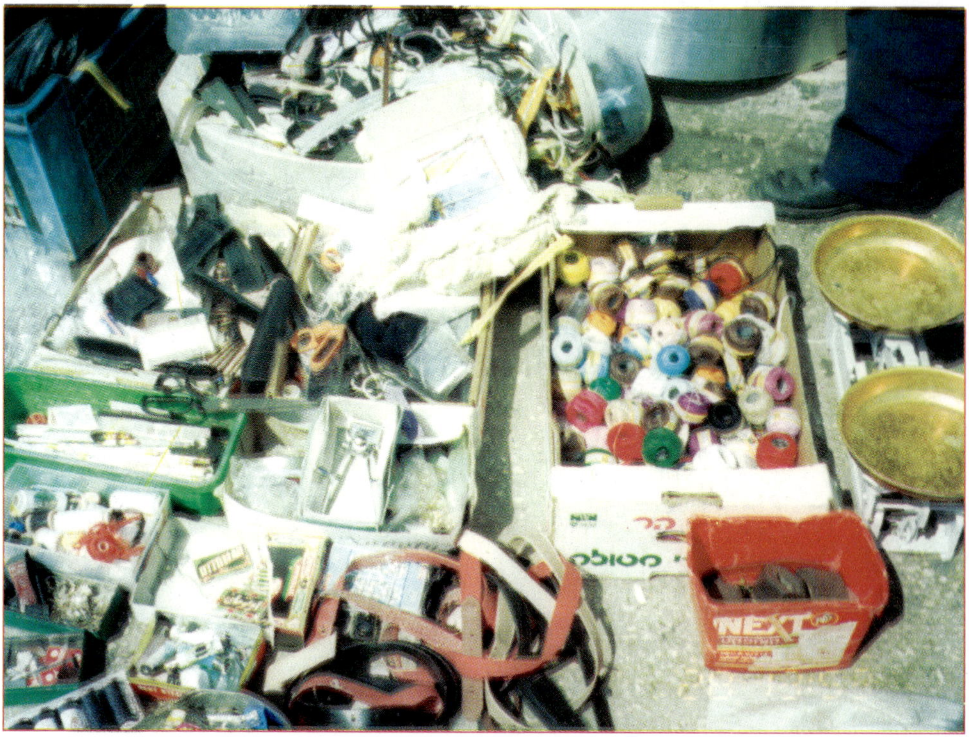

Plate **8**

Father to Son

"I was 12 when I started in diamond business in Rangoon", he began. "My father was in diamonds".

Kirtilal's father died and he was apprenticed to his father's firm. Having acquired the expertise, he went to Belgium in 1933 to spend 15 years there. "Before 1947, I used to come here to buy diamonds", he said.

Kirtilal's expertise and business acumen proved a formidable combination and as his business grew, so did his family. As he opened and expanded offices in New York, Hong Kong, Antwerp and Bombay, he could place one or more family members in each office.

"I have four sons and three daugters", he revealed. "Two of my daughters are married and one is in New York. All are in the diamond business. I have 15 grandsons".

He continued: "I export rough diamonds to India and import polished diamonds from there. All deals are made by word of mouth. Here they are sealed with the expression *mazal-u-bracha*, or *mazal* for short, a Yiddish word.

"There is no competition between Israel and India. There is good technology here and Israel is good in big and fancy diamonds. India sells well in small diamonds because labour is expensive here. We have the manpower. Ninety-five per cent of all Indian diamond merchants come from my ancestral home, Palanpur near Mt. Abu. The sea is big. Everybody can swim".

Being the first Indian diamond merchant to set up shop in Israel, Kirtilal's office complex had extensive facilities. In the lunch room adjacent to his office, I was treated to a Gujarati vegetarian meal.

He was a relaxed host. Million-dollar deals could wait as his thoughts flitted to India. Yes, it was his grandson's wedding in Bombay which had caught media attention. Kirtilal was building a Rs. 25-crore hospital at Bandra, Bombay, to give back something of the good fortune he has enjoyed. One of his proud possessions was the 1972 "outstanding importer from Israel" award, presented to him by the President of Israel.

I put my camera, which had got me into trouble with one of the armed guards, to use to catch Kirtilal's genial expression. But he wanted his souvenir and got an assistant to take a picture of us at his spartan dinning table, sporting two kinds of Gujarati pickles. An Israeli guest could hardly believe that he had been served a principal meal.

Land and People

Human nature has an extraordinary capacity to adjust to abnormal situations. During the big American phase of the Vietnam war in the sixties, I marvelled at the insouciance of the people living in the midst of war and devastation. And any visitor to Israel 1990 would be struck by the air of normality that prevailed in most parts of the country as the intefada in the occupied territories took its mournful daily toll.

The air of normality in Jerusalem was unaffected by the stabbing of an Israeli girl soldier—all girls are required to do two years' military service from the age of 18—in East Jerusalem, annexed by Israel after the 1967 war. There was no barrier any longer between East and West Jerusalem and the Israelis, with their diligence and attention to detail, had rebuilt the eastern sector, history willing. Almost everywhere one dug, ancient history peeped out and the historical sites had to be left undisturbed.

The Israelis might have decimated the partition between the eastern and western parts of the city, but the Arabs—Palestinians to be precise—still lived in the East. The intefada reverberated there in the curfew imposed by the underground on shops. All shops closed at noon and Israelis tended not to go to the East too often. It is an irony of history and the development of religious faiths that the Wailing Wall, so sacred to Jews, stands cheek by jowl with the impressive main dome of the mosque on the rock.

Even outside the occupied territories, there were tensions underneath. Israelis smoke a lot—to release tension, an Israeli suggested to me—and conscripted boys and girls carry rifles as others their age would carry knapsacks. Israelis had much to show for their determination and faith. The smiling fields and orchards were a testimony to Israeli hard work and innovation. The desert bloomed and the highways and motorways of Israel had an almost European air of ordered placidity, but for the palms that suggested that one was not exactly in Europe. And there were the relics of the various wars— derelict military vehicles strewn around the country, much as the bombed church in West Berlin has been left undisturbed as a stark reminder.

Israeli Paradoxes

In the forty-second year of their independent existence, Israelis were facing many of the paradoxes of their life. Starting out as a pariah nation, except for the support of the United States and some other Western powers, Israel was now recognised by an increasing number of countries, with the East European nations vying with one another to extend recognition. Yet the cancer of war and insecurity the country had faced since its birth was gnawing at its vitals as the people faced the disturbing problem of the Palestinians.

The Palestinian issue, as the world knew it, brought Israel face to face with the dilemma of the Israeli state. In the tempestuous history of the nation, Israelis wanted nothing more avidly than to be accepted in the region. Yet the manner in which the state was founded and the peculiarities that made up the Jewish nation had meant an almost eternal period of conflict.

As the Israeli Deputy Foreign Minister, Benjamin Natanyahu later to become Prime Minister, explained to me in Jerusalem, his people were unique in that they neither reconquered the territories they had lost—circa B.C.—nor were they willing to be assimilated with the people of the countries they lived in. These characteristics gave Israelis their strength and their weakness. They had the capacity to survive in a hostile environment and they were tortured by a sense of insecurity even when there was a chance for peace.

Apart from the political circumstances that brought Israel into being, the romance of building up a modern nation state on the strength of the diaspora had been unique in the annals of recent history. The kibbutz movement—the nearest thing to socialist egalitarianism—brought people of diverse cultures together and as the state developed and a people's army took shape, Israelis laboured and reaped some of the rewards of innovation and hard work. Its security and financial underpinning by the United States in a hostile Arab world had been a necessary attribute of Israel's survival.

The irony of historical circumstances and Jewish tenacity was that although the Israelis desired nothing more than secure peace, their temperament and history posed difficulties for them in making the necessary concessions to achieve it. Israel's continuing occupation of the West Bank and Gaza Strip was a patently untenable position. Even as sections of the right wing sought to appropriate these territories, with around a million and a half Palestinians, they were making things more difficult for themselves. "Security" was a holy cow in Israel for understandable reasons, and the desire to redraw the map in keeping with the maximalist demands of the right wing was compounded by a process that was necessarily tortuous.

Israel's problems were accentuated by the fact that it remained an ideological state in an age in which ideology was being thrown overboard by the communist world. Israel's political mosaic was reflective of the pulls of what an astute Egyptian political analyst has called the historical and security views. The young in Israel tended to be less ideological and should move the political pendulum away from an apocalyptical view of history even as the country's politics moved towards the right.

The intefada in the occupied territories was raising the costs of Israel's defence while winning the country much opprobrium around the world. Israelis smarted under what they considered unfair criticism. For the right wing, which came in many shades, the world's criticism merely hardened its resolve to achieve maximalist solutions. The absurdity of the prospect of an ideological Jewish State with a significant Arab population was never faced squarely, except at a universally unacceptable cost.

Siege Mentality

A people who set such great store by its suffering—over the centuries and longer—inevitably became more firm in its resolve to battle the world. A siege mentality came naturally to a people who bears the burden of a deeply unhappy history. But in the all-pervasive indoctrination of the Israeli state, the surprise was that the young tended to strike out a new path. Perhaps the influence of the non-ideological world and their hankering for a more normal life served to take youth to a less apocalyptical view of history, and their place in it.

The intefada had shaken Israelis out of the belief that the process of the occupation would, in course of time, become a fact of life. However Israelis might explain their security needs, the concept of ruling a million and a half Palestinians in perpetuity made little sense. The autonomy plan of the Prime Minister, Yitzak Shamir of the right-wing Likud Party, was a concession to propitiate Washington and the rest of the world. Yet the wrangle over the nature of the Palestinian delegation and the indirect role the Palestine Liberation Organisation should or should not have in its selection exposed the vulnerability of the Israeli right. Logically, elections in the occupied territories should lead to a form of independence, a prospect the right abhors.

The political stalemate in Israel was compounded by the near parity of the two main parties, Likud and the Labour Party, each with 40 per cent support, and the stranglehold the system gave to religious parties. Some of the religious parties are not as obscurantist as they might appear, but any realistic political solution had to cross the hurdle of securing the agreement of diverse groups. Likud and Labour both blamed the system without uniting to bring about a change. With some feeling, the Israeli President, Chaim Herzog, told me in Jerusalem that India should avoid the proportional representative system like the plague. The Israeli political system, he said, was rotten.

The intefada and the United States had combined to jolt the Israeli political establishment out of its reflex reactions. Apart from the divisions in Israeli opinion these two factors had brought to the fore, the political system in the country gave full play to politicians to bargain for short-term advantages. Shamir's attitude was understandable because he was part of, and represented, the right constituency. The conduct of the Labour leader, Shimon Peres, was more reprehensible in that he had failed to take the high moral ground. Petty politicking, rather than the broader picture, seemed to be the guiding force in Israeli politics.

Political analysts in Israel were waiting for the elections, due in one and a half years, for "the princes" to take over from Shamir and Peres.

They are the younger and second rung politicians who were competing furiously among themselves. Some like Ariel Sharon, the feisty leader of the right, were expected to survive the anticipated generational change. But the assumption was that the new crop of leaders would be more pragmatic and more willing to trade territory for peace.

The pity is that in Israel's hour of need, when there was a real chance for peace, which all Israelis desired, statesmanship was in short supply. The hope of many in Israel was that the young would show the country's squabbling and ambitious politicians the way out of the present impasse. It is a consummation devoutly to be wished.

"You can learn from your neighbour Burma", President Chaim Herzog told me in the Presidential House in Jerusalem. "Both Ne Win and U Nu before him had told their critics when threatened that recognising a country was for Burma alone and no one else to decide".

President Herzog added, "India's approach doesn't make sense. Diplomatic relations don't mean that you agree with other countries. They are a function of a country's independence".

Indo–Israeli Relations

Time and again during a visit to Israel the discussion reverted to the issue of Indian-Israeli relations. Buoyed by the queue of East European countries seeking relations with Israel and the prospect of resuming full diplomatic relations with the Soviet Union, Israeli ministers and officials expressed a measure of exasperation, tinged with regret, over New Delhi's refusal to open full diplomatic relations. Israeli officials readily conceded that one objective of their foreign policy was to end their country's isolation.

Israelis were not unaware of Indian compulsions in keeping Israel at arm's length—the importance of the Arab world for economic and political reasons, the latter in the context of Pakistan in particular, and the large Muslim population and the sympathy that exists in the country for the Palestinian cause. But they made no secret of their bewilderment at what they viewed as Indian pusillanimity. On a more minor and deeply felt note, officials expressed dismay over the pinpricks Israelis had been subjected to.

A Foreign Office official told me that an Israeli academic invited to a conference in India had refused to participate in it because of New Delhi's refusal to treat him as an Israeli delegation, unlike the other participants. The same official said a television interview conducted with the Prime Minister, Yitzak Shamir, a year ago for "The World This Week" programme had censored his views on Indian-Israeli relations.

Benjamin Natanyahu tried another tack. He suggested that far from being a disadvantage, India would discover that having full diplomatic relations with Israel would be to its advantage. President François

Mitterrand had found out that France was more in demand in the Arab world after he had warmed up to the Israelis. The Arab nations, in his view, would woo India more, not less, if India and Israel exchanged ambassadors. He regretted the prospect of India being among the last countries to recognise Israel, after China. "In a year, we'll have diplomatic relations with 130-odd countries", he said.

In Natanyahu's view, there would be full diplomatic relations with the Soviet Union, followed by China. Warming to the theme, he declared: "The situation has changed with the disintegration of the Soviet empire. Non-alignment has lost its relevance. What is India waiting for? I am at a loss to explain the Indian stand. We have so much in common".

The Chinese approach to Israel was, for many Israeli officials, a telling foil. China had opened an eight-member "tourism" bureau in Israeli and Jerusalem would reciprocate by opening an "academic" centre in Beijing. It was perfectly well understood by both countries and rest of the world what this transparent camouflage implied. And officials said they were somewhat surprised by China having stolen a march over India.

Ari Rath, former editor of the *Jerusalem Post*, told me that Indira Gandhi had agreed in a meeting with him in New Delhi during her tenure as Information Minister in the Shastri cabinet that she would permit an Israeli to be based in New Delhi as an agency correspondent for South-east Asia "provided he was a genuine correspondent". Yet nothing materialised. In fact, the point of having an Israeli consulate in Bombay, rather than Delhi, was that it should not block the opening of the Israeli embassy in the capital.

Joseph Hadass, a senior Israeli official, informed me that he had put off his planned visit to India last year after the dust it had raised in the Indian media. A seasoned diplomat, who has served as ambassador in many countries, said he found it surprising that the Pakistani ambassador was more interested in exchanging views with him than his Indian counterpart in Brussels. He described Indian diplomats' conduct as "timid".

At least one official in Jerusalem was more specific in suggesting that as two non-Muslim nations in the region, there was an obvious convergence between the two countries. Other themes ranged from the pluralistic nature of the two societies against the background of the regimes that existed in the Arab world to a natural affinity in the common thrust for modernisation through science and technology.

Ethnic Indians in Israel added their own voice to pleading for full diplomatic relations. There were around 50,000 Indian Jews settled in Israel. Noah Masil, secretary of the Indian Jews Association and a television technician by profession, said he was seeking to revitalise the Indian-Jewish Friendship Society and was hoping for some dignitaries to attend the Independence Day celebrations in Israel in August. "India should invite the first ethnic Indian member of the Knesset, Ben-Meachem", he suggested. He wanted India to give Israel full diplomatic recognition.

Indians' Demand

Other Indians, prosperous Gujaratis who were doing a roaring trade in diamonds and lived in Israel, suggested on a more practical plane that New Delhi should open a legation in Tel Aviv. Obtaining visas for India meant going to Cairo or sending passports by courier to Antwerp, another world centre of diamond trade, to be processed by the Indian embassy in Brussels. The doyen of Indian diamond merchants, Kirtilal M. Mehta, whose grandson's recent wedding in Bombay was the event of the year, agreed that India should have a representative in Israel.

The jurisdiction of the Israeli consulate in Bombay had been extended to Kerala, the home of the majority of Indians Jews who have migrated to Israel. Besides, Cochin has fine synagogues. But Israeli officials chafe at being kept out of Delhi; the consul is not received officially in New Delhi during his visits to the capital.

Most visitors to Israel from the subcontinent are from Nepal and Sri Lanka. Yet a trickle of Indians found its way outside the intense activity of the diamond merchants. Israelis emphasised that they played their part in helping the developing countries.

Two of the institutions taking foreign students or specialists are the Weizman Institute of Science and the Rupin Institute. At Weizman, I met Venkatesh Ramakrishna of Bangalore pursuing membrane research. A vegetarian, he was delighted by the range of fresh vegetables available in Israel.

At Rupin, B. M. Sharma, a teaching faculty member of the Agriculture University of Rajasthan, was just settling down to a three-week course in agricultural support systems. He was full of praise for the drip irrigation system developed by Israel. Rupin mostly caters to Israelis but groups of between 20 and 30 students from abroad were given a chance to interact among themselves and with Israelis to resolve specific problems.

The point Israelis wished to make was that they had the will and the capability to share their experience with others, particularly those belonging to the Third World. A leaf India could take out of Israel's book is the use of solar water heaters. They cost the equivalent of $ 500 apiece and dot the roofs of houses and apartment buildings across Israel.

Developments in East Europe had been a bonanza for Israel in two ways. There was a rush of Jewish migrants from the Soviet Union and the avidity with which East European countries were pursuing the promotion of relations with Israel was pleasing to the Israelis. Given this setting, Israelis were more forthright in giving expression to their feelings about India's diplomatic stance.

I could give Israelis little cheer. The National Front government was inward-looking, I told them. Dependent as it was on communist support for survival, reviewing relations with Israel was at the bottom of its agenda.

Chasing Peace in 1990

Israel lived on several planes. It is a modern nation striving for excellence. On another planes, a nation in almost perpetual war of one sort or another looked at the future with hope and foreboding. Beyond the specific planes and a peace process that seemed entangled in five-point and 10-point plans, there was the first glimpse of peace. Peace would not break out tomorrow or the day after, but for the first time since the troubled founding of the Israeli state about the same time India achieved its independence, the real questions were being discussed.

Israel was divided down the middle not over the desire for peace but over the price that had to be paid for it. The margin of error, all Israeli acknowledged, was excruciatingly small and the question really boiled down to the kinds of risks Israel could afford to take to secure peace. The majority of people, it would seem, believed that it should accept a Palestinian entity.

One of the problems was that Israel was governed by the so-called National Unity government, a phenomenon that led to perpetual inter-party warfare and a measure of immobility. Even as the painful process of adopting a presidential form of government proceeded in fits and starts, the leaders of the right-wing Likud party of Yitzak Shamir and the Labour party of Shimon Peres adopted postures of defiance or reconciliation.

President Chaim Herzog told me in his Presidential House in Jerusalem that he was optimistic about peace. "I have the feelings that things will move", he said. "The distance is not so great". He believed that sooner, rather than later, the three foreign ministers (of Israel, Egypt and the US) would meet and eventually Israel would talk with Palestinians. Yasser Arafat's Palestine Liberation Organisation the President still described as a terrorist organisation and he said that the charter of the organisation called for the destruction of Israel.

There were, of course, any number of hawks. Shamir himself had ruled out the territory for peace concept. When I suggested to President Herzog that I could not envisage Shamir signing a peace agreement with the Palestinians, he demurred. He answered by pointing out that it was Menachem Begin who signed the Camp David peace agreement with Egypt. Begin's son, Benjamin Begin, a respected Member of Parliament, was, however, as hawkish as they come. I asked him if he saw the proverbial light at the end of the tunnel. A geologist by profession, he answered, "What is the point if the light at the end of the tunnel is of a train hurtling towards us?"

Netanyahu's Views

Benjamin Natanyahu explained to me how the West Bank—Judea and Samaria to Israelis—was vital to the country's security. Anyone sitting on the hills in the West Bank could threaten Israel at will. His solution had a familiar ring. He wanted the border with Jordan to stay where it was, along the river, with minor adjustments. The Palestinian population, he suggested, could vote in the present state of Jordan, if it so desired.

Shamir's autonomy plan for the occupied territories offered "full autonomy," short of control over defence and foreign affairs. The sticking point over the composition of the Palestinian delegation—the Israelis want to keep the PLO and outside Palestinians out—arose out of Jerusalem's fear that once the principle of outside participation was accepted, Israel would have to accept the "right of return." Instead of around one-and-a-half million Palestinians in the occupied territories, there could be twice as many in the future Palestinian entity.

Men like Ariel Sharon opposed Shamir's plan because they believed that it would be the thin end of the wedge. In other words, once the occupied territories were granted autonomy, it would be an irreversible process that would lead to an independent Palestinian entity, whatever form it took. The Palestinians, on the other hand, looked askance at the autonomy plan because they wanted to assure themselves of the end result.

As Israelis often emphasised, Israel's was a pluralistic society, unlike the situation in the Arab world, and they were particularly sore that the world has been less than fair to them. Down in the Gaza Strip during a visit, I discovered a ghost town, with the Palestinian underground movement having ordered a general strike, a common phenomenon.

The commander of the area, Colonel Giora, sat at his desk in his headquarters behind a posed picture of a hooded terrorist to answer questions. He was clear that he was performing his duty but he decidedly left open the question of what military power alone could do. Professional soldiers were learning the difficult task of coping with essential riot duty and he said he had punished an officer who had "overreacted" about three months ago. According to him, there were more Palestinians killed by other Palestinians than by the Israeli army. He said that in the half of the Strip area he controlled, including Gaza City, there had been three avoidable deaths in the last four months.

As I was driven around the city in an army jeep, I asked a young second lieutenant who was riding with me, a rifle casually slung across his shoulder, how he liked his work. "I don't like it," he answered, and his unhappy expression was proof enough that he would be happy to get away from it all. Military service is compulsory for all Israelis from the age of eighteen—three years for boys and two years for girls.

Crisscrossing Israel—a small country even counting the occupied territories, as Israel emphasised—it was difficult not to be impressed by three aspects: the almost universal desire for peace, the compulsions that went to make the Jewish nation and the innovative and go-ahead nature of the people. Each of these aspects impinged on the future of West Asia.

Some Israelis despaired of ever seeing peace in their lifetime, as a noted women biologist told me in Jerusalem. Others pointed to the Arab view of Israel as a cancer in the region. A young woman who had spent half a year travelling round the world, including India, after her army service, said, "Please tell Shamir that we don't want war. We don't want to fight."

Peace in Years?

Others more in tune with the gyrations of Israeli politics were more sanguine. "I am optimistic," said an analyst. "How soon will there be peace?" I asked. "It is a question of years," he answered. "A new generation of leaders will take over after the next general election in one-and-a-half years and we are now discussing the real question— the Palestinian question. Even Palestinians desire peace as they are tortured by the fear that the Israeli nation cannot accept any but watertight guarantees."

Israel lived as much in the past as in the present. "We are paranoic," an Israeli analyst of the Arab world told me. "Half of us come from the holocaust and the other half from persecution in the Arab world." The moving holocaust memorial in Jerusalem was a constant reminder of the past as is the Diaspora museum in Tel Aviv recounting the older tragedy of the Jewish people. The young in Israel could not forget how they came to the land of Israel and how, over the ages, their people had suffered at the hands of Christians in particular.

"But even a paranoic people," an Israeli told me, "can have reason to be paranoid." The world's image of a mighty Israeli fighting machine looked different in the Israeli setting. It was as if the nation was afraid that if it let down its guard for one instance, there would be the danger to the very life of the state and its people.

Young soldiers with slung rifles were a common sight in much of Israel. Many of the conscripts stood on the road to hitch rides to their destinations. But despite the fears and foreboding, there was a thrust forward into the future. This was apparent as much in the everyday use Israel makes of solar water heaters as in pushing forward in innovative agriculture, science and technology.

The story of Israeli agriculture is a recognised phenomenon and if the Israelis had not created the Biblical world of milk and honey, they have had a good shot at it. Israelis were basking in the glow of the reforming countries of East Europe seemingly competing in opening diplomatic relations with their state. Hungarians, in particular, were very active, and in the words of a philosophy professor of Hungarian origin, tinged with cynicism: "The Hungarians think that the Jews have money and America will also come to their rescue."

But the big news for Israel was the prospect of welcoming some half million Soviet Jews over the next few years. Hundreds arrived in Israel each week, Israeli resources being taxed to the maximum to cope with the flood. They were both a challenge and an opportunity.

The challenge was clear enough. The opportunity was provided by the induction of a largely qualified class of people who would provide fresh blood to strengthen the sinews of the Israeli state.

A Famous Victory

The dramatic results of the Israeli elections in 1992 brought about a Labour victory under the leadership of an old war horse with impeccable credentials. Yitzak Rabin was 70 and was chief of staff in the Israeli victory of 1967.

The significance of the Israeli election results was two-fold. It represented a swing towards a more pragmatic and less doctrinaire policy. Second, it brightened the prospects of the West Asian peace process. The Israeli nation still remained divided down the middle, but the results confirmed the impression I formed during my visit that given a chance, a majority of Israelis would accept a separate Palestinian entity. And it was the young, together with a substantial section of the Soviet Jewish emigrants, who tipped the balance in favour of Labour.

Yitzak Shamir and his Likud party lost because their policies had led the country to an impasse. Relations with the United States, the guardian of the Jewish state, were at an all-time low and building new settlements in the occupied territories while talking peace in the US-initiated peace process begun in Madrid did not make sense. High unemployment levels and inflation and the US refusal to give loan guarantees until the settlement process was halted had led to gloom and uncertainty.

Rabin, unlike Shamir, had promised to freeze settlements, opening the prospect of obtaining $10 billion in US loan guarantees, and give autonomy to Palestinians within nine months. The future of Jerusalem was not on the negotiating table nor Palestinian statehood.

A Sea-Change

As an opening gambit, Rabin's stance represented a sea-change from the previous official position and no one could have expected more from him at this stage. Rabin had also made a distinction between "strategic settlements" and "political settlements" in the occupied territories—a distinction the Palestine Liberation Organisation and Palestinian negotiators at the peace talks did not accept.

Even as Israelis desired peace, "security" was a holy cow for them, given their troubled beginnings and the wars they had fought with their Arab neighbours. The Israeli dilemma was that they could not have an ideological democratic state while keeping one and a half million Palestinians as a subject people in the occupied territories. How Rabin would set about resolving this dilemma at the peace talks—the next session was scheduled in Rome—and otherwise would determine the shape of his country and prospects of peace.

Rabin's credo as an Israeli war hero was an essential ingredient in his victory because it gave his people the assurance that he would not sell his country short. He had therefore to proceed with great caution in the concessions he would offer, but the importance of the Labour victory was that the stalled peace process could discuss substantive issues. Peace was now on the agenda.

Against this backdrop, the contours of a peace formula could take shape. The future of Jerusalem could not figure in the immediate agenda because it raised too many politico-religious issues; unlike the occupied territories, it was annexed by Israel—an annexation the world did not accept. And the issue of the Golan Heights seized from Syria would have to be addressed separately.

As an attainable goal, autonomy for the West Bank and the Gaza Strip was on the cards, with Israel retaining control over defence and foreign affairs. For the Palestinian negotiators, the key questions would be the time-frame for the autonomy experiment and their under-standable insistence that it would not foreclose statehood for the Palestinians.

As the peace negotiations inched their way to progress, Rabin's main tasks would lie at home. The hardliners in Israel represented a major constituency and they had set their hearts against the concept of territory for peace. Indeed, they had a point in believing that the granting of autonomy to Palestinians could lead to only one result: an independent Palestinian state, allied through it might be with Jordan.

Economic Problems

Rabin would need to expand his constituency beyond Labour supporters and the young by convincing his people that in the longer term, living in a garrison state was no solution, that both peace and security had become attainable goals. Partly, his success would depend upon how he resolved the economic issues. They concerned high unemployment rates, the serious housing shortage, with hundreds of thousands of Soviet Jews waiting in the queue, and inflation. Other political questions lay in the future. Behind the Israeli reservations about accepting the PLO and outside Palestinians in the negotiating process was the fear that once the principle of outside participation was accepted, they would have to accept the Palestinian refugees' "right of return".

Beyond these issues lay the question of what the future Israel would be. Was Rabin's victory the beginning of a process of marginalising the religious parties which had traditionally obtained their pound of flesh from the two main parties? Could Israel retain its basis as an ideological state in an increasingly de-ideologised world?

Judging by the reaction of a cross-section of young people I met in Israel, the old beliefs did not have the same resonance. All Israelis above the age of 18 had to do army service, except for the dispensation obtained by the religious parties. After their stints, the young went wandering round the world.

The indoctrination by the ideological state proceeded apace. The young were constantly reminded about how their people had suffered over the ages, particularly at the hands of Christians. The holocaust museum in Jerusalem and the Diaspora museum in Tel Aviv are monuments to an unhappy past.

But the kibbutz movement had lost its earlier *élan*; the young were drifting away from the settlements. More than anything else, the young in Israel wanted to live like the young elsewhere in the world and were more than willing to grasp an opportunity for peace.

The diaspora culminated in the founding of a Jewish state. It is an irony of history that this had led to what might be described as the Palestinian diaspora. In the power play among states and the dramatic changes in the world, the dream of a Palestinian state might be nearer fulfilment.

It is another irony of history that the two most vital peoples in West Asia are Israelis and Palestinians. The Israeli genius was apparent in what they had made of their troubled land. And Palestinians say with justifiable pride how they had contributed to the making of Arab states with their sinews and brains.

The wandering Jew had been replace by the wandering Palestinian. He lived in camps under the close surveillance of his Arab masters. He taught and ran government ministries in several states. His devotion to acquiring knowledge was second only to his propensity to take the gun to fight for his cause.

With Rabin's victory in the Israeli elections, the wandering Palestinian was one step nearer securing a home.

Rabin's Assassination

Revolution, it is said, devours its own children. What had been happening in West Asia was far from a revolution, but the halting, incomplete and imperfect steps towards peace between Israelis and Palestinians had met their defining moment. The murder of the Israeli prime minister, Rabin, at the hands of a Jewish extremist in 1995 was a stark reminder of the polarisation in Israel and left a host of questions on carrying on the peace process, such as it was, up in the air.

Much of the world mourned Rabin's passing away in the brutal way it happened although there were some in the Arab world and in Israel who were rejoicing. There is the human tragedy of the assassination even in a part of the globe where countless persons have been experiencing countless such tragedies. But Rabin was a key player in the moves towards an accommodation between Jews and Arabs and even as the world sought to come to terms with his abrupt departure, the one question that was being mulled over was how it would affect the rickety and incomplete structure of peace that had been constructed thus far.

In immediate terms, it was easy to see that the opposition Likud party, which had vociferously opposed the moves Rabin's government had made with the encouragement and support of the US admini-stration, would lie low for a time. The shrillness of the political debate in Israel was best exemplified by the extreme right but the Likud played its part in seeking to define the peace process as something approaching treason. This was regrettably not the first political assassination in West Asia, or elsewhere for that matter, but it was the first assassination of a prime minister in Israel.

Shimon Peres, Rabin's foreign minister and veteran of many portfolios in many cabinets, had been among the main architects of the Oslo process and temporarily took charge. The conventional wisdom was that, in Israeli terms, he was perceived to be too much of a dove to be able to carry out a process which would get tougher by the day. Rabin was a man of war who chose to strike out on a different route. Israel was divided down the middle between those who would trade land for peace up to a point and others who believed that maintaining occupation and the garrison state of Israel was the only answer.

How the Oslo process had been implemented was loaded against the Palestinians. The travails of the second stage and the new concessions Yasser Arafat had to make to get it going were vivid indications of the trumps in Israeli hands, thanks to the long-standing support of successive US administrations. Yet the PLO leader maintained his faith, even as many Palestinians lost it, that however halting the peace process, it could have only one conclusion: the establishment of an independent Palestinian entity. In the end, Israeli settlements on the occupied West Bank and in the Gaza Strip would have to go because there could not otherwise be peace. Nor could there be peace in West Asia as long as Israel occupied the Golan Heights and a portion of Lebanon.

Israeli Divisions

Rabin's assassination highlighted the deep divisions in the Israeli camp. Both the Likud and the religious right were convinced that the imperfect peace that was being offered to the Palestinians could only lead to an independent Palestinian state. The opposition's efforts to stop the process had not succeeded because Rabin had credibility as a leader who would not barter away Israel's security and he enjoyed the full support of the Clinton administration. Ironically, the Jewish lobby in the United states was itself divided between the pro-peace and anti-peace flanks and Rabin had occasion to complain that a section of American Jews, primed by the Likud, was making the task of his government more difficult.

The umbilical cord between the United States and Israel remained intact. Israel had been viewed as the primary strategic ally of Washington in West Asia by every US administration, whatever its stripe, although Democratic administrations had been more gushing in their support. The Clinton administration was no exception. What changed was the realisation in the Bush administration that after the anti-Iraq coalition won a victory in the Second Gulf War, an attempt had to be made to try to reconcile the traditional blank cheques American administrations had been giving Israel with the Palestinians' just demands. The result was the Madrid peace initiative which began the secret Oslo conclaves.

The end of the Cold War and the disintegration of the Soviet Union also persuaded Arafat and his Fatah followers that the American-blessed plan was the only option open to them, imperfect and loaded though it was. And the Palestinian National Authority had to live with the anachronism of its antonomous zone closed at Israel's whims and fancy, with Palestinians exercising little authority on who could come in or go out. And even as the chequer-board of compromises of the second phase was beginning to be implemented, Capitol Hill believed it was its prerogative to announce to the Palestinians and the world that as far as the United States was concerned, Jerusalem, including the eastern Arab part of it, had been given to the Jewish state. The Clinton administration disliked only the timing of the move, not its substance.

The shock of Rabin's assassination could accelerate the implementation of the second phase. But first the interim nature of the government had to be decided, whether Peres could carry on till the scheduled elections next year. Given the polarisation in Israeli society, a national coalition government seemed hardly conceivable. And since the present government had a paper-thin majority in parliament, Peres had to tread carefully.

The test would come in the planed last-stage negotiations in the middle of 1996: the problem of Jewish settlements and the all-important question of Jerusalem. The likely stalemate on these issues would inevitably take time to resolve but there could not be peace in the region until Israel agreed to a time-table for the settlements' withdrawal. Second, the US might have awarded Jerusalem to Israel but Palestinians and the Arab world could not rest, short of a just solution of an issue that touched their religion and hearts.

The United States had moved into the election mode although the presidential election was one year away. The Clinton administration would be even further restricted in the moves it could make in West Asia. Shortly before Rabin's assassination there were credible reports that he had told President Bill Clinton that the Syria track would be put on ice until after the Israeli elections because he could not jeopardise his chances by agreeing to withdraw from the Golan Heights. There seemed to be even less likelihood of any significant moves to bring Damascus into the peace process.

Enter Netanyahu

In 1990, as a member of Israel's Likud government, Benjamin Netanyahu explained to me at great length why his country should keep all the gains of the 1967 war. "Otherwise," he told me, "if you were to run across the country from one end to the other, you would reach it in a few hours." In other words, the giving up of occupied territory was not an option open to Israel, in his view.

That was, of course, before the start of the Madrid peace process, Rabin's triumph, the secret Oslo negotiations, the handshake on the lawn of the White House in Washington and the fitful implementation of what had been agreed to. Fitful and flawed. Because even as the status of East Jerusalem was left to the final status negotiation as well as the fate of the Israeli settlements on occupied land, the Labour party government decreed that East Jerusalem was not negotiable and the process of nibbling at more land around Jerusalem and on the West Bank proceeded apace.

Soon the loaded word "security" came to acquire an all-consuming dimension. The territories of the West Bank and Gaza strip were shut off, this time longer than before, the agreed redeployment of Israeli troops from Hebron was put on hold until it had come to acquire a totally new character with the victory of Netanyahu with the support of the religious right. The new prime minister went to the Wailing Wall in Jerusalem to give his thanks to those whose support made the difference between victory and defeat.

Washington and the Netanyahu camp were burning the wires and making the right noises in favour of "peace", but the sense of shock felt by the Arafat camp and the wider Arab world was a truer expression of the consequences of a Likud victory when the chance of real peace was hanging by a fragile thread. No amount of diplomacy or backtracking by Netanyahu would change a stark fact. Peace was farther away than at any time since the Madrid process began. In West Asia, if there was no land for peace, there was no peace at all.

Let us take the best construction that could be placed upon Netanyahu's pragmatism. The agreements already made would be honoured, the Israeli troops would not be redeployed from Hebron, the settlements were to be expanded, with more houses and more roads and more fortifications eating up more occupied land. The Palestinians would be given little more than municipal rights and the Likud was envisaging to convert the Palestinian areas into settlements so that Israelis had a free play, and the Israeli state would, of course, have the freedom to send troops into any area it desired.

For more and more Palestinians and Arabs, the last hopes of extracting a measure of dignity and self-respect from the Oslo accords titled against them had vanished. Facing a pro-Israeli Clinton administration and a West that seemed only too willing to accept the marginalisation of Palestinians, few choices lay ahead. And whatever option they chose to take, it would add up to one thing: there would be no peace in West Asia. There comes a time in the life of a people when their patience snaps and the results of their impatience can only be unpredictable.

It was pointless blaming Netanyahu or his Likud supporters because the results of the election revealed starkly that the Israeli nation was roughly divided between those who wanted peace on total Israeli terms, placing Palestinians in a humiliating and subservient position, and others who would take a measure of risk in seeking genuine peace. The country remained thus divided despite Madrid and Oslo and the White House handshake so favoured by CNN and the interminable confabulation among Israelis, Palestinians, Egyptians and almost everyone else. The shock of Rabin's murder by an extremist Jew seemed to have been balanced by the bombing runs of extremist Palestinians in Israel. As Rabin's widow bitterly complained, the assassin, who was allowed to vote, had the last laugh.

Or did he? That was the question.

Eating Crow

For the hardliners in Israel, Netanyahu's triumph could not have come at a better time. After President Clinton gave everything but his official endorsement to Shimon Peres, he had to eat crow by inviting Netanyahu to the White House and getting his secretary of state,

Warren Christopher, to field embarrassing questions from reporters. Even if the US president were to be less partisan than he had been on West Asia, his re-election bid placed an immediate constraint. Jewish votes and support were too important to be trifled with.

The United States had to think of salvaging the Palestinian track before it could think of reactivating the Syrian track, which had stopped dead with Netanyahu's blunt rejection of giving up the Golan Heights, taking away any Syrian incentive for making peace. Netanyahu might well be a pragmatist but it was open to question whether his present supporters such as Ariel Sharon and the extreme orthodox right would permit him to backtrack. And a succession of Israeli leaders had shown over the decades how the tail wagged the dog, as far as American policy towards Israel was concerned.

The likely stalemate and possible break-up of the West Asian peace process were destined to have wider repercussions. For one thing, it remained to be seen whether the new respectability Israel had sought to achieve in the region in trade and commerce could continue to flower. Second, the entire American exercise of winnowing the extremists from the moderates could have little credibility in West Asia if a different yardstick was used to judge Israelis. What was going for the Americans was that the painful set of agreements arrived at between Palestinians and Israelis made it difficult entirely to reverse course, but a new conflagration could, if unchecked, make nonsense of the entire process that started in Madrid, itself born out of the Second Gulf War.

Many Arabs had realised that the luck of the draw was against them. The United States was a partisan arbiter while the balance the Soviet Union gave in a bi-polar world had disappeared. The US was a necessary bulwark against possible threats for countries in the Arabian Gulf and West Asia. But peace could not be made at the expense of one side in reordering the consequences of an unjust occupation. You could not put down as vital a people as Palestinians by humiliating them and denying them all vestiges of statehood and dignity. It was a question far more important than the political fortunes of Clinton because it could come to haunt America and the world for a long time to come.

There was pathos in the appeal of the Palestine Liberation Organisation to the mythical international community to make Israel observe the rules. The international community meant the United States and Israel had never been a respecter of rules, as far as Palestinians were concerned.

Netanyahu's Illusion

What does the world do when one of the two principal parties to an ongoing peace process wins an election in his country on the promise of wrecking that very process? The reactions to Benjamin

Netanyahu's victory varied. Washington was pretending that nothing much had changed, as far as promoting the peace process was concerned, and the Arabs should give the Netanyahu government a chance to tame its policy.

The Arab world called a summit, for the first time in six years, and made a pertinent point. The process of normalising relations with Israel was directly dependent upon its adherence to the postulates of the Madrid peace process. This self-evident verity was unwelcome to Netanyahu for two reasons: it was a joint Arab stand and it was a warning that if his government repudiated the process or stopped it dead in its tracks, the West Asian region could revert to political turmoil and worse.

Few wanted to see that happen. Only in peace could the nations of West Asia build their prosperity and happiness. And only in resolving the central problem of the Israeli–Arab confrontation could there be a chance for peace. It was the only silver lining of the Second Gulf War that it spawned the Madrid peace process in 1991, leading to the Oslo accords and their halting implementation on the ground. These agreements were titled towards the Israelis but accepted by the mainstream faction of the Palestine Liberation Organisation for two reasons. In the post-Cold War world, there was little option to accepting an arbiter who was blatantly pro-Israeli and the hope was that even this imperfect peace would lead to a Palestinian state.

The main parties to the Arab–Israeli conflict had reached the crossroad because President Bill Clinton, locked up in his re-election bid, was a prisoner of Israel even more than US administrations normally were, and Netanyahu plainly repudiated the concept of a Palestinian state. If it is a case of the tail wagging the dog, Netanyahu was happy to be that tail. What was worse, a new confidence trick was being tried on Palestinians and the wider Arab world. A Netanyahu–Yasser Arafat meeting was being billed as a great Israeli concession as was the redeployment of Israeli troops from Hebron. Whether the new Israeli prime minister met Arafat or not was entirely irrelevant as long as he made the agreements he should and Israel remained in default by not withdrawing from Hebron.

Arafat's hopes of the peace process being revived were understandable because he had invested much in the process. Washington was almost equally anxious to try to prevent a collapse of the Madrid conference and all it had spawned because its vital strategic interests were involved even as it was unwilling and unable to sever the umbilical cord with Israel. In immediate terms, Washington's policy was to try to keep talking until after the presidential election in the US. The new president was likely to have a little more room for manoeuvre although Clinton's return to office would only strengthen Netanyahu's hands and return the region to turmoil.

The wafer-thin majority Netanyahu gained over Shimon Peres showed that Israel was split down the middle. The hardline Likud was in the ascendant because a series of suicide bombings had made a sufficient number of Israelis doubt the efficacy of the path the Labour Party had chosen. Depending upon how the question was posed, a majority of Israelis would opt for land for peace. Netanyahu's belief was that peace could only be imposed on the Palestinians and Arabs on his terms and he had sufficient influence over President Clinton or a future US administration to try his experiment while, in effect, refusing to give his people the chance freely to exercise their option.

Grim Scenario

It was a grim scenario because it would be foolish to believe that the Palestinians would be satisfied will remaining a subject race content with exercising municipal powers. And as everyone knew, the Israeli–Palestinian confrontation was at the heart of the larger Arab–Israeli conflict. In other words, without resolving the core issue, there could be no genuine peace in West Asia. Netanyahu seemed to be using his "window of opportunity" to bully Washington while the Clinton administration lay prone subject to the slings and arrows of a presidential election.

The Clinton administration believed that it had enough levers of power to keep the lid on West Asia's troubles. It was the guarantor of security for several states. The asymmetry in individual Arab states' relations with Israel was common knowledge, with two of them having signed treaties and others having gone some way towards an accommodation with Israel. The Cairo Arab summit's message was, therefore, significant in holding out the threat of a diplomatic retaliation if Netanyahu were to carry out his threats. It does not take a Sherlock Holmes to realise that the more united the Arabs are, the greater their effectiveness.

The bombing in Saudi Arabia, the second time American serviceman have been targeted in that country, should be condemned. But Netanyahu was quick to use it as a lever for his purposes: a joint resolve to fight terrorism everywhere, his code for terrorism against Israelis. If the US bought his argument that the Israeli–Palestinian problem was basically one of fighting terrorism, we could bid good bye to the whole Madrid process. Homilies on land for peace from the Group of Seven industrialised countries were irrelevant. What was needed was a new initiative from the non-American component of the G-7 countries to ensure that the achievement of the peace process, paltry as it had been, was protected and carried forward. Given European supineness in the face of American power, there was little prospect of a new European move.

On the face of it, Netanyahu seemed to be in a strong position to defy the Arabs and the wider world in demanding that, contrary to the winds of change everywhere in the world, his law of enforcing and solidifying a colony in the heart of West Asia must take effect. Captured land would be annexed or built over at Israeli will, the Palestinians would remain second-class citizens, if that, and could not be allowed to anything more than running municipal affairs. If that was the Israeli vision of happiness, they were living in a fool's paradise.

The pity of it was that a majority of Israelis would be perfectly happy to give Palestinians their land and state if they were to be left in peace. It was the intention of politicians and others of Netanyahu's ilk never to let the people answer this question in a straightforward way. So Israelis and Arabs alike had to suffer as the region descended into further bouts of turmoil while Washington sought to reconcile its interests in the Arab world with its very special strategic ally and friend, Israel, in the only way it knew how to—by siding with Israel.

The Victor of Wye

The ghosts of Oslo were present at the signing ceremony in Washington in October 1998 of a deal between Israelis and Palestinians that was a caricature of what was envisaged in 1993. That it was being greeted with relief, if not joy, around the world was an indication of how dramatically Israeli Prime Minister Benjamin Netanyahu had won and how much a defensive Palestinian leader Yasser Arafat had to concede in the name of peace. And in a supreme sign of contempt for his American hosts, Netanyahu held President Bill Clinton hostage for eight hours over a totally unconnected demand for the release of an American convicted of spying for Israel.

It had been a singular triumph for Netanyahu. Palestinians who were vowing not to sign a partial deal had done just that. And the Israelis could continue to build new settlements and expand the existing ones because the injunction against such acts was couched in double-speak—the two sides agreeing not to take "any step that will change the status of West Bank and Gaza"—that had permitted the Israeli prime minister to say that Oslo did not ban new settlements.

And at the end of the day, assuming that Netanyahu would keep his word, the Palestinians would receive a total of only 40 per cent of occupied West Bank land out of which a princely 14.2 per cent (including the notorious "nature reserve") would be under total Palestinian control. The remaining portion would have Israeli security supervision. And, in a final triumph, Netanyahu had succeeded in jettisoning the promised third Israeli troop redeployment under Oslo—

it had been pushed into a committee—while "final status" talks were to start forthwith.

CIA's New Role

Palestinians would naturally ask the question: What had they gained? In an ironic twist, the US Central Intelligence Agency, the buddy of the Israeli Mossad, was made the arbiter of overseeing Palestinian fulfilment of security commitments. It did make a change from eliminating difficult foreign leaders and subverting foreign governments. And only 750 of the 3,500 Palestinian prisoners in Israeli jails were to be released.

What then had the Palestinians gained? President Clinton said, "The Palestinian people can at long last realise their aspirations to live free, in safety, in charge of their own destiny". This was certainly not the case, and the Palestinian leader Hannan Ashrawi was nearer the mark in suggesting that "you are not going to see dancing on the streets". Netanyahu was candid in declaring at the signing ceremony. "I am today brimming with some confidence". Yes, the Palestinians had been promised some crumbs, those crumbs promised long, long ago: a sea-port and an airport in Gaza, the forgotten "safe passage" between Gaza and the West Bank and a new American promise of economic assistance.

Yasser Arafat had reportedly promised not to declare the formation of a Palestinian state on May 4, 1999 if no agreement on the "final status" was reached. It would be a miracle if such an agreement were to be sealed by then.

During 19 months of stalling, Netanyahu began an entirely new settlement in occupied Arab East Jerusalem and had undertaken an expansion spree of existing illegal settlements, creating the proverbial new facts on the ground. And he insisted on his pound of flesh at Wye by getting Arafat formally to call the Palestine National Council to excise the covenants seeking the destruction of Israel when the old charter had already been superceded by the Palestinian executive's decision. President Clinton himself planed to be among the cheerleaders at the session.

A foretaste of the "Wye River memorandum", as it was described, was the detention of journalists who went to the home of the Hamas leader Sheikh Ahmed Yassin in Gaza city to seek his reaction to the deal signed in Washington. Palestinian police had surrounded his house in order to gag him.

There were time-limits and time-tables galore and the almost military precision with which they were mentioned could only mock a process begun in Madrid in 1991 and consigned to the deep freeze by Netanyahu until revived after a fashion at Wye by the American midwife. Final status talks were to begin 10 days after the memorandum entered into force.

What then were the Palestinians to look forward to, Arafat having been finessed by President Clinton and Netanyahu? There were loopholes enough for the Israelis to exploit, "security" for Israel having been elevated to a podium above peace. Indeed, the victor of Wye was Netanyahu and, after him, President Clinton whose impeachment by Congress had momentarily been forgotten.

Barak to the Fore

The best thing that could be said for the revised Wye agreement between Israelis and Palestinians was that it separated the Ehud Barak regime from that of his predecessor Benjamin Netanyahu. Beyond that, the staggered transfer of minute portions of land and the rationed release of Palestinian prisoners were more important for their symbolism than for any great concessions Tel Aviv had made.

The goal of a framework of final peace talks had been moved to February 15, 2000 and the signing of an accord to September 2000. As so often before, the prospect of an independent Palestinian entity had proved to be a mirage in the desert; the only constant theme since the luckless Oslo agreements were signed had been the relentless building of new settlements and the expansion of existing ones on occupied land. These then became non-negotiable or were bargaining chips in Israeli hands.

Even before he became leader of the Labour Party and won the election to become prime minister, Barak had exulted before an international press gathering in Jerusalem that the cards were stacked in favour of Israel in the post-Cold War world, with its patron emerging as the sole surviving superpower. The implication was that the Palestinians better take what the Israelis were prepared to offer. Thus far, it had been precious little.

Barak had, indeed, proved to be as tough a negotiator as his predecessor, with the difference that his toughness carried greater credibility with Washington and the West. Thanks to Netanyahu's calculated adventurism in annexing more occupied land, his successor now appeared to have come to the conclusion that sufficient new facts have been created on the ground to begin "final status" talks with Palestinians. And his admonition to the Americans to play a less prominent role in the talks was a shrewd move to insulate the Clinton administration from the fall-out of the kind of lopsided peace Israel was seeking to impose.

Lancing the Boil

The initial agreement with Palestinians was essential to Barak's larger objective of resuming talks with the Syrians, also to lance the boil of the occupied zone in Lebanon. US Secretary of State Madeleine Albright, who was seeking to thaw President Hafez Al Assad's attitude to Israel, had a more useful role to play than she did in the Netanyahu era when she was administered a slap in the face by the Israeli regime on her appeal to take "time-out" on building new settlements.

But now that the Israelis had as strong a hand as they would ever get to play, short of victory in a new major war, it was time for the Palestinians to turn their attention to the final status talks. The release of Palestinian prisoners was important as were the building of a sea-port at Gaza and safe passage between Gaza and the West Bank (typically, decisions that should have been implemented long ago were being presented as Israeli concessions).

The principal issue the Palestinian leadership had to decide, after broad consultations, was the shape and nature of the future Palestinian state. Barak would have few problems in conceding such a state while seeking to annex as much of the occupied land as possible and making the future entity toothless by barring it from raising an army in the real sense. How much land were the Palestinians willing to lose at the altar of peace?

Second, what would be the Palestinian leadership's decision on occupied East Jerusalem? The Israelis had annexed the occupied part and Barak was as firm as Netanyahu in declaring that an undivided Jerusalem would remain the capital of the Israeli state. Israel's flexibility would extend only to naming an outlying part of the city as the Palestinian state's 'Jerusalem'. Would the Palestine Liberation Organisation buy this make-believe?

Next was the question of refugees, generations of whom had been born in refugee camps dotted in the Arab world. The Israelis would seek to bar most of them from returning to their homes, in the present occupied land or in Israel, perhaps agreeing to let in a symbolic handful. Israel did not want inordinately to increase the population of the future Palestinian state.

It was to be expected that if the Israeli–Syrian track could be reactivated, Barak would seek to inject an element of competitiveness in peace-making between Syrians and Palestinians. The Israeli-occupied zone in Lebanon was an albatross around its neck and the prime minister had to deliver on his promise of withdrawing his troops from there in 2000 on the best terms possible. He needed Syrian help to be able to do so.

Yasser Arafat was in an unenviable position as he fought an uphill battle to secure a measure of land, dignity and independence for his people. The last laps would be the hardest of all, even if the new deadlines did not prove to be a mirage. The strongest card he had in his hand was that, at the end of the day, a patently unjust final agreement imposed by Israel with the support of its mentor the United States would not bring about peace but would lead to a new conflict.

Barak's Folly

The main loser in the deadly game of Hezbollah attacks on Israeli soldiers in occupied South Lebanon and Israeli warplanes knocking out Lebanon's key power stations and bombing suspected guerrilla hide-outs was Israeli Prime Minister Ehud Barak. For after a dream resumption of the so-called peace process, negotiations on the two tracks had screeched to a halt and the number of Israeli soldiers killed had restricted the Labour leader's room for manoeuvre at home.

But the question Barak needed to ask himself was whether his strategy for "comprehensive peace" was flawed in any case. He was betting on making peace with Syrians first in exchange for the Golan Heights—he had probably not decided whether it would involve the whole of the Golan back to its 1967 borders or less—and then taking on the Palestinians and fobbing them off with as little as possible of the West Bank, retaining Jewish settlements and cutting what remained into ribbons by Israeli highways.

There were two problems with this approach. In an effort to win concessions from Syria, Barak overplayed his hand and lost the initiative. There was no reason to believe that Syria's President Hafez Al Assad would have settled for anything less than all of the Golan. Second, even if the prime minister's strategy had worked with his interlocutors, would he have been able to sell both deals to a divided Israel?

Above all, the basic contradiction between Barak's concept of peace and genuine peace was that if Arafat were to accept the parody of a Palestinian state that was on offer, the injustice of it would make Palestinians rebel, sooner than later. This was quite apart from the influence Hamas exercised over events because no self-respecting Palestinian could countenance a "state" consisting of fragments of territories, supervised by Israeli armed forces, without the right to raise an army.

At an international gathering of journalists in Jerusalem, Barak had outlined his assessment of how the cards were stacked in favour of Israel. In the post-Cold War world, he said in essence, there was only one superpower left and it was a close friend and ally. The ball game had therefore changed radically in favour of Tel Aviv and the Palestinians had better take what they were offered. With the United States in Israel's pocket, the Palestinians had nowhere to go.

A Grand Scheme

Against this backdrop, Barak, once in power, set out to implement his grand scheme. In addition to getting together as large a coalition as he could, he employed the last year of the Clinton presidency to impose a deadline for deals to be signed in the two tracks. Given the American political calendar, a new president in the White House would mean a hiatus in Washington's foreign policy-making ability. Not only was Bill Clinton the most pro-Israeli American to occupy the White House but he also had a vested interest in helping Barak in order to leave a legacy in West Asia that would wipe out his impeachment ignominy.

First, Barak was reminded by the Syrians that he had to pay the full price for peace, and the Hezbollah upset his apple cart by their success in killing Israeli soldiers in an area they should not be in in the first place. The Israeli prime minister had promised to leave South Lebanon by July 2000, a year after assuming office, but he wanted to synchronise a withdrawal with an agreement with Syria. Tel Aviv's charge that Damascus was using the Hezbollah as a lever to prod the negotiations might or might not be true, but Barak's vulnerability to losing Israeli lives had changed the scenario.

While no one expected peace-making in West Asia to be simple or smooth, the new turn of events represented a major setback to Barak's capacity to negotiate. How long he would have to show his fellow countrymen that he was the tough guy remained to be seen but he would be viewed differently by the Arab world. And President Clinton would be breathing down his neck to get him to make some kind of peace in at least one of the two tracks.

The broader issue of peace-making between Israelis and Arabs seemed beyond the grasp of either Barak or President Clinton before the latter would leave the White House. The Israeli prime minister was right in his assessment that peace-making with Syria was easier than with Palestinians, once he bit the bullet. But real peace could not be built on the basis of suppressing Palestinians by giving them the trimmings of a state without sovereignty and pockmarking the West Bank with fortresses of Jewish settlements.

There was irony in Israel and Lebanon sending letters to UN Secretary-General Kofi Annan accusing each other of escalating attacks which could undermine the so-called peace process. The United Nations had been kept at arm's length by the United States because it wanted to be the sole arbiter between Israelis and Arabs. The European Union's efforts at attempting mediation had been rebuffed, Brussels having been given the privilege of being the largest donor of the Palestinian Authority. In this respect, Israelis lived in the best of both worlds because the only serious mediator was their special friend and ally.

Bombing Lebanon, 2000

Perhaps the biggest instant killings in human history were effected by the atom bombs dropped over Hiroshima and Nagasaki by the United States in World War II. Yet the progress of mankind had been determined in part by distinguishing combatants and non-combatants in wars and strife. The international covenants and agreements that came into force, particularly enshrining the work of the Red Cross, were attempts at more humane warfare, if it could be so described.

In recent times, the genocide in Rwanda emerged as the most senseless and horrific killings of innocent civilians. The mythical international community was still mulling the culpability of the United Nations and its most powerful members in turning a blind eye to them. Weapons of mass destruction were, by their very nature, indiscriminate in killing soldiers and civilians alike and the self-appointed guardians of nuclear power had been busy seeking non-proliferation goals for decades.

Everyone paid lip-service to protecting civilians in war although more often than not, they become targets or get caught up in the fighting. In psychological terms, it was important to maintain this distinction, no matter how often the benchmark was breached. That psychological barrier was shattered by Nato's eleven-week bombing of Yugoslavia and the world had been witnessing its chain effect ever since.

Nato bombed civilian infrastructure such as bridges, power stations and even television stations, apart from causing "collateral damage", a euphemism for the unintended killing or wounding of civilians or destruction of civilian property. Serbians were still paying the price of the air war because electricity was fitful, the homes were unheated and bridges lay in ruins. The bombing of petroleum complexes and storage tanks released polluting substances that remained in the atmosphere.

A report took Nato to task for the destruction of civilian targets and the killing of civilians. Nato's underlying theme in selecting many of the targets, particularly in the later stages, was to spread panic and fear among the civilian population so that it might rebel against the regime of Slobodan Milosevic. That is what the warlords were supposed to do in the bad, old days. Mankind, it seemed, has not progressed so much after all.

Russian Retort

Nato's bombing had been repeated on a larger scale by the Russians in Chechnya. While the war of words between Moscow and the West intensified, Russians had a point in arguing that the United States in particular had lost the moral right to castigate the leaders of the Russian Federation after what was done to Serbia. There was the additional point Russians made: they were trying to safeguard their country's integrity whereas Nato had disregarded national frontiers to bomb Yugoslavia without UN sanction.

Chechnya was not the end of the story. In response to the Hezbollah killing of seven Israeli soldiers in occupied South Lebanon, Israelis bombed three of Lebanon's key power stations, wounding 22 civilians and cutting 50 per cent of the country's electricity supplies. Tragically, Lebanon had been painfully recovering from its 16-year civil war. Tel Aviv's logic seemed to be that if Nato could do it to Serbia, why couldn't Israel to Lebanon.

But a strange thing then happened. The initial American support for the Israeli bombing so outraged the Lebanese that massive anti-American demonstrations were held outside the US embassy in Beirut. Frustrated by a solid phalanx of soldiers and policeman who kept them away, the demonstrators, mostly students from American-funded universities, attacked other American targets, including the CNN network, a day later to express their anger.

The explosive potential of the anti-American wave in Lebanon was only too apparent in further stymying Israel's negotiations on the Syrian and Palestinian tracks. Madeleine Albright was reportedly engaged in a damage-limitation exercise and Egypt's President Hosni Mubarak had been sufficiently alarmed by events to make the first ever visit to Beirut by an Egyptian head of state.

The United States and the West in general had a penchant for dividing the world into the good guys and the bad guys. Milosevic was the bad guy, so his power stations, bridges, and television stations could be bombed. Russia was the bad guy, so it could not bomb Chechnya. Israel was a good guy, so it could bomb Lebanon's power stations. But the danger in reducing the world to such simplistic categories was obvious and the even greater danger of legitimising the destruction of civilian targets and infrastructure was staring the world in the face.

There cannot be a selective determination of when civilians can be killed and their support infrastructure destroyed. All the good work done by men and women of humanity to safeguard civilians from war's cruelties was in danger of being unravelled. It was no coincidence that in the post-Cold War world of one superpower, we had regressed in some respects. Human suffering, it would seem, had come to take second place to geopolitical strategies and needs.

A Retreat

In a curious way, the inglorious hasty retreat of Israelis from South Lebanese territory they had occupied for 22 years could prove a defining moment for West Asia and the future of the region. Because even as the Israeli media were comparing the retreat to the last helicopter that ferried Americans out of Saigon with the Viet Cong at the city's gates, an evacuation without completing any of the objectives for which Israel invaded Lebanon and took over a self-declared security zone had portentous psychological implications.

The comparison to Vietnam cannot be taken too far, but in both cases the military adventures became highly unpopular at home and in both cases the objectives were far from clear-cut. If the Israeli objective was to protect northern Israel from guerrilla attacks, the Hezbollah guerillas showed that they could extract an unacceptable price, and in the end Prime Minister Ehud Barak's election promise to leave within a year became an undignified stampede.

The Lebanese, in particular the Hezbollah, were celebrating and ordinary Lebanese belonging to the occupied region were the happiest of all because they could claim back their roots and return to their families. For the Israelis, it was a time for soul-searching even as there was relief over putting an end to a continuing drain of blood and tears. Like all mercenary armies, the allied South Lebanon Army disintegrated once it realised that the Israeli paymasters were leaving for good.

Given their history and how the state of Israel came to be founded, Israeli strength—doggedness for a cause—had also been its weakness because the country's alignment with the West, in particular the United States, gave it the technological and financial edge in the confrontation with the Arabs. And after the string of victories they won, Israelis came to believe in their invincibility. South Lebanon had shown that they were no longer invincible.

Inevitably, Israelis changed since the foundation of their state. The idealism of the kibbutz had given way to a desire to live like a modern nation state. Israelis were divided not merely between the secular and the conservative but between those pining for a normal life and others who placed security above all else. Israelis found it hard to understand that placing security on a pedestal had precisely the opposite effect to the one intended. Because security had to be related to the physical and political environment.

Price of Peace

Even those Israelis daring to go beyond the security mind-set did not realise that peace came at a price, and the price the so-called doves were prepared to pay was parsimonious. It was accepted in Israel, as elsewhere in the world, that a Palestinian state was in the offing. The dispute was on the kind of Palestinian state it should be and the maps and conditions on offer by the Israelis were so outrageously unjust that the Palestinian Authority would dig its own grave were it to accept them.

If the ugly manner of Israel's departure from South Lebanon would persuade Israelis about the virtues of humility, it would make them happier and help towards resolving the central issues of the historical confrontation in West Asia. To begin with, any realistic discussion had to be on the basis of a Palestinian state that would look like one and had the attributes of statehood. Second, an imaginative formula had to be devised to resolve the issue of Jerusalem. Third, a realistic and calibrated scheme had to be found for the return of Palestinian refugees, those who wanted to return.

It took the Americans many years to get over the Vietnam syndrome. A whole generation was scarred by it and even after the American-led victory in the Second Gulf War, US presidents' freedom of action in coping with regional crises remained circumscribed by their fear of "body bags" coming home. As the 11-week Nato bombing of Yugoslavia demonstrated, future American-style wars had to be surgical (from the American point of view) and so one-sided that they precluded US casualties.

For the Israelis, the withdrawal from South Lebanon might have a more salutary effect. Israel, in common with any other country of the world, cannot choose its neighbours (indeed, the neighbours never welcomed its emergence as a state in their midst in the first place). Thus the obsession with security had to give way to the realisation that it should be balanced with trust built on the basis of a fair settlement.

For the Arab world, the symbolism of the Israeli retreat was something to savour. The Lebanese authorities were left with the task of effectively controlling the occupied area that had been vacated. But celebrations were certainly in order as long as the Arab world realised that Israel had still to leave the Golan Heights and make a fair peace with the Palestinians.

Israeli Dilemmas

The question everyone was asking in West Asia at the end of the Clinton presidency was: where do we go from here? Hopes had alternated with despair and violence as Israeli–Palestinian confabulations, with and without US mediators, had lurched from one crisis to another. Till the very end, President Bill Clinton seemed determined to snatch success from failure. He did not succeed.

In essence, the question was simple. How could Israeli co-exist with Palestinian and other Arab neighbours without having to man a garrison state? Much store was set by the Oslo accords, flawed as they were. Bit by bit the accords unravelled as deadlines were observed more in the breach by Israelis and the basis of trust was shattered by the building of more and more settlements on occupied land. What was the point of "final status" talks when one of the parties was busy altering their basis? And the deadline for these talk was, unsurprisingly, not observed.

Clearly, the Oslo accords were titled against the Palestinians. Yasser Arafat accepted them in the end on the assumption that the step-by-step approach would lead to the formation of a viable Palestinian state. It was a difficult decision opposed by some important members of his Fatah movement, apart from such opposition groupings as Hamas. While Hamas was more than willing to queer the pitch at crucial moments, the Israelis were divided down the middle and were for a time riding high on the powerful American patronage they enjoyed.

Given the strategic relationship between Israel and the United States and the influence of the American Jewish lobby, the Palestinians were at a great disadvantage. It was partly because of this set of circumstances that Arafat embraced Oslo; partly, it was to win international recognition.

Despite the cards stacked in its favour, Israel's Achilles' heel was that the colonial situation it found itself in was eroding the basis of the Jewish state and becoming increasingly untenable. Painfully, it extricated itself from the occupation of southern Lebanon. And as the new intefada raged on the streets, Israel's declared policy of retaliation by answering stones with bullets was becoming counter-productive. Prime Minister Barak went as far as he thought he could go by agreeing to give up nearly 95 per cent of occupied West Bank, give Palestinians sovereignty over their holy places in occupied East Jerusalem while refusing Palestinian refugees the right of return to Israel.

Too Little too Late

In the end, it proved to be too little too late. After more than seven years of negotiations, it was ironical to be told by the two sides that time was too short to make a deal in view of the approaching end of the Clinton presidency and the February 6 Israeli elections. The basic problem was that Israelis were still wrestling with the kind of peace they wanted and the price they would have to pay for it.

Two threats made were more in the nature of tactical ploys than serious proposals. Barak's threat of a unilateral separation of Israelis and Palestinians, placing the latter at an even greater disadvantage, would make Israel's plight worse than it was. It would invite more terrorist acts and increase the hostility of the Arab neighbours. Similarly, Clinton's threat of his proposals being valid only as long as his presidency lasted was a pressure tactic. Before he left office he reiterated the validity of the proposals that were left on the table. Nor did the Likud leader, Ariel Sharon, have the freedom to disregard what Barak had offered.

Israelis needed to realise that giving the Palestinians something less than a contiguous viable state would serve no one's interests. The occupied West Bank had been shred into ribbons of roads, carved out of appropriated Palestinian land, leading to fortified Jewish settlements. They would have to go. Second, Palestinians had to have sovereignty over Muslim holy sites in East Jerusalem. Third, while Israel could not accommodate the more than three million Palestinian refugees spread over many countries inside Israel, it had to accept its moral responsibility and make a significant gesture in this regard.

There were a host of other questions a final deal would involve such as water usage, the right to raise Palestinian forces and Israel's stationing of troops in the Jordan valley on a temporary basis. But the crucial answer lay inside Israel. How long it would take to persuade a majority of Israelis that the country's salvation lay in a peace deal Palestinians could live with? Would the dynamic of Israeli politics continue to work against a reconciliation?

While the very nature of the state rules out a multi-religious dispensation, normality for Israel would mean co-existence with neighbours. Barak had the distinction of spectacularly increasing Jewish settlements on occupied land while offering terms to Palestinians no other Israeli prime minister had articulated. And if the Israelis moved towards an accommodation with Palestinians, could a settlement with Syria on the occupied Golan Heights be far behind?

In the dying days of the Clinton presidency, Palestinians put out a memorandum decrying American mediation, suggesting that they and the Israelis could best solve the problems themselves. Was the memo anticipating the more laid-back style of the George W. Bush presidency? If Oslo was anything to go by, Palestinian–Israeli efforts under Norwegian, rather than American, auspices had not proved conspicuously successful.

The new political dispensation in Israel was unlikely to have the luxury of the previous Likud regime of Netanyahu stonewalling a new effort to make peace. The Palestinians' frustrations had grown and would prove more difficult to contain. Nor could the US look kindly on a political stalemate leading to a greater accretion of strength to Hamas and other groupings opposed to the Oslo version of peace.

If the Bush administration could present a less partisan face to the Palestinians than its predecessor, it would help improve the chances of peace. Finally, Israelis had to come to terms with reality.

Sharon in a China Shop

The Palestinian tragedy has taken on a deeper hue because it is based on Ariel Sharon's illusion that the harder he strikes at Palestinians, the sooner they would cry uncle. The Israeli prime minister is propitiating his domestic constituency, rather than addressing the real problem. His predecessor Ehud Barak discovered that though he went far by his lights in seeking a solution, it was not far enough and Israelis sought the hardliner to gain the elusive goal of security.

Seven years of talks between Palestinians and Israelis under the umbrella of the Oslo accords had resulted in a curious quilt of ostensibly autonomous Palestinian areas and other territories under Israeli or alleged joint control. By entering and destroying Palestinian structures in supposedly Palestinian autonomous areas, Sharon was thumbing his nose at Oslo, demonstrating to the world how fragile and unjust the basis of the original accord was.

In a flash, the world saw the Israeli–Palestinian problem for what it is: a colonial occupation of Palestinian land. We had moved a long way from the early days of a Palestinian refusal to accept the nation state of Israel, and a succession of wars won by Israel against Arabs strengthened Tel Aviv, with the 1967 war serving as a benchmark. The Oslo agreements were premised on the bargain of Arab acceptance of Israel on the basis of land for peace.

In this instance, the devil not merely lay in the details but in the great gap between the two sides on how much land to give for peace and on the emotive questions of restoring the captured East Jerusalem with its holy sites to the Palestinians and the return to Israel of millions of refugees. With Syria, the problem was relatively simple, the return of occupied Golan Heights, except for a strip of land Israel claims for security and the water rights it desired.

For the first time, Barak attempted to grapple with the crux of the problem with the Palestinians, even privately conceding partial Palestinian sovereignty over East Jerusalem; the return of the refugees proved almost impossible to resolve. But his time, as also President Bill Clinton's, was fast running out and as a tortured Israeli nation sought to wrestle with the question of war and peace, a growing majority felt that it was getting the worst of the bargain: continuing insecurity despite what Israelis saw as radical concessions.

An Internal Debate

While more Palestinians and some Israelis continued to be killed and yet more Palestinian homes were destroyed, Israelis were essentially fighting a battle among themselves. Having tried Barak the peace-maker, they were now letting hardliner Sharon crack the whip. It was all part of an internal debate at the cost of more innocent lives, more Palestinian anger, with the new Bush administration having publicly intervened only once to rebuke Israel for rubbishing Oslo. The less interventionist approach of President George W. Bush sat well with Israeli hardliners and might even have the benefit of giving Israelis time to clarify their differences.

The truth is that Israeli society was deeply split between the hardliners and doves, between the orthodox and the secularists, between the young and the old. Israel's safety net is the United States, its mentor and protector, and it is only when the US administration realises that its larger interests are being harmed that it can bring itself to criticising Israel's policy.

As Israel's new hardline policy provoked more Palestinian violence, as it could, a majority of Israelis would realise that the Sharon way of doing things was no answer to their problems. The disastrous Israeli invasion of Lebanon in the eighties and retention of a southern occupation zone for 22 years were the handiwork of Sharon, the then defence minister.

Barak, will help from former President Clinton, might have served his country better than his people realised because he articulated the essence of a formula that could show the way to peace. Palestinians should be granted sovereignty over their holy sites in East Jerusalem. The right of return to Israel should be conceded in principle although in practice it could only be of a symbolic nature. Third, Palestinians should have a viable state—settlements on occupied land should go, with clusters around Jerusalem allowed to remain as long as the Palestinian state was compensated with Israeli land.

How long it would take the nation state of Israel to reconcile itself to a realistic formula for securing peace remained to be seen. It is, above all, an Israeli problem for two other reasons. Israel is an ideological state in an era in which pragmatism, rather than ideology, is the rule. Second, permanent colonisation of the Palestinian people even if it were possible in a post-colonial era, is not an option for a nation founded and justified on the basis of its Jewishness.

As long as this dispensation continued, Palestinians could not but rebel at the inequity of a system under which they were boxed in at Israeli will unable to go to work or even visit one another in demarcated Palestinian areas. Collective punishment was the rule, rather than the exception. And many Palestinians returned only to rubble where their homes stood because they were allegedly built without Israeli permits or were described by Israelis as source of hostile fire.

War is never a pretty picture, but when a colonised people are humiliated and made to suffer fresh privations each day, the ruling colonial power builds an immense amount of hatred against itself. Before parts of Gaza Strip were handed over to the Palestinian Authority, I took a ride in an Israeli military jeep with Israeli soldiers barely in their teens. I asked one of them whether he liked what he was doing. He turned to a senior officer for his approval before answering. "No, I hate it."

The teenage soldier was Israeli's peace constituency.

Violence without End, 2001

Something changed irreversibly in the world's view of the Israeli–Palestinian problem. Stemming from the furious debates and walk-outs at the Durban UN conference on racism, it was not the wording of the final declaration that was important but the recognition that the suffering symbolised by the Holocaust could not wash away the sins of the state of Israel. And Israel's role and methods as a colonial power are an anachronism in this age.

To an extent, the Palestinians and their Arab supporters were expressing their frustration with the situation as it had developed in the region. With the Bush administration's hands-off approach and Ariel Sharon's assumption of prime ministership, the cards were even more heavily stacked against the Palestinians. Adding to the economic hardships of curfews and blockades were Israeli armed incursions into Palestinian areas to raze buildings, the use of F-16s to strike terror and the assassinations, mostly by helicopter gunships, of marked Palestinians.

The cycle of violence never ended because suicide bombers struck Israeli targets to seek revenge and they, in turn, propelled Israeli strikes with their impressive weapons of war. The Oslo peace process was in tatters and efforts by Israeli Foreign Minister Shimon Peres and Palestinian leaders to meet to talk could yield little but momentary relief. We were in a new phase of the Israeli–Palestinian confrontation because hopes of a negotiated settlement, riding high during Yitzak Rabin's time and the relatively brief tempestuous reign of Ehud Barak, seemed remote. In essence, the Sharon government disowned the land-for-peace formula of Oslo and both Likud and Labour governments had negotiated in bad faith because they had been busy expanding and building new settlements on occupied land and failed to observe deadlines while making a mockery of the "final status" talks.

A Distant Goal

The Israeli goal of security and peace was more distant than it had been for a long time. If Sharon believed he was fighting a war of attrition, he was going up a blind alley. And by deliberately destroying the infrastructure of the Palestinian Authority, poor as it was, he was destroying Yasser Arafat's ability to rein in the more radical Palestinian elements. Indeed, Sharon's very posture was making it impossible for Arafat to appear to be doing Tel Aviv's bidding.

Would Israel then remain a garrison state for all time? The deaths of civilians through suicide bombings muted the voice of the peace constituency but could not entirely stifle it. The hawks in the Israeli political spectrum were in the driver's seat and each new incident of violence helped their cause.

The irony is that the separate existence of Israelis and Palestinians mooted by some got stuck on a fundamental problem. One had to define the contours of the Jewish state before it could be walled off. And what would Israel do with its more than a million ethnic Arab citizens inside Israel? Partitions, as we know from the Indian subcontinent's example, can be a massy business, and incorporating conquered territory and people into an ideological state is particularly hazardous.

The trend set by Oslo for the gradual integration of Israel into the region had been abruptly halted. Israel could not for ever live like an island in an Arab sea. True, Israel had the full support of its protector, the United States, and could count on European countries in its hour of need. Tel Aviv also expanded its relations with other countries around the world. But there was no substitute for intercourse with neighbours, particularly because a significant number of its own citizens are Arab, whatever their status at home.

There were, indeed, a host of weighty arguments in favour of Israel seeking a fair accommodation with the Palestinians. The search for a sane solution had, in effect, been postponed, and the prospect was for much blood and tears on all sides before they could pick up the threads again. The hope of the hardliners in Israel was that the longer violence reigned without the Bush administration spending sleepless night over it, the greater would be the "facts on ground" and the better bargain Israel would be able to strike at Palestinians' expense.

Diplomatically, Palestinians were chipping away at the sympathy of a large part of the world for Jewish suffering in another age by juxtaposing what the Jewish state was doing to Palestinians. Could occupation justify the methods Israelis were using to subdue a people rebelling against their plight? How could an occupying power arrogate to itself the role of a judge and executioner? Could F-16s and helicopter gunships and tanks be employed to try to cow down a people who had stones for weapons or must rely on suicide bombers?

The implicit goal of the Arab world at Durban was to register its outrage over Israeli behaviour and to get the world to reflect on this outrageousness. That was more important than the language included in the final compromise declaration.

The Palestinians

Arafat in Exile, March 1988

Tunis, lapped by the Mediterranean, has a pleasant, placid, provincial air about it. It is a symbol of the many contradictions of West Asia that this charming Tunisian capital was the host of the Palestine Liberation Organisation, complete with a bureaucracy of nearly a thousand persons. And the multi-storey Arab League headquarters in the city was guarded by gun-toting sentries and functionaries equipped with walkie-talkies.

The headquarters was moved from Cairo to Tunis after Egypt signed the Camp David agreement with Israel.

In between his constant travels to various Arab capitals, Yasser Arafat resided in Tunis, protected by double posses of guards with Kalashnikovs and automatic weapons, provided by the Tunisians and his own organisation.

After a thorough search of all equipment, journalists were led into his heavily guarded room in a bourgeois house. A large portrait of a smiling Arafat was duplicated by the smiling leader fielding questions from journalists with aplomb.

Arafat dismissed the Shultz Plan for West Asia as one determined by "five no's". It was against self-determination, against independent Palestinian development, against an independent Palestinian state, against an active and decisive international conference and against the PLO. Arafat said he had not received the plan, which bypasses the PLO.

"We are for international legality", Arafat declared, responding to questions about the PLO's acceptance of United Nations resolutions. He was firm in the conviction that the Palestinian cause would succeed. "Peace needs courageous men", he says. "We are ready". He called the young fighting Israeli troops with stones "my new generation".

Arafat said he would want to go back to being a civil engineer after an independent Palestinian state was achieved. Born in Jerusalem 59 years earlier, he believed he would visit Jerusalem again. "The revolution will succeed", he says.

A National Front

It was of a piece with the contradictions of West Asia that while the second in command in the Arab League, under secretary-general Adnan Omran, breathed fire and brimstone in his headquarters, talking about the Palestine problem in apocalyptical terms, Tunisian Foreign Minister Mahmoud Mistiri presented a suave rational front, suggesting that the Palestinian problem had evolved.

The stark contrast between these views was brought home to us through separate meetings with the two functionaries in a single day. The central point of interest was the Shultz Plan which "envisages" a tight framework granting limited autonomy to the occupied West Bank while leaving the substantive questions to the second phase. The Arab League had yet to take a collective stand on the plan, but Omran dismissed it as almost an insult to the Palestinians and a proposal made in the Camp David style, a pejorative expression in West Asia.

Mistiri, on the other hand, found positive elements in the Shultz Plan for three reasons. It came from the United States, it acknowledged the problem, reflecting a new realism on the part of Washington and envisaged some solution. According to the foreign minister, the plan was a starting point so that Palestinians and Israelis could talk to each other.

I asked Arafat about the Tunisian foreign minister's declaration. His cryptic answer was, "I respect his point of view".

The contours of a phase of intense diplomacy were already clear, whatever the fate of the Shultz Plan. Everyone was conscious of the fact that this was an American election year and its dictates had priority over US policy. The fasting mouth of Ramadan would start on April 18, thus limiting the active phase of Arab diplomacy for a time.

The Palestinian question came to the fore thanks to the spontaneous uprising in the occupied territories, which had brought the Palestinians the world's sympathy while posing a problem for the Arab states.

Beyond the Palestinian question hung the Iran–Iraq war like a dark cloud and the wave of Islamic fundamentalism the Iranian revolutions had created. Egypt still remained outside the Arab League, having been suspended after it signed the Camp David accord with Israel, although a number of Arab League members had resumed diplomatic relations with it.

Omran drew comfort from the fact that President Mubarak of Egypt had suggested that Camp David was something whose time had come and gone. Egypt was not quite ready to return to the Arab League because its Camp David obligations conflicted with those of the League charter. But Egyptians remained important players in West Asia.

Stark Reality

Beyond the posturing by the hardliners and the moderates lay the stark fact that the Palestinians, by capturing world attention, had reminded the Arabs and the world that the problem would not go away. Shultz's diplomacy in West Asia, leading to the formulation of his plan, was dismissed by Arafat as a "Kissinger-style shuttle mission" to bail out Israel. But the several months' long uprising in the occupied territories posed a crisis not only for Israel and its superpower supporter, but also for the Arab states.

The Arab League summit was scheduled for the first half of April. Relations between Yasser Arafat and Jordan were far from normal after the breakdown of their joint efforts in another phase of diplomacy although Arafat confirmed that he had in principle accepted an invitation from King Hussein.

He planned an early visit to Moscow. Arafat said no country in West Asia was his enemy, and he called differences among the Arab states as being in the family. But the varied orientations of the Arab League members, each with its interest to protect, made the problem of arriving at a consensus that much harder.

Rhetorically there was, of course, total Arab support for the Palestinians' cause and the Arabs gave financial assistance to the Palestinians. Arafat made the point that a new scheme had been put into operation whereby three families among an estimated three millions Palestinians living abroad would support one family among the one-and-a-half million Palestinians living in occupied territories. This attempt to reach a measure of self-reliance was meant to strengthen the main Fatah faction of the PLO.

All that was being offered the Palestinians so far was limited autonomy, which could later be expanded. Jordan's association with the West Bank was a key question because it was a mechanism to deny the Palestinians an independent state while posing political problems for the Jordanian monarchy, with the increase in Palestinian population it would involve.

Conservative monarchies were juxtaposed with radical regimes in the region, and the Palestinians had proved to be an intelligent and enterprising people. Apart from the problem on its own doorstep the new phase of interest in the occupied territories posed for Jordan, Egypt, which administered the Gaza Strip until the Israelis took it through a war disastrous for the Arabs, was not too keen to be drawn into playing a central role, conscious as it was of its alignment with the United States. And Syria, the home of many dissident PLO factions, had its own scores to settle with Arafat.

The previous Arab summits and Yasser Arafat and Arab League spokesmen were one in demanding a substantive international conference under United Nations auspices, as opposed to Shultz's symbolic conference which would give way to discussions between Israelis and a joint Jordanian-Palestinian delegation.

Arafat, of course, was justly angry with the American decision to close down the PLO mission in New York, describing it as "shameful" and a repudiation of international agreements. But the Arab accent on a UN-sponsored conference to decide on the fate of the Palestinians should bring some cheer to the beleaguered United Nations.

Coalition Building

It needed the psychological push of the murder of Abu Jihad to make Arafat's dramatic meeting with President Assad in Damascus possible. But a reconciliation between the mainstream Fatah faction of the Palestine Liberation Organisation and Syria had been in the making for some time and was determined by internal and external compulsions.

The uprising in the occupied territories refocussed the world's attention on the Palestinian question, bringing to the fore the need to show Arab solidarity. Syria's problems in Lebanon and its need for American diplomatic help led to a more flexible policy on the part of Damascus. Besides, the public Soviet advice to Arafat on the need for the recognition of Israel and its security concerns was a pointer to Moscow abandoning its earlier radical posture.

The symbolic reconciliation did not mean that differences in the PLO, or among the Arab states, had been resolved. It meant that Syria as one of the most radical of the Arab states had chosen to relegate its reservations about Arafat to the background to be able to present a united front on the issue. This represented a triumph for Arafat and would inevitably mean greater pressure on the Israelis and their American allies.

Symbols are particularly important in the Arab world, and symbolically, the Arabs had crossed the Rubicon. The Arafat-Assad meeting also mitigated to an extent the Palestinians' anger over the Arab League states' failure to call a summit meeting on the uprising. This had already provoked George Habash, leader of an important PLO faction, to make the charge that some Arab states were hoping to postpone the holding of the summit until the Israelis had succeeded in putting down the uprising.

On March 30, 1988 in Damascus, Vice-President Abdel-Halim Khadam had told us — a group of nine journalists from around the world — that there were efforts at rapprochement with the PLO. "There are political and organisational differences among them. But they have now frozen their differences". He did not add that Syria harboured the radical PLO factions nor did he allude to the unceremonial exit from Syria of Arafat and his faction five years earlier.

Arafat, Khadam said in answer to a question, could open an office in Syria "when he returns to the constitution of the PLO". "Even Arafat's antagonists speak in the name of the PLO", he explained. "The dispute is not about the PLO but about its tasks and behaviour".

Radicals' Stance

Spokesmen of the radical PLO factions in Damascus spoke about Arafat's alleged dictatorial tendencies, but at the heart of their dispute with Arafat and his Fatah faction lay the Egyptian question. Arafat sealed a reconciliation with Egypt a few weeks after the Amman Arab summit; even worse, from the radical factions' point of view, was the abortive agreement between King Hussein of Jordan and Arafat. The radicals also looked askance at Arafat's contacts with "progressive" Israelis. According to Arafat, "There are progressive and democratic forces in Israel. We have many contacts with these groups."

Arafat made no apology in telling us in Tunis that "Egypt has a big role to play" on the Palestinian question whereas for the radicals, an Egypt which signed a separate peace with Israel remained an anathema. There were strains between Arafat and Jordan after the abortive Amman agreement. Spokesmen of the Fatah faction acknowledged that "Palestinians are most at ease with Egyptians, but it is very difficult to ignore Jordan".

There was one common position all Arab states took: the PLO was the sole representative of the Palestinians. And the PLO commitment to an independent Palestinian state was accepted by all factions in the organisation. Since the Israelis were nowhere near returning the occupied territories to a Palestine even in a confederation with Jordan, differences in the PLO on this issue were of somewhat academic interest. But they remained a potent source of conflict and trouble.

Criticism of Arafat was not confined to the radical factions of the PLO. An independent Palestinian like Jawad Saleh, a deported mayor from the occupied territories, was a moderate. But he spoke in terms of the PLO having "neglected" the occupied territories and an organisation using "remote control tools". "If the PLO does not change its methods and contracts", he said in Cairo, "there will be disregard for the PLO leadership".

It was one of the attributes of Arafat as a leader that, despite the criticism and controversies surrounding him, he remained supremely confident. "We are mature", he told us in Tunis. "We have come of age. We are one body—the Palestinians".

As the Palestinians' confidence grew, the future was beginning to assume a more real shape. And the Arab states' dilemmas increased even as they paid lip-service to the cause of Palestinian self-determination. One of the quarrels the Jordanians have had with the Soviets was Moscow's alacrity in signing joint declarations on an independent Palestine state with the PLO. As a minister put it in Amman, "Can the Soviets get the Americans to accept such a state? Will Israel agree?"

The new Soviet moderation on this question was naturally to Amman's liking. But Jordan was chary of suggesting that it had a plan for the Palestinians—what Crown Prince Hassan suggested was like putting the cart before the horse. Arafat acknowledged, "I accept the partition plan although I do not like it personally". His reference was to receiving back the occupied territories, rather than the whole of Palestine. Even the radical PLO faction in Syria said that they would accept the return of the occupied territories in the first stage.

Arab Ambivalence

The reluctance of some Arab states to take a collective stand on an elaborate blueprint for the Palestinians' future was understandable. Egypt, of course, was still outside the Arab League and had little interest in the summit being held. But even Jordan, and perhaps Saudi Arabia, would not be too keen on grasping the nettle of the Palestinians' future at this stage.

It was universally agreed in the Arab world that Camp David was a dirty phrase. Egypt itself was distancing itself from the agreement it had signed with Israel even while observing the bilateral part of the Camp David accord by suggesting that "Camp David is no longer on the agenda". Cairo blamed Israel for repudiating the commitment for achieving a comprehensive peace, but was undoubtedly grateful that it could say so to re-establish its credentials in the Arab world.

For the small Israeli peace camp, the Palestine Liberation Organisation is "a very democratic movement, like Israel". Crown Prince Hassan called the PLO a coalition having different patrons in the Arab world. For Jordan's Minister for Occupied Territories, Merwan Doudin, the PLO was basically a revolutionary movement which should not be required to behaved like a state. In his view, the PLO factions had a hard time working for a consensus. He explained: "We contributed to the establishment of the PLO. We thought it was too early to talk about the PLO being the sole representative of the Palestinians, but we accepted the Arab consensus ... If the PLO has a say in what is happening in the occupied territories, it is good. But what is happening there is excellent".

The PLO was still hovering between being an incipient state and a revolutionary movement. It had to be both in order to keep the loose coalition together and to enthuse the faithful. Few leaders other than Arafat could perform the task of being a friend of President Mubarak and, after a fashion, President Assad.

Algiers Declaration

Bit by bit the jigsaw puzzle in West Asia was falling in place. It would still take much time, effort and blood for the full picture to emerge. But more than 20 years after the Israelis had captured the West Bank and the Gaza Strip and had been trying to make their conquest permanent, a Palestinian state was emerging out of the shadows of war and defeat.

The credit for the more hopeful scenario must go, in the first instance, to the Palestinians in the occupied territories. For more than 11 months they had defied Israelis to make their point. They nudged the Arab states, each preoccupied with its own problems and ambitions, and the world to heed their voice. Indeed, the intefada, the uprising, brought the Palestinian issue many would rather forget to the centre stage.

Next only to the intefada, Arafat and his mainstream Fatah faction in the PLO deserved credit for bringing about a denouement that took the whole process forward. It was Arafat's political acumen that was responsible for his success in bringing round the hardliners to accept Israel's existence.

The *deus ex machina* for the historic Algiers declaration was no other than Jordan's King Hussein, who administered the bitter medicine of waving all claims to, and dissociating himself from, the occupied territories. It took Arafat months of constant travel and interminable discussions with Arab leaders to be able to achieve what he did in Algiers, with some help from President Mubarak. The latter helped in reconciliation moves to bring Arafat and King Hussein together. Arafat thus proved equal to the challenge posed by the King.

The Algiers meeting of the Palestine National Council (PNC), the PLO's parliament in exile, accepted UN resolution 242 implicitly recognising the state of Israel. The hardliners among the PLO factions and Syria remained unreconciled. But, conscious of the wishes of the Palestinians in the occupied territories, they chose not to walk out of the PNC meeting.

All the Arab states except Syria and many members of the Non-aligned Movement, including India, had recognised the Palestinian state. Despite Israeli warnings, Egypt had accepted the PNC declaration. There was some ambiguity in the Soviet acceptance of the declaration but not specifically the state, presumably because it had a role to play in the final resolution of the crisis.

Marking Time

The US administration, in its final months, was marking time. Some praise for the PLO move had been interspersed with criticism that recognition of Israel was not made explicit and there was no formal renunciation of terrorism.

Although the PNC stated specifically that it "rejects terrorism in all its forms", Arafat made a distinction in suggesting that acts of violence committed in lands controlled by Israel were permissible. It would be up to George Bush to steer his country towards a more realistic position.

What the PLO move meant in essence was that one of the major hurdles to the movement towards resolving the Palestinian issue had been crossed. Many other hurdles remained before an international conference with the participation of all parties concerned could be held.

The United States remained a key to the resolution of the problem because of its strategic alliance with and support for Israel and its presence in the area. Once the new administration was convinced that the Algiers declaration offered the best hope for moving forward, it would have to summon the will to put enough pressure on Israel to see reason.

Arafat was setting his sights on the United States. He declared at Algiers: "Our political declaration contains moderation, flexibility and realism, which the West has been urging us to show. We feel now that the ball is in the American court."

Israeli itself remained a deeply divided nation, as the election results showed. The likely assumption of office of the hardliner Yitzak Shamir of Likud could be a blessing in disguise because the contradictions between Likud's desire to retain the occupied territories for all time on the one hand and the growing political, financial, manpower costs and the world's opprobrium on the other would become starker by the day.

Western European nations had failed to recognise the Palestinian state, to no one's surprise. But the pressures of the European Economic Community on Washington and Israel to move forward would grow under pain of individual nations recognising the new state. At the very least, Washington would have to show that it was heeding the new realism displayed by the PLO.

The calling of the international conference would, of course, be a preliminary step to eventual peace. Even the size of the new state and its capital would present problems.

Resolution 242 refers to the pre-1967 war boundaries of Israel; resolution 338 merely reiterates the older resolution and urges talks. There is the even earlier resolution 181 which would give the new state additional area which had been incorporated in Israel. Arafat specifically and emotionally referred to Jerusalem as the capital of a free Palestinian state: the eastern part of the holy city was a booty of the 1967 war.

American Hedging

Unlike the occupied territories on the West Bank and in the Gaza Strip, Israel had incorporated the whole of Jerusalem and the Syrian Golan Heights. The US had suggested the conversion of Jerusalem into an open city because it has religious connotations for three of the world's religions. Besides, Washington had thus far not conceded the whole of the occupied territories to a new Palestinian entity.

Past American policy, specially under the guidance of Henry Kissinger, had been to deny the Soviet Union a role in West Asia. This was not a realistic policy and had been altered to the extent of acknowledging that the mechanism of an international conference could not be activated without the participation of the Soviet Union.

The new thaw in superpower relations was a good augury inasmuch as the American and Soviet leaders could talk to each other on regional conflicts. The United States would have to persuade Syria, a key state, to join in, but the superpowers would have to agree among themselves on the format of a conference as and when it took place. There were differences on how substantive the role of the conference should be.

However, the complexities of the West Asian scene would also have to be taken into account. Iran had so far refused to give up its rejectionist line and Syrian sensitivities on the Golan Heights would need to be addressed. While King Hussein was content that the shock he administered to the PLO had a salutary effect, President Mubarak had bigger plans.

Egypt was the only Arab country to have made a separate peace with Israel. Its position would have been untenable if it had not recognised the Palestinian declaration. Having done so, President Mubarak was positioning himself to play a mediator's role in the prolonged and Byzantine negotiations that would precede an international conference.

The evolving West Asian scene, indeed, offered Bush an opportunity and a risk. The opportunity was that he could build on the historic Algiers declaration to begin the process of ending the Arab–Israeli divide, which was at least as old as the United Nations in its present form. If he succeeded in accomplishing this task, in cooperation with the Soviet Union, he would find an honoured place in history.

The risks arose out of the minefield West Asia was. President Ronald Reagan was given a taste of Lebanon and chose discretion, rather than valour. And for any American President, there were obvious problems in dealing with Israel, in view of the political and economic clout the Jewish lobby exercised. But, in a sense, Bush had no real choice. American inaction in West Asia would mean that a new stage for violent conflicts would be set, threatening the very strategic interests Washington was seeking to protect.

A Beginning, 1994

Now that the Palestine Liberation Organisation was on its way to governing Jericho and the Gaza Strip, despite hiccups, the focus should shift to the future of the large remaining part of the Israeli-occupied West Bank and East Jerusalem. For the Israeli hardliners were right in one respect: Palestinian autonomy over a limited part of the territories was the thin end of the wedge for Israel. From here on the process of an independent Palestinian state was irreversible; the uncertainties related only to the time it would take and how the process would be completed.

Problems and difficulties lay ahead. Some of these related to the task of governing as the PLO shifted gears from a revolutionary movement to a government. Others would arise out of the inevitable turmoil in the still occupied territories and its repercussions on Israel and yet others on how soon and fully Israelis reconciled themselves to giving up all the occupied territories. As we had seen in the implementation of the September 1993 accord between the PLO and Israel, achieving the goal of an independent Palestinian entity would not be smooth.

Judging by the comments of members of the Israeli government, Rabin seemed to have made a strategic decision to give up nearly all the territories barring East Jerusalem. But he had to convince his people that he had made the right choice, and to do so he would need to build on the success of the "Jericho-Gaza first" option. But Israel suddenly found itself in a position of weakness because even if the process of autonomy for the limited area went against perceived Israeli interests, it had no option but to give up the occupied land.

The contours of the West Asian map were, therefore, set to change, a change accelerated by the end of the Cold War and the consequences of the Second Gulf War. Indeed, it would be surprising if the process of self-governance for all the occupied territories took as long as the stipulated five years. Jericho and Gaza would set off a momentum which would become progressively more difficult to control and the task of Israeli policing of the occupied land next to impossible, except at an unacceptable cost. It would be in the interest of Palestinians and Israelis alike that the question of moving the settlements out be completed early, rather than late. As it was, the settlements in the Gaza Strip and Jericho represented a time bomb.

Obviously, Israel's task of accepting the inevitable would be easier if it could reach a settlement with Syria on the Golan Heights. The circular arguments on this issue were well known and the role of the United States would be a key factor not only in giving Israel the kind of guarantees and financial assistance it wanted but also in convincing it on leaving the whole of the Golan. The settlements presented less of a problem because, unlike in the West Bank, they concerned relatively few Israelis.

Intefada's Role

As we look back on the saga of the Palestinian struggle, the failure of Israel's grand plan to change the demography of the occupied territories in order to incorporate them was due to the growing realisation of sections of the thinking population that their country could not secure peace by subjugating millions of Arabs. The intefada played a notable part in this process and the stone-throwing boys were in the front ranks of the struggle in showing the Israelis and the world that brute force was no answer because, despite the deaths and suffering, it merely fuelled the people's opposition.

In the end, Israel's ally and patron, the United States, came to realise that the longer Israelis stayed on as occupiers, the greater would be the threat to peace in the region and the more nebulous its own position. There was no way the Palestinians could be subjugated by a country seeking to derive its justification from a dim past. Inevitably, the process of reaching the first stage of the goal took long, with the secret parleys in Oslo forming an essential link in the chain.

Palestinian opponents of the Gaza-Jericho option were wrong because they did not see the inevitability of an independent Palestinian entity short of an armed struggle. Some opposed the deal for ideological reasons, but the vast majority in the opposition camp did so because of their fear that Palestinians would be fobbed off with a symbolic stump of a state. They failed to see the larger picture and a growing realisation among Israelis that continued occupation of the West Bank and the Gaza Strip was becoming a liability. If they wanted to seek peace with their Arab neighbours, force was not the answer.

In the event, Palestinians in the autonomous areas had regained their dignity, despite the question marks that plagued them. The joyous scenes of people welcoming Palestinian policemen in Gaza and Jericho were witness to their sense of relief; the stone-throwing boys rode police trucks waving Palestinian flags as the new law enforcers humoured them. For many, born outside or forced to leave after Israeli occupation, it was an emotional homecoming. A new era had dawned even though many were conscious of the uncertainties that lay ahead.

There was not much point in dwelling on the problems facing the PLO in governing Jericho and the Gaza Strip. There would be difficulties and foul-ups in administering areas that had been under occupation for more than a quarter century, but the Palestinian leadership would get its act together and begin tackling the endemic problems of unemployment and poverty. In this task, they would require the goodwill and financial assistance of their Arab neighbours.

Strategists were inclined to look at the future place and shape of an independent Palestinian state, whether the so-called Jordan option would provide the answer. But for the next few years, Palestinians and the world would be involved in the process of the complete dismantling of Israeli occupation. As we witnessed the Yemen tragedy, peace was not quite breaking out in West Asia, but the beginning of Palestinian administration of Jericho and Gaza was evidence of an emerging new dispensation which could, over time, remove a central cause of conflict in the region.

For the Palestinians, it was still too early to run up their flag of independence in the manner the reborn South Africa did. But in their difficult task of translating their long struggle into the realisation of their dream, Palestinians should know that they had arrived at a crucial point in their journey.

The Roadblock, 1995

Behind the angry exchanges between Palestinians and Israelis, most recently in Paris, lay a simple truth: meetings and get-togethers could not resolve the problems until the basic contradiction between the two sides could be tackled. And that contradiction was that the Israelis could not have peace while they helped themselves to more occupied land. The Cairo summit among Egypt, Israel, Jordan and the PLO and the follow-up meeting at foreign ministers' level in Washington were exercises in futility because conference bonhomie could not substitute a just basis for pursuing the peace process.

What had happened in recent months was a conjunction of two phenomena: The plummeting popularity of the Israeli prime minister, Rabin, consequent upon a series of suicide bombing attacks on Israelis and an Israeli decision to intensify its hold on occupied land and expand it. Fencing in the autonomous areas of Jericho and the Gaza Strip was a reflex action, the building of industrial parks abutting the autonomy areas was a tentative step in the direction of separating Jews from Palestinians and the public posture of holding Arafat responsible for ensuring Israelis' safety was a convenient way of stalling the whole peace process.

Rabin had apparently come to the conclusion that Arafat held a weak hand and had no alternative but to acquiesce in the humiliations the Israelis chose to pile upon him—in other words, the PLO leader was trapped by the autonomy agreement. One of Rabin's compulsions was domestic politics, but beyond that, as the continued surreptitious building of new settlements revealed, was the Labour Party's agenda to expand the scope of Israeli settlements, buttress occupied Jerusalem with a new periphery of settlements and present the Palestinians with a *fait accompli*. Not only would the Israelis continue to claim the whole of Jerusalem as their undivided capital, but also an expanded area around it and whole areas of settlements with guarded roads on the occupied West Bank.

Israelis were betting on their belief that a beleaguered President Bill Clinton had no option but to go along with whatever they did. Support for Israel cut across the two parties in the United States; apart from the celebrated Jewish lobby, there was bipartisan support for Israel as the main American strategic ally in West Asia. And Egypt was being faulted in the US because it pierced the camouflage of the patently unjust demand that Arabs should sign the Nuclear Non-Proliferation Treaty extension while Israel continued to exercise its privilege of remaining out of it. Despite the rhetoric, Washington did not want Israel to sign the NPT even as the US openly gave it a strategic military edge over its neighbours.

What Israelis, and perhaps Americans, did not realise was that there would come a breaking point in the tolerance level of even the most moderate Palestinians. Rabin was not helping himself or his country by placing impossible burdens on Arafat and his Palestinian Authority. If more and more Palestinians were convinced about the picture that was emerging, that Israel had a hidden agenda in agreeing to the Oslo accord, opposition would not be confined to the Hamas movement, and the scale of violence when that happened could well be imagined.

Israel was quite pleased with the peace treaty it was able to sign with Jordan and the quasi-diplomatic recognition it had won from some other Arab states. Perhaps Rabin had forgotten that these successes were built on the shoulders of the PLO, and as the Oslo agreement began to unravel, they could prove to be illusory gains. There cannot be peace in the region without giving Palestinians their just due and no amount of rhetoric or hype can change that.

American Bias

Arafat has been pleading with the United States and West Europe to help in breaking the deadlock by pressuring the Israelis. Washington remained the key player and was obviously interested in preventing the peace process from imploding, if only to safeguard its own security concerns. But the American agenda was weighted in favour of Israel and it could only offer palliatives to the Palestinians. If not the Clinton administration, the majority in the US Congress seemed to have decided that the whole of Jerusalem belonged to Israel; the administration's appeal to the legislators was to wait till 1996 when the question was ostensibly to be discussed. Israel won a diplomatic victory by making Jordan's King the guardian of Muslim holy sites in occupied Jerusalem to outflank the PLO.

The hope was that the dangers of a new conflagration in West Asia would make the Clinton administration pause to consider the risks of its strategy. The answer was not to hold public conferences with Palestinian and Israeli representatives and retail the fiction of a mere hiccup in the peace process. If it had the will, or acquired it, the US had to pressure Israel in private to give up its hidden agenda. Washington should not settle for being fobbed off by Rabin's plea that he needed to bend with the prevailing Israeli wind to stay afloat politically. If he could not pursue a peace policy that would ultimately benefit his own country, he should make way for another. The future of the region and of countless lives depended upon statesmanship.

Without doubt, the United States had great leverage in pushing the peace process forward, despite Israel's ability to manipulate the

American system. If it employed that leverage only to get the Arab states to sign the indefinite extension of the NPT without Israel, it would fail in bringing about peace to the region. Merely harping on Arafat's responsibility to prevent attacks on Israelis from the autonomous areas was to address the symptom, instead of the cause. Such a posture could only help to breed cynicism among Palestinians and lead them to those who offered a different route to success. Rabin had chosen to get out of his dilemma by simply disregarding the Oslo agreement (it was not written in stone, he once suggested). If Arafat were to follow a similar course, we would see the end of the Oslo edifice.

For once, the cliché of peace hanging in the balance was true.

Resurgence of Violence

The new upsurge of violence in the occupied territories had taken the problem a stage closer to a cataclysm most of the protagonists were seeking to avoid. Yet the logical end of the renewed flare-up following the shooting of seven Arab labourers by an Israeli was that something had to give.

Of the two main protagonists, the Israelis and the PLO, pressures were mounting on Arafat to abandon his peace strategy for a harder line. The Israelis, on the other hand, were caught up in a government crisis, a recurring phenomenon, with the result that there could be no forward movement on the only peace proposal on the table, the Baker Plan.

The Americans, on their part, had stepped up the pressure on Israelis, but such pressures had traditionally been of limited value. And the Israelis had a perfect alibi, that because of the government crisis, with Shamir still wrestling with putting together a majority, decisive action was out of the question. The so-called unity government broke up over the Baker peace plan.

The United States was continuing its dialogue with the PLO, but as the intefada in the occupied territories had re-ignited with old fury and the PLO and the other Arabs increasingly exercised over the settling of Soviet Jews in Israel and the occupied territories, a new stage had been reached. Debates in the United Nations Security Council and other fora could help up to a point but could not be a real substitute for meaningful steps towards a resolution of the Palestinian question.

Arafat was following a two-pronged strategy to cope with the crisis: seeking to mobilise world opinion and to get the Arab world to speak with one voice, particularly on the dangers of settling Soviet Jews in the occupied territories. In the latter objective, the projected summit had met the political fault lines in the Arab world.

Any real beginning of a solution to the Palestinian question lay with Israel. The Baker Plan was, in itself, a modest proposal and called for starting an Israeli–Palestinian dialogue. The right-wing opposition to the proposal symbolised by Shamir and much of his Likud party stemmed from their belief that any such process, once started, could only lead to an independent Palestinian state in the end.

During a visit to Israel in January 1996, I formed the distinct impression that given propitious circumstances and much quiet diplomatic work, the majority of Israelis could ultimately accept a separate Palestinian entity. But two conditions seemed necessary to achieve this objective: a change in leadership in both the Likud and Labour parties in the next general election, and suitably camouflaging the independent Palestinian state of the future.

The problem such an optimistic scenario presented in the near term was how to prevent the crisis from boiling over in the meantime. Arafat had proved to be a highly skilful leader and had managed to surmount a host of crises involving himself and his organisation with his head above water. But the new intensity of the intefada and the seemingly inexorable march of Soviet Jews into the occupied territories, as the Arabs saw it, were placing immense pressures on him.

Arafat's Dilemma

Arafat had to continue justifying to hardliners his tactic of making concessions for the peace process without any result to show for it. On the contrary, Palestinians continued to be killed in the occupied territories and by settling hordes of Soviet Jews on them—the bulk of them thus far in East Jerusalem—the Israelis were seeking to change the demography in their favour.

A further complication had been added to the Palestinian crisis by the dramatic events in the Soviet Union and East Europe. Mikhail Gorbachev's *glasnost* and *perestroika* and a non-ideological foreign policy had led to the free flow of Jews to Israel after the United States imposed a quota on their number for settlement. And as the East European countries had thrown away their communist clothes with alacrity, they had joined the queue in recognising Israel.

Apart from the demographic changes Arabs feared the Soviet Jews would bring about, the East European developments had given a decided boost to the right wing in Israel. For one thing, the obvious ideological contradiction in absorbing millions of Arabs in a Greater Israel was less menacing. Second, Israel's aim of receiving *de jure* recognition from most of the countries of the world had moved a step closer to fulfilment.

The key elements of a solution remained where they were: primarily in the United States' ability to put pressure on Israel and a hoped-for change in Israel itself. With the superpower *entente* in place and the new Soviet tendency to avoid entanglements in the Third World, the Arabs were inclined to be on the defensive. And each Arab state had its own set of problems and ambitions. Sometimes, these ambitions clashed, exemplified in the prevailing Iraq–Syria discord.

In this complex situation, Egypt was seeking to find a path out of the minefields. Now that it was securely rehabilitated in the Arab world, and President Mubarak's visit to Moscow was an indication of how far he has normalised relations with the East, Egypt had stepped out to try to reconcile differences in the Arab world as it kept its fancied role as a bridge between Israel and the Palestinians.

The new turn the Palestinian crisis had taken meant that when tampers and tensions were high, Egypt's moderation and flexibility had to take a back seat. It thus reverted to the United States to help temper the Arab rhetoric and do some plainspeaking in public for the benefit of Israel. The latter President George Bush had attempted to do by calling for Israeli restraint while suggesting that the political processes be speeded up to get on with the peace agenda.

If international diplomacy consisted of a series of balancing acts, many of the principal players were doing precisely that. The United States was duly mindful of its strategic interests in Israel in addition to the pulls the Jewish lobby exercised even as it tried to move Israel towards the negotiating table. Egypt had to zealously guard its Arab credentials as an honest broker between Israel and the Palestinians.

In Arab eyes, the Soviets had largely opted out of a major role on the Palestinian issue. But the greatest balancer of all remained Arafat. He had to satisfy those undertaking the intefada in the occupied territories that he was working zealously on their behalf. At the same time, as he gathered international support, he had to send the right signals to Washington, that he was open to concluding a reasonable peace.

The question that remained to be answered was whether the re-ignited intefada and Israeli immobility would severely impair Arafat's ability to keep the Palestinian struggle going while leaving him enough room for conducting meaningful negotiations when the time came.

Cloak and Dagger

If they were not so tragic, developments in the Palestinian–Israeli confrontation seemed to assume comic proportions more suited to second-rate pulp fiction that to the real-life world. Imagine the pantomime. We had two spooks in Amman following their quarry in a car, with their accomplices riding separately. They overtook their target and sprayed him with a mysterious poison out of a stick they took out of a bag. The bodyguard of the Hamas leader Khaled Meshal gave chase and held the spooks long enough to enable them to be arrested.

The spooks' cover was blown off almost immediately because they did not want Canadian consular assistance despite allegedly being Canadian. And then followed frantic efforts in several capitals to bring the improbable story to an end, with Jordan's Prince Hassan dispatched to Washington with a letter. The founder of the Hamas movement, Sheikh Ahmed Yassin, languishing in an Israeli jail, was released at the dead of night and sent to Jordan.

There was no deal, said King Hussein.

And yet miraculously the spiritual leader of Hamas was transported by helicopter to an adoring crowd in Gaza. The two Israeli secret agents, who deserved medals for their genius for bungling, were put in another helicopter and sent to Israel at about the same time.

There was no deal.

But 20 more Palestinian prisoners were released from jail, with the promise of 40 to 50 more to be released in weeks.

And Israeli Prime Minister Benjamin Netanyahu, flanked on either side by the acknowledged hawk Ariel Sharon and the defence minister, in his trademark rapid-fire prose, told a press conference in effect that it was his job to send assassination squads to hunt for men he considered enemies. There was an edge of desperation to his acting, with combativeness emerging as braggadocio.

And to complete the improbable nature of the second-rate pulp fiction story, the lanky American Dennis Ross with the lean and hungry look, a veteran of many failed missions to the region, arrived. His brief was to begin the esoteric work of committees in an exercise Washington still referred to as the peace process.

Israel Bungling

Leaving aside the bizarre and entertaining aspects of the drama we had witnessed, the bungled Israeli murder attempt had damaged its relations with Jordan, with Canada (Israelis tended to dismiss it as a country of little consequence) and other nations baffled by the workings of Netanyahu's mind. No one expected the United States to condemn what was in effect an Israeli-authorised attempt at murdering an opponent and the tortuous reaction of the State Department spokesman was hardly a surprise.

Whatever the comic and tragic elements of Netanyahu's method of pursuing "peace with security", the West Asian game would change radically. The Netanyahu government had helped the Hamas movement greatly by depriving the PLO leader Yasser Arafat of credibility through using the structure of the flawed Oslo agreements to build more settlements, including in occupied Arab East Jerusalem, refusing to pull back Israeli troops from the West Bank or implement any of the other agreements such as secure passage between Gaza and the West Bank or allowing Palestinians a sea port and an airport.

The popularity of Hamas grew by leaps and bounds as Israeli actions produced more and more suicide bombers, and as even the long-suffering Arafat could not countenance the whole of East Jerusalem, the declared capital of the future Palestinian state, being swallowed up by new Jewish settlements, the so-called peace talks ground to a halt. After a calculated attempt at doing nothing, the US secretary of state, Madeleine Albright, did came visiting and set up a Washington meeting between the two sides. Yet again, the PLO was forced to swallow its pride and return to the conference table which Netanyahu was offering as a concession. It would appear that for Israelis of Netanyahu's ilk, even talking to the PLO was a condescending privilege offered to a serf.

As Ross began his ritual exercise, one effect of the dramatic developments was that there were suddenly two power centres among Palestinians. Israeli demands that the PLO suppress Hamas and arrest the militants among them sounded rather hollow in the new context. Significantly, Sheikh Yassin's first public call on his native soil in eight years was to maintain Palestinian unity, and many would have observed that in the hero's welcome the Hamas leader received on arrival in Gaza, Arafat was missing.

There is a hoary old theory that a complicated situation should be made more complicated before it can be resolved. In this instance, it is arguable whether Netanyahu was forced into releasing Sheikh Yassin or whether he used his own impetuousity and the incompetence of Mossad agents to pose a new challenge to Arafat. By all accounts, the Israeli prime minister was a reckless player, and, given the impasse he had led his country into, he was playing double or quits to escape the hopeless debts he had incurred.

For their part, Palestinians should welcome the new development because it moved the discussions between them and Israelis from the familiar old grooves which had been gradually leading them to impoverishment and political decimation. What had been the record thus far? Palestinians lived in little enclaves that were called autonomous. They were often cut off from the world or even from fellow Palestinians. Their livelihood had frequently come to an end at the whim of the Israeli rulers. Arab East Jerusalem was being transformed before their very eyes. They are not given direct sea or air access.

There would in future be a stern spiritual voice in Palestinian ranks warning Arafat not to accept defeat, that talks in themselves could not be an end, that there had to be not only a time-frame but also substance. How long could Israel fool Palestinians and the world by agreeing to something, refusing to implement it, and then offering its partial implementation as a concession? If Netanyahu had learned this technique from a succession of US administrations, he was a good pupil. The parallel was obvious.

The US did not pay its United Nations dues as a lever to force through its agenda. Once it secured the agenda, it wanted more. Then it offered to pay a part of what it owed the UN and its agencies in instalments on the further condition that future dues should be reduced by a formula devised by itself and other Washington-imposed conditions met.

To Netanyahu's discomfiture, Sheikh Yassin would now be watching.

A Pervasive Gloom

Leaving aside the theatricals and posturing that were so much a part of what was once a peace process, the United States and the world needed to ask hard questions before West Asia would be sucked into a new major confrontation. First, the hold the American Jewish lobby had over US policy on West Asia, quite apart from strategic interests, had never been demonstrated as clearly. Second, using Arafat as a prisoner of the Madrid process spawning the Oslo accords, which had been rejected by Israeli Prime Minister Benjamin Netanyahu, could only encourage Hamas to take over the effective leadership of Palestinians.

If the much debated American plan calling for Israeli withdrawal from a ludicrous 13 per cent of the occupied West Bank was any indication, the Clinton administration had settled on the Jewish state retaining the bulk (some US reports suggest as much as 60 per cent) of the occupied West Bank and the whole of occupied Arab East Jerusalem in the "final status" talks that Washington and Tel Aviv wanted soon, spiking the agreed third phase of Israeli troop deployments. The American expectation obviously was that Arafat would finally cave in to American demands.

No measure of public relations tactics, such as Hillary Clinton's studied call for the creation of an eventual Palestinian state with few attributes of national sovereignty on what crumbs of occupied territory the Palestinian Authority was given, would resolve the central crisis in the Palestinian–Israeli equation. Netanyahu had already rejected the land-for-peace basis of the Madrid process.

By any standard of justice or fair play, the Americans, who were the main supporters and protectors of the Israeli state, should be the last party to mediate between Palestinians and Israelis. But the power of the United States (and the American Jewry in it) became unchallenged after the end of the Cold War. The Israelis, both Labour and Likud, exulted and used the new status of their friend and protector to demolish the Palestinians and their right to a viable state.

In recent times, Europeans had tried to have a look in on the Israeli–Palestinian equations, but their efforts had been half-hearted and timid, conscious as they were of the Israeli approach, supported by the US, to rebuff any but partisan American mediation. The European moves, largely symbolic as they had been, had veered between the outspoken French stance to Britain's almost total identification with the American recipes. Europeans said that as the main economic aid-givers to the Palestinians, they should have a greater say in the unravelling of the Madrid process, but the Americans brushed off such statements with contempt, knowing that the European Union had a long way to go before it could influence political and strategic events in West Asia.

Russian Weakness

Russia, which was beginning to look at its interests in West Asia, if only for the longer term, was woefully weak and was in no position to be an effective brake on American partisanship for Israel. President Boris Yeltsin's moves had been largely symbolic, in helping halt a new threatened American attack on Iraq, in dealing with Iran and in speaking out in the UN Security Council. It was, however, not lost upon the Palestinians and Arabs that Russia was only too prone to cave in to US fiats in the end, as the placing of Russians troops under American and Nato command in Bosnia demonstrated as well as bowing to Nato's eastward expansion at Moscow's expense.

The burden thus fell on the Palestinians' neighbours, the Arab world and Iran (Turkey's relations with Israel would seem to rule it out) to rescue the region from a looming confrontation.

What the Arab world could do was to help extricate Arafat from the impossible situation he found himself in. The Hamas leader Sheikh Ahmed Yassin was seeking to place the problem in perspective by his current tour of the region. The truth is that the basis on which Arafat accepted the Oslo agreements had been entirely repudiated by the Israeli government and by participating in the charade of Israeli withdrawal from 13 per cent of occupied land Netanyahu was making a show of rejecting, he was giving credence to a phony American ploy.

The problem before the Palestinians and the larger Arab world was what kind of a Palestinian state would come into being. Would it be a cartoon state enjoying little more than municipal powers lying supine at the mercy of Israeli guards and army, a Bantustan to wit? Even the Labour leader Shimon Peres had suggested that an eventual Palestinian state had to be demilitarised. Would Israel alone have the right to armed forces? And if a genuine Palestinian state enjoying sovereignty was to come about, it could not be like Swiss cheese.

Arafat had been warning that the failure of talks would lead to grave consequences. Both Tel Aviv and Washington seemed immune to these warnings from the PLO leader. Only when this warning was supported by the Arab world and the Hamas movement, now gaining in popularity among Palestinians, would the US and Israel sit up and take notice.

War and 'Peace'

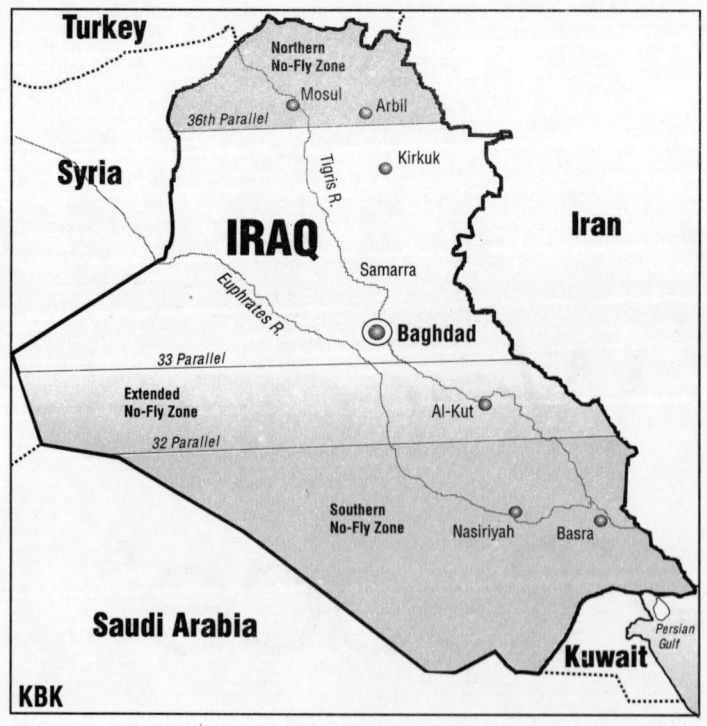

A Time Bomb

More than two months after the Iraqi invasion and annexation of Kuwait, the prospects of war had receded. But all the peace formulae being floated had an implied, if not explicit, linkage with the Israeli occupation of the West Bank and Gaza Strip.

Diplomatic moves on the Gulf crisis continued and we were treated to new doses of propaganda. The key to a resolution of the crisis was President Saddam's withdrawal from Kuwait, the French having stretched the point by suggesting that initially he declare his intention to withdraw. But much as President François Mitterrand feared that a direct link between the Iraqi withdrawal and a resolution of the Israeli occupation of Palestinian territories would complicate the problem, such a linkage had already come to exist.

Indeed, Yasser Arafat might have bet on the right horse after all, despite displeasing the Egyptians and angering the United States, from his point of view. The intefada in the Israeli-occupied territories was showing signs of tapering off. All the concessions Arafat's mainstream Fatah faction had made to move the peace process forward had led to a dead end.

The United States suspended its dialogue with the PLO over its failure to condemn the attack on Israeli targets. And it seemed that Arafat had run out of options, with nothing to show for his concessions and the radical wings of the PLO gathering strength. Arafat saw his opportunity in Saddam's invasion of Kuwait and even as he peddled peace formulae, he had hitched his bandwagon to Saddam's for his own purposes.

Arafat had also divined the mood of the bulk of the Palestinians as the pro-Saddam demonstrations in the Israeli-occupied territories and in Jordan revealed. The fact that Saddam, in an effort to get out of the corner he had painted himself into, sought to link his indefensible action to the Israeli occupation of Arab lands was an added bonus for Arafat. And as it happened, the killing of Arabs over the temple controversy in Jerusalem brought the Palestinian agenda to the world stage.

There could be no two opinions about the fact that by invading and annexing Kuwait, Saddam had indulged in a totally unacceptable action. But in the process, he had caused enough ripples to change the contours of the West Asian scenario. In addition to unfreezing the Palestinian issue, he was banking on the adverse Arab reaction to the large Western, particularly US, military presence in the region. That American troops were in the holy Muslim state of Saudi Arabia, was a particularly evocative issue. And the Iraqi rhetoric—on how the wealthy Arabs, specially in the Gulf states, used their money—was combustible stuff.

Israeli Distance

Israel had been careful in keeping its distance from the Gulf crisis and the United States had been equally cautious in not involving Israel. There was no profit for either of these two countries in linking Arab anger over the continuing Israeli occupation of the West Bank and Gaza with the question of the Iraqi annexation of Kuwait. But the link was in the process of becoming firmer.

Thanks to the new equations between the superpowers, the United Nations, in particular the Security Council, was working more effectively than it had done for a long time. This meant that if the succession of Security Council resolutions slapped on Iraq had to be implemented, so should the resolutions asking for Israeli vacation of the occupied territories. A continuing PLO offensive on this front was to be expected.

Besides, if peace was the preferred option in getting Iraq to withdraw from Kuwait, a face-saving formula for Saddam had to involve a commitment to move the Israel–Arab question to the front burner. One way of accomplishing this would be to call a West Asian peace conference, a concept bristling with problems because the role of such a conference and the Palestinians' representation on it were contentious issues.

The Israeli right wing had been strengthened in its belief that Saddam's action was part of an Arab pattern and no concessions on territory could be made. Indeed, a legitimate question that could be asked was why a wrongdoer who had "stolen" a country should be given a face-saving formula. The answer was that, given the complexities of West Asia, the repercussions of Saddam's action had taken in a wider gambit and the unresolved problems of the Arab–Israeli divide would merely exacerbate an already explosive situation.

The War Option

Perhaps the Americans had reduced their room for manoeuvre by hesitating to undertake a "surgical" strike on Iraq in the first week after the invasion. The UN Security Council's moves on Iraq had been a striking demonstration of the world organisation's ability to act in unison. By the same token, Washington would be breaking ranks if it were now to adopt the war option without the sanction of the Security Council. And there were divisions in the ranks of the five permanent members.

Some good would have come out of evil if Saddam's misadventure were to lead to the beginning of a resolution of the Arab–Israel enmity. Israeli society was split down the middle on making peace with the Arabs, and Kuwait's annexation had understandably strengthened the hardliners' hands. The doves in Israel were for the land-for-peace formula, but it would be wrong to underestimate Israeli fears.

The main Israeli fear was that hemmed in as it was by Arab states, its original borders were insufficient to offer protection. Second, Israelis believed that though the Arabs might formally accept their country's inviolability, the desire to throw them into the sea was ever present.

Obviously, any ultimate solution must comprise major powers' guarantees for Israel, but the Israelis must first resolve their internal contradictions. In the longer term, Israel's future could only lie in trading territory for peace because the continuing occupation of the West Bank and Gaza Strip was sapping its moral strength and posing impossible ideological problems.

A West Asian conference was the answer inasmuch as it could be a generally acceptable starting point. Besides, such a conference should have a referral role although Israeli sensitivities over giving it too much power had to be accommodated. Individual talks between Israelis and Palestinians and others could then move ahead. Israeli fears over including outside Palestinians posed problems, but they were not insurmountable.

The Israeli right wing's fear was that once the peace process started in earnest, it could only go one way: towards a loss of territories Israel occupied. This was true, but the other option, of hanging on to the territories, would become increasingly counter-productive for the moral and material well-being of the Jewish state. The question of East Jerusalem's future was somewhat different from that of the West Bank and Gaza.

So, while the Gulf time bomb was ticking away, Arafat's gamble of siding with Saddam might still pay off. With the world changing as dramatically as it had, even West Asia might see some peace in the years ahead. The explosive mix of mountains of gold in the form of oil, the minority nature of most regimes in the area and the major world powers' interest in ensuring supplies of oil did not give much cause for optimism. Perhaps Saddam might still go down in history as the Arab leader who helped give the Palestinians their land.

The Score Card

When Iraq walked into Kuwait to seize it and annex it, it triggered a series of wide-ranging consequences. First, there was the question of one country's conduct in overrunning and capturing another without provocation. Then there was the danger it represented to the United States and the West and Japan of an Iraqi regime with regional ambitions seeking to corner a large slice of the world's oil. Third, Israel and its protector, the United States, feared that the balance of forces would be tilted against them.

It was clear that President Saddam had overplayed his hand. Having fought the eight-year war with Iran, which ended in a stalemate, Saddam was left with a million-strong army and a large debt. The simplest solution, he thought, was to grab the prize of Kuwait, with hundreds of billions of dollars to its credit and a bountiful oil wealth. Iraq sought to justify its seizure by its historical claims to the territory.

Where Saddam miscalculated was to underestimate the consequences of his reprehensible action on the post-Cold War world. Thanks to the dramatic changes in the Soviet Union and Eastern Europe, the superpowers were no longer adversaries in the old sense. In the intricate web of relationships President Mikhail Gorbachev was building with the United States and the West, he had no option but to condemn the Iraqi action and go along with the US in a series of resolutions passed by the United Nations Security Council to bring Iraq to heel.

The Soviet Union had been the traditional ally of and supplier of arms to Iraq. But in the new era of *glasnost* and *perestroika*, Moscow could not but criticise the indefensible Iraqi action underlining President Saddam's isolation.

The US response to the Iraqi action was immediate and severe. Saudi Arabia and the other Gulf states were sufficiently frightened of Iraq to permit the stationing of American troops. Over the weeks, since the Iraqi invasion of Kuwait, the Americans had built up an impressive array of forces in Saudi Arabia and, together with the other Western powers, the biggest armada in the Gulf and surrounding seas since the end of the last war.

But the American action, even as it sought to enforce the United Nations-mandated sanctions against Iraq, had received a wider acceptance by virtue of Washington's ability to take the Soviet Union and the other three permanent members of the Security Council with it at each stage of the calibrated offensive against Iraq. The UN Security Council had condemned the Iraqi invasion, had asked it to withdraw from Kuwait, had imposed mandatory sanctions against it and had finally given the member countries with forces in the region the right to use force to implement the sanctions.

Divided Arabs

The Arab League was split down the middle by the Iraqi action. Kuwait's ruler in exile was understandably exercised, and it was left to Egypt's President Mubarak to try to ward off the inevitable. At an emergency Arab summit called by him in Cairo, he failed to avert a split and had to remain content with a majority decision authorising an Arab force to go to the aid of Saudi Arabia.

In view of Egypt's close economic and military relationship with the United States, President Mubarak was under pressure to provide the Arab component of a multinational force in aid of Saudi Arabia. Apart from Egypt, Morocco and Syria had chipped in with token forces of their own.

Indeed, the crisis caused by Saddam's action had made strange new alignments in the Arab world. Syria, considered the scourge of the West, had sided with Egypt and, indirectly, the United States. King Hussein of Jordan, viewed as the traditional ally of the United States, titled towards Saddam until brought in line by the United States. And Arafat, leader of the mainstream faction of the Palestine Liberation Organisation, had sided with Iraq, rather than Egypt.

Saddam took two important steps in seeking to surmount his isolation. He sought to contrast the West's reaction to his action to its continuing tolerance of the Israeli occupation of the West Bank and Gaza Strip and asked for the withdrawal of Syrian troops from Lebanon. Second, he sought to neutralise Iran's hostility by giving up captured territory and prisoners of wars and its claim to the whole of the Shatt al-Arab waterway. He thus swallowed the humiliation of telling his country and its army that the eight-year war and the millions dead were a futile adventure.

Saddam was seeking to exploit two evocative themes in trying to win popular Arab support over the heads of the leaders of their countries: the anti-Israel feelings and the anti-American sentiments. That he had succeeded in this task in a measure was revealed by the pro-Iraqi demonstrations in the Israeli-occupied territories, in Jordan and in other Arab countries. Besides, the stationing of American forces in Saudi Arabia was unpopular with Arabs.

Iraq's muscle-flexing and invasion and annexation of Kuwait had been particularly unfortunate for countries like India. There were half a million Indians in the Gulf countries—170,000 in Kuwait alone. Forty per cent of the Indian oil imports came from Kuwait and Iraq and India's political relationship with Iraq had been traditionally close because Saddam, for India, represented a secular force in a region increasingly coming under the sway of fundamentalist forces. For all these considerations, as also because of the minority character of the National Front government, India's official reaction had been muted.

India was worried on another count. Pakistan had been quick in agreeing to provide a token military contribution for the multinational force in Saudi Arabia. With the withdrawal of Soviet troops from Afghanistan, Pakistan had lost its status of a frontline state in American eyes. The Indian apprehension was that it would again stake its claim and receive new American weapons as a reward.

The Israeli Link

What of Israel? Israel was initially pleased with the deeper divisions in the Arab world, but it did not take its leaders long to recognise the dangers. Saddam's ostentatious linking of Israeli occupation of Palestinian territories with his own blatant disregard for international law meant that the Arab–Israel divide had again come to the fore.

With Israel being ruled by the rightist Likud government, the US-sponsored peace process had stalled for some time. Arafat was placed in a particularly difficult position because he had made a series of concessions which yielded precious little. Besides, the Americans suspended their dialogue with the Palestine Liberation Organisation on the plea that the organisation had not condemned a PLO-sponsored terrorist act and had not taken the necessary disciplinary measures.

With the kind of military presence the United States and other Western countries had in the region, a war was an ever-present prospect. But the efforts of the UN secretary-general and many of the Arab leaders were directed at finding a peaceful way out.

Iraq would have to withdraw from Kuwait either way. The Arab effort was to find a face-saving formula for Saddam which might gave him some fringe territorial concessions. It seemed unlikely that the United States would agree to any formula which sought to reward Saddam, in however symbolic a fashion, for his blatant aggression.

Much of the world's attention was directed towards future American aims in the region. The maximalist American position was to see the political demise of Saddam, but if he agreed to withdraw from Kuwait unconditionally, the US could hardly insist on Saddam going. The hope, of course, was that the inner dynamics of political forces in Iraq would see Saddam ousted.

But once the US had succeeded in achieving its objective of seeing Iraqi troops out of Kuwait and the restoration of the old regime, would it insist on keeping its forces in the region on a long-term basis? Judging by the kind of force build-up, it was taken for granted that a significant American military presence would remain in the area for a considerable time.

If there was a war, its aftermath would necessitate an American presence to help reorder relations. But even in the event of the resolution of the Gulf crisis without resort to force, the process of readjustments in the region would take time—a period during which Americans would prefer to remain in the region.

The oil wealth that had brought unprecedented prosperity to West Asia has also brought with it the attention of the United States and the other major powers. It was in the interest of the West to cut to size the ambitions of Saddam as it was formerly in its interest to help Iraq against Khomeini's Iran. But Iraq as a regional superpower would not find favour with Iran or Egypt, to name two countries of the region.

What Saddam might have succeeded in achieving, whatever the fate that awaits him, was the reopening of the Israel–Arab issue and in highlighting the precariousness of the thrones many of the traditional rulers in the area occupied.

On the Brink

Two facts compelled attention as the world teetered on the brink of war in the Gulf. President Saddam Hussein had bitten off more than he could chew. Second, whatever the tortuous paths events in the coming days and weeks would take, West Asia could not revert to what it was before Iraq's totally unacceptable invasion of Kuwait.

However distressing Iraq's original action, the near universal condemnation of the move and the induction of a United States-led armada in the Gulf, in addition to American soldiers, now joined by those from Egypt and Morocco, in Saudi Arabia, meant that this was a hand President Saddam could not win. Apparently, the Iraqi President underestimated world reaction and the consequences of changes in the Soviet Union and the end of the Cold War.

Saddam's two recent moves showed his dilemma. One was to seek to link Kuwait with an Israeli withdrawal from the occupied territories. The other was his dramatic decision not only to withdraw from the occupied Iranian territory and release its prisoners of war but also to accept the division of the Shatt al-Arab waterway, the ostensible reason for starting the eight-year Iran–Iraq war.

President Mubarak's desperate last-minute effort to ward off the inevitable—the induction of a large American and Western military presence—served merely to deepen the divisions in the Arab world. Egypt's compulsion in responding to the American demand for a multilateral force for Saudi Arabia was all too apparent. The resolution in the hastily convened Arab summit in Cairo was the fig-leaf for sending Egyptian troops to Saudi Arabia.

President Saddam, on the other hand, had few cards to play. There were the evocative salience of the large-scale American military presence in the region and the Palestinian issue. He had now used both cards to advantage by calling for opposition to the alleged desecration of holy Muslim places by American troops and by suggesting that the United States in particular and the West in general had double standards, doing little to get the Israeli-occupied territories vacated while coming down on him like a ton of bricks.

Throwing a Hand

It was ironical that the Iraqi regime which, despite its nature, was in a measure a modernising influence vis-à-vis the fundamentalists should appeal to the Arab world in the name of religion. And it was a measure of President Saddam's vulnerability that he should throw away his hand in Iran's favour after eight years of war and millions of deaths in order to neutralise, if not befriend, his old enemy.

As the pro-Iraq demonstrations in several Arabs countries had shown, Saddam had a constituency. And to a Palestine Liberation

Organisation on the verge of desperation in failing to move the peace process forward, he had brought new hope by taking the issue again to the front burner, admittedly for his own reasons.

Although President Saddam could hardly hope to keep his Kuwaiti prize, his actions and the world's reaction had consequences far beyond the issue of Kuwait. The invasion of Kuwait was a wrong move because, despite Iraq's historical claims, capturing a country by force without any provocation was not an option open to any nation in the post-World War II world. At the same time, the vulnerability of ruling families sitting on mountains of oil wealth had been brought home.

The world had acknowledged that after Iran sued for peace in the eight-year war, Iraq had emerged as a formidable regional player, with a million-strong battle-tested army. By his impulsive move, Saddam had contributed towards nullifying his country's advantage. He could not expect to win a hot war and any peaceful solution to the crisis could only be on the basis of a total Iraqi withdrawal from Kuwait.

But the shock of the Iraqi action had destroyed the fragile stability of the Gulf states which would have to widen public participation in governance and perhaps devise merger plans among themselves. The Gulf Cooperation Council had proved to be a broken reed. It could not protect a member country from being annexed, and its most important member, Saudi Arabia, had itself to seek the protection of the United States.

Bonus for Iran

Iran, which had received a bonus out of the crisis created by Iraq, could perhaps proceed with building bridges to the West with a greater measure of confidence. Inevitably, Iran would be largely domestically oriented in the immediate future. The ruling elite remained divided and the Khomeini revolution, which stirred the Muslim world, had also left a bitter legacy incompatible with the building of a powerful modern state.

Egypt's dilemma had perhaps been the sharpest in the Gulf crisis. President Mubarak achieved something of a miracle by rehabilitating his country in the Arab world, which had ostracised it for years after its separate peace with Israel. That he could achieve it in tandem with a continuing close arms and economic relationship with the United States—still the Satan for many in the Arab world—spoke of Mubarak's political acumen.

The cruel dilemma Mubarak had to face was that given the inevitable escalation of anti-American feelings in the Arab world and being on one side of the Arab divide, he would find it increasingly difficult to retain the middle ground he had chosen to enhance Egypt's profile. After Camp David and the close military and economic relationship with the United States, Mubarak could not be another Nasser; in a rather novel way, Saddam was trying to take on that mantle for his own purposes.

What of Syria, the lone Arab supporter of Iran in the eight-year war? An evolution of Syrian policy had been in progress for some time; witness Damascus' publicised role in the release of Western hostages. It seemed that the Syrians had decided that flexibility, rather than hardline anti-Americanism, was a better approach for winning friends and influencing people. The Israel issue concerned Syria in a very direct manner because the Israelis had annexed the Golan Heights and Syrian troops remained in Lebanon.

The Israelis, for their part, could derive little comfort. Whatever Saddam's motivations, his linking the invasion of Kuwait to the continued Israeli occupation of Palestinian territories had brought the Arab–Israeli divide to the fore. There could only be further pressures on Israel to make meaningful moves towards resolving the core issue, once the Gulf crisis was resolved.

Second, the Israelis had to take into account the growing radicalisation of the Palestine Liberation Organisation. Arafat possessed an enviable political acumen and could change his stance again if it suited him. But the fact that he had chosen to go with Iraq, rather than Egypt, and the widespread pro-Iraqi demonstrations in the occupied territories showed that the pendulum was moving away from moderation in the PLO.

President Saddam could claim that he had set in motion a chain of events which would change the face of West Asia. True, but the costs would be incalculably high for himself, for Iraq, for the region and the world.

Alice in Wonderland

As the United Nations' imposed deadline for Iraq's withdrawal from Kuwait had only 24 hours to go, an atmosphere of unreality prevailed in the capital of Iraq. Many Iraqis believed that a miracle would happen and there would be no war despite the apparent failure of the Perez de Cuellar mission. Our long-delayed flight from Amman had arrived just before the UN secretary-general left Baghdad.

The National Assembly session met the next morning to hear standard perorations. There was no give in the Iraqi position although some sign of flexibility was apparent in the official *Baghdad Observer* bringing up the question of Iraqi withdrawal from Kuwait in the context of President Hafiz Assad's appeal to President Saddam to defuse the crisis.

The atmosphere in Baghdad had an eerie feeling of normality. Bright lights and neon signs lit up the shopping districts and malls. The profusion of Saddam's immense portraits and an over-sized statue were flood-lit at night. Government-run television had adulatory sequences of the President and the righteousness of his cause.

Indeed, on the surface it had appeared to an outside observer that foreigners, rather than Iraqis, were afraid of the morrow although some reports suggested a movement of Iraqis to the mountains and the desert. Many diplomatic missions had closed down or had a nominal presence while a small staff at the Indian mission was coping with anxious inquiries from those wanting to leave.

Two French correspondents arrived with gas masks. Indian professionals were searching for ways to get out before the deadline. The 10-member team from the National Building Organisation was sent back home from Jordan and was almost in tears. Jordan had imposed new restrictions on transit stay. A 16-member Indian component of a peace team to join an international group on the Iraqi–Saudi border was sent home and not allowed to stay another night in Amman.

An Alice in Wonderland atmosphere prevailed. It was as if the world had been turned upside down. Ask any Iraqi and he would tell you how unjust the world was and how the West in particular, led by the United States, was observing double standards in relation to Iraq and the Israeli occupation of Palestinian land.

In a mirror image of how the West, the US in particular, looked upon President Saddam, a popular perception in Baghdad was of a particularly evil George Bush leading the world to war.

A Media War

Until the bombings started, the eighth floor of the Information Ministry in Baghdad was where all the action was. There in a room plastered with the mandatory photographs of President Saddam sat a thick-set man who went by the simple appellation of Saddoun. He performed his job with panache. Like some of his colleagues, he was overworked as the world's press descended on him to seek interviews with dignitaries, permission for television crews to operate and for extension of visas.

Earlier requests for interviews made through the Iraqi embassies were dismissed out of hand. One was required to make a fresh application for meetings and requests for interviews with the President were invariably turned down. One of the mysteries of the Iraqi information effort was the press room that never materialised. We were put up in the Al Mansour hotel next to the Information Ministry, rather than at the Al Rasheed where most of the international press was staying, because we were told that a press centre with all communication facilities would be set up in our hotel.

Days went by and there was no press centre, which would be set up, we were later told, in the Information Ministry. The only way to get reports out was by long-distance telephone or the telex facility in Al Rasheed hotel. Other non-official telex and fax facilities had been withdrawn. Al Rasheed accepted dollars in cash or American Express cards; it did not honour international telex credit cards. Except for American Express, all travellers' cheques were taboo. Much as the United States, in particular President Bush, was the hated symbol of Western might, the dollar ruled Baghdad.

Like much else in Iraq, the Information Ministry was a bundle of contradictions. At one level, it was an efficient propaganda tool, but there was surprising inattention to the needs of the press. There was no system of periodic briefings, no official communiqués for the visiting press. The official *Baghdad Observer* was our bible unless a dignitary was trotted out as the spokesman. The day of the first bombing raids and on subsequent days the *Observer* failed to appear although Arabic language newspapers continued to be published.

Poor Relations

The print media were poor relations in the information war. All attention was paid to television networks and even when we were included in interviews, we became mere adjuncts to the television anchormen in jackets and tie, as opposed to the rest of the media dressed for the most part in unkempt jeans and windcheaters.

It was again for television cameras that the one event of the day was chalked out. On January 15, the UN deadline for Iraqi withdrawal from Kuwait, television crews had a field day as massive staged demons-trations were held in Baghdad and other cities to carry the messages of defiance and peace. Effigies of Uncle Sam were burnt as was the American flag as peace volunteers from the West helped the Iraqi propaganda effort by cheering the blood-curdling calls for a holy war.

The Cable News Network was as much of an ubiquitous presence in Baghdad as the peace groups. Australians, Germans, Americans and men and women from many other nationalities would sidle up to the press in Al Rasheed to present their naïve peace formulae or to get messages out to their relations at home. We called them "peace loonies" because one could have little respect for people who willingly became tools of a government propaganda effort.

On January 16, when the deadline passed and nothing happened, the Speaker of the National Assembly, Sa'adi Mehdi Saleh, was the spokesman for the day as he reiterated the official line of defiance while giving the news that Saddam would personally lead the military operations in the event of a conflict. He was speaking for the benefit of television cameras as crews rearranged furniture and bric-à-brac for the best angle shot.

Outside, in the streets of Baghdad, it was as if a plague had decimated much of the population. The streets were empty, apartments forlorn and the most sought after vehicles were taxis as they sped loaded, taking all who could leave to the mountains or the desert, as far away from the capital as possible.

The routine was tending to become repetitive—calls on Saddoun on the eighth floor of the Information Ministry, the trek to the hotel, the taxi rides around a city still guarded by portraits of President Saddam dotted like mushrooms after copious rains.

War Begins

Then everything changed. The American air raids on Baghdad in the early morning hours of January 17 and the rattle of the anti-aircraft batteries pockmarking the city signalled the beginning of the Gulf War. After spending the night in the shelter of the Al Mansour, we discovered that there was no water in the bathrooms nor was there electricity.

Al Mansour was emptying by the hour. Journalists packed their bags either to head for the Jordan border or move into Al Rasheed. In view of its location, Al Mansour was simply too dangerous to be in.

Many journalists left. A friendly Spanish reporter came up to me to say: "It is a warning for us that we should get out". Those who left after the first bombing raids took two days to get to Amman. The border was closed for the day by the time they got there and the great exodus slowed down the caravans. On the way, air raid sirens caused further delays as cars detoured to the villages until the all-clear was sounded.

We journeyed to our mecca, the Information Ministry, that morning only to find the eighth floor out of bounds. After a time, Saddoun appeared in the reception room to announce that a bus would take journalists who wanted to leave up to the border. At the end of the morning, there was no bus, and reporters scrambled to hire taxis at exhorbitant prices to get out. Like the mythical press centre, the promised bus had vanished into thin air.

Telephone and telegraph connections were cut, censorship was imposed, and the only link to the world the privileged journalists had was through satellite link-ups, one belonging to the Cable News Network and the other to the BBC.

The Information Ministry moved to Al Rasheed hotel, in a sense. Saddoun was to be found in the hotel bomb shelter, his stubble growing by the day. He censored copy before television and other reporters journeyed to the hotel garden, where the dish was set up, to phone in their copy.

The Al Rasheed bathrooms were without water, the rooms were dark. For about $ 120 a day, we had the privilege of sleeping on the floor in the basement shelter.

The first bombing raids had won the admiration of all visiting journalists. The Defence Ministry headquarters had been bombed with precision and even more amazing was the surgical strike at the telecommunication tower, which had been sliced as with a knife. There had been no effective Iraqi counter-attacks, the anti-aircraft batteries seemingly firing to little purpose.

The fortunes and the mood changed on the next and subsequent days when the Iraqis demonstrated that they could bring down raiding planes and capture some pilots. The Information Minister, Latif Nusayyef Jasim, appeared in the foyer of the Ministry sporting a military cape and looking larger than life with his impressive moustache, to give the message: "We have demolished the myth of a short war".

Bomb Shelter

The Al Rasheed shelter had become our home. There was light, thanks to the special generator, although the bathrooms were inadequate and filthy. Television sets were turned on day and night for the entertainment of all. We did not have to watch them to know what was on. Every so often, a lilting tune showed a boy in a squeaky voice extolling the virtues of the great leader, Saddam Hussein, in song as the screens flashed images of the President with a child in his lap, the President being sung hosannas. One gesture of the President we found particularly endearing. It was a jerky hand movement in tune with the music, encouraging the people to go on singing his praises.

Al Rasheed was falling apart. The meals were skimpy, there was often no coffee at breakfast and bills had to be paid instantly to ensure that the diner would not disappear into the shelter when the sirens sounded. As an Indian journalist, I got special treatment from the Indian hotel staff, almost all of them now pining to return home.

Outside, in the streets, we were kings of the road. Except for an odd car and a taxi, the city had gone dead as we surveyed the damage caused by the latest raids. A tottering building partially caved in, neighbourhoods hit by a deflected bomb or cruise missiles, shops boarded up and the children who remained played on the deserted streets.

The fortunes of the war were apparent enough at Al Rasheed. On the morning of January 19, a notice went up. No credit cards of any description were accepted; even American Express cards had been given the go-by. Only dollars in cash were the accepted commodity. Western journalists were fully equipped; an Italian television anchorman had declared $ 30,000 in cash on arrival at Baghdad airport before it was closed.

Our travellers' cheques were little more than useless paper. A letter from the Indian embassy offering to settle our bills was treated with contempt. The embassy apparently did not have enough funds to give the two of us a few hundred dollars in cash in exchange for the dollar travellers' cheques we were carrying. I sought the help of a television crew member to change travellers' cheques for cash to be able to pay the hotel bill.

We had received our marching orders, the Iraqis having decided that international journalists were doing little good to the Iraqi propaganda effort. The television networks packed their mountains of equipment to leave behind as they headed for the border. They would probably never see their expensive equipment again. Only the CNN won a reprieve, its lone reporter phoning in censored copy from the garden of Al Rasheed.

This war, unlike any other, was the CNN war as the marvel of satellite television brought live coverage to homes in the world. The Iraqi Information Ministry was closely monitoring the CNN—a large dish in the Ministry's compound was a conspicuous sight—but after a time "The Gulf War Live " on CNN began to pall, as I discovered in Amman.

In propaganda terms, the Iraqis had the best of both worlds. They had maintained a world presence while tightly controlling what went out of Baghdad on CNN. But then censorship was a game all sides were playing.

My great regret on leaving Iraq was that Saddoun had turned hostile, presumably because of what I had been writing from Baghdad. For the press corps, before it was thrown out, Saddoun rather than Saddam was the symbol of an unnecessary war, despite his failure to keep his promises. Ultimately, there was no need for a press centre.

One of the treasured memories I have of the war is of Saddoun consoling a woman photojournalist who had been grilled by the security police. With his sardonic wit, he was telling her: "The trouble with you is that you give priority to your job, rather than your husband".

In a Bomb Shelter

In the shelter of Al Rasheed hotel in Baghdad during those first days of bombing by American and allied forces, it had become something like home. You carved out a few square feet of space and settled down to spend the night as best you could while the inevitable sirens blared and bombs fell outside.

Al Rasheed's shelter is an immense complex of rooms. Fate had brought a motley crowd of people together. There were hotel guests of various nationalities. Ambassadors still resident in Baghdad had foresaken their homes temporarily to seek the security of the shelter. The inevitable clutch of journalists tried to make their stay in the shelter each night as short as possible because they wanted to go out and observe.

The richer Iraqis had made the shelter their home, with several generations bunched together in groups. They wore a lost and forlorn look. And there were the hotel staff, many of them from the Indian subcontinent, whose families had left their quarters to live in the shelter. Mercifully, they were safe because a portion of the Al Rasheed staff quarters was burnt from the fragments of a missile or debris from Iraqi artillery fire. All that the staff lost was some property.

Inevitably, the subcontinentals stayed together—Indians and Bangladeshis and Pakistanis. A group of richer Indians living in Baghdad had finally moved to the hotel and had preferred to be in the section allotted to the hotel staff and their families, instead of the demarcated guest rooms. In the exceptional circumstances of Baghdad of those days, men and women from the subcontinent sought comfort in each other's company.

For the last day in Baghdad, Ramesh Chandran of *The Times of India* and I—the only Indian journalists left in the Iraqi capital—spent the night in the staff section to share experiences and exchange gossip. A Bangladeshi, wife of the non-functioning laundry in-charge, had prepared the evening meal and the family ate it with relish in their little corner.

The Indian group—most of them professionals or in business—was playing cards. Indians' passion for cards marks them out in any international setting. A sturdy Sikh told me he had lived 10 years in Baghdad and he lamented what had been lost as he and his group made plans for their trip out of Baghdad, Iraqi and Jordanian authorities permitting.

"Iraq was the best and richest country in the area", he said. "There was money to be made and there was wonderful law and order".

I plied him with questions on the kind of law and order he had in mind.

Iraqi Order

"I'll give you one instance", he said, warming to the theme. "A woman was driving her car and it stalled. A beat policeman or security man was soon on the scene—they are everywhere—and he tried to act funny. She reported the matter to the authorities. She happened to be an army man's wife and they do a lot for the army here. The man was traced and she was escorted by an official to the place where he was held. Her escort gave her a loaded revolver and asked her to shoot the man. She did not have the heart to shoot, so the escort took the revolver and shot the man dead".

There was no question that my shelter companion considered it exemplary punishment which had made the capital so safe for womenfolk. It was safe in other ways as well, I discovered—so safe, in fact, that the Indian community considered it prudent never to refer to President Saddam by name. He was called Uncle and everyone understood the code.

My interlocutor had his views on Kuwait as well, he being fully sympathetic to Iraqi positions. "I'll tell you something", he said. "A member of the Kuwaiti ruling family, when he came on a visit to Baghdad, used a 25-dinar bill, which had Uncle's picture on it, to wipe his shoes. That's how arrogant the Kuwaitis were. Leave aside the Kuwaitis, our Indians who lived in Kuwait thought they were superior to us here. They treated us like poor relations".

For the first time, a note of bitterness entered my shelter campanion's account. "Iraq is the richest country. It did not need Kuwait", he suggested.

The hotel staff from the subcontinent had other thoughts on their mind. It was how to get out of Iraq, with only a very few wanting to stay on in Baghdad till the bitter end. But they were, in a sense, prisoners of their employers. It was standard practice for employers in Iraq and the Gulf to retain the passports of their employees. The passports were kept locked up until an employee is permitted to leave, and he must obtain an exit permit from the authorities.

For employees on various rungs of the hotel hierarchy, the attraction of their jobs was the handsome bonus they received in free exchange they could remit home. After Iraq's invasion of Kuwait, the bonuses had been suspended and few placed reliance on the vouchers they received instead. And so many Indian and other employees hovered between hope that the hostilities would end soon and their desire to forget about their losses and retrieve their passports to head for home.

Outside the shelter, for us journalists, the clutch of Iraqi Information Ministry officials presided over by the looming presence of Saddoun and the taxi drivers hovering outside the hotel entrance were our main companions. The taxi drivers were demanding anything up to $ 5,000 to take us to the Jordanian border, and the rates went up as the Iraqi authorities gave us our marching orders.

I felt rather sorry for the Iraqi officials. They were minor functionaries in the hierarchy and were not authorised to give out news, even if they knew what was happening. The English-language *Baghdad Observer* failed to appear after the first night of bombing and on subsequent days and thus we were forced to rely on the Arabic-language press, suitably embellished with immense pictures of President Saddam and full of the rhetoric of defiance.

Empty Streets

On the empty streets outside, we toured the city in taxis—becoming scarce and more expensive by the day—to spot the buildings that had been hit in the latest bombing runs. The Defence Ministry headquarters and the telecommunications tower were the objects of the first day's strikes, but each successive bombing run left more buildings in ruins, some ordinary housing blocks also standing bent, with iron girders sticking out like entrails in a human body.

One early morning, we saw the spectacle of a huge fire lighting up the sky outside the hotel. It was a refinery which had been hit, and the flames rose higher as we marvelled at the precision of the missiles. The nearby conference hall, across the road from the hotel, had also been hit, presumably on the assumption that it was a communication centre. The hotel itself was safe, we all felt, because the CNN was there.

It was, for the most part, an unreal war. The bombs and missiles rained from the skies, usually in the hours of darkness, and those left in Baghdad through compulsion or circumstances—the journalists were there by choice—tried to go about their chores as best they could. Although the aim of the missiles was usually uncannily precise, there was often the odd civilian building hit, and people were killed.

Uncertain Bureaucrats

As the bombings continued, the Information Ministry officials looked more bedraggled, more preoccupied, more uncertain of what their jobs were. Before all but Peter Arnett of Cable News Network were told to leave, the CNN and British television were the major preoccupation of Iraqi officials. The rest of us did not count. For the Iraqis, pictures were more important than words. From their secure bunkers, Iraqi officials saw precisely what CNN was beaming to the world from Baghdad and how they could fine-tune their propaganda offensive. It seemed to us from the print media that the war was being fought as much on television as it was in the skies.

Before the bombings started in the early hours of January 17, we saw the city empty by the hour. The mood of the people who remained was one of resignation. Despite the brave words over the air waves and in the Arabic-language newspapers, there was little enthusiasm for the war. It was as if the people were helplessly playing their preordained roles. They had been through the eight-year war with Iran which had left half a million Iraqis dead out of a total population of some 18 million, and now the great leader and God had willed that Iraq must fight against the might of the United States and 27 other allied countries.

As I cruised round the city in a taxi after each night's bombing runs to see the new devastation, I felt sorry for President Saddam for the first time during my week-long stay. The immense portraits of the President standing in such profusion at every street corner were not floodlit, as they had been each night. It seemed that by plunging the omnipotent symbol of the Iraqi state into darkness, the Americans and their allies were making a political point more powerful than their bombs and missiles.

I was on one of the last Iraqi Airways flights from Amman to Baghdad before the war, and I asked a spirited Iraqi girl of Kurdish origin during the flight to explain to me how President Saddam could give up all he had won in the eight-year war with Iran. "Sometimes", she answered, "one has to make a smaller sacrifice for a bigger cause".

And what were her feelings about the Iraqi regime's use of chemical weapons on her people, the Kurds? I asked. Her answer was evasive. "I have not been there to find out what actually happened". she said.

I did not meet that girl again to ask her where the "bigger cause" had led Iraq. Perhaps she could not have answered that question.

Ordered Out

After being ordered to leave Iraq, I stood at the entrance of Al Rasheed hotel in the city, unshaven and unwashed for two days, waiting to negotiate with a taxi driver on the astronomical and rising prices for the five-hour ride to the Jordan border. I had by then spent three nights in the hotel bomb shelter, huddled with a motley group of people. Every inch of space was taken as we spread ourselves on the floor, with official security men carrying gas masks and guns ordering the impatient to remain in the shelter.

The expulsion order had come because of the general tenor of reporting which did not match the Iraqi rhetoric of defiance and victory. Although I could not get my reports out after the January 17 initial American bombing raids, my dispatches could hardly have pleased the authorities.

It was around 2.30 p.m. All but two cars holding correspondents and television crews with equipment had gone when a powerful blast right in front of the hotel brought the plate glass of the hotel entrance crashing down. I had flung my raincoat over my luggage and it was covered with glass fragments. All of us ran for our dear lives into the basement shelter, the faces of some Iraqi women ashen white; others, including an English woman reporter, were shell-shocked.

For us, marooned in the hotel for the most part, the war had never come closer. Chandran and I did not go right down into the shelter but waited behind its door to rescue the baggage, including the precious typewriter, a subversive commodity in Iraq. We took our courage into our hands and brought the luggage into the basement, but a box containing mineral water for the road journey remained standing. Finally, in a lunge, Chandran brought the box in. "Imagine, losing our lives for mineral water and luggage", Chandran remarked.

Neither of us was in a cheerful mood, but that was for other reasons. Apart from the distress we were causing our families by remaining in

Baghdad, we had not been able to send out our reports. All telephone and telegraph communications with the rest of the world had been cut and the only method of reaching the newspapers was through the satellite links of the Cable News Network and the BBC, which were horrendously expensive, ranging up to $ 500 for a short telephone message. And the price of leaving Baghdad was simply beyond our reach—the $ 215 a day granted by the Reserve Bank of India looked pitiful, compared to the thousands of dollars spent by Western newspapers and television networks at the drop of a hat. The Indian embassy, with a depleted staff under a chargé d'affaires, had not proved particularly helpful even when its telex line was working. After the morning of January 17, the embassy telephone and telegraph lines were not working, but it continued to maintain a wireless link with Delhi.

On the afternoon of January 19, it was an American cruise missile apparently aimed at the Islamic conference centre and the refinery behind it. Iraqi officials were quick to claim that they had downed an American aircraft. It was, of course, a morale booster for the Iraqis fighting a messy and unnecessary war.

Exit Order

Those correspondents who could not leave were given a night's reprieve—"leave at six in the morning", we were ordered. Driving at night on the road to Jordan was particularly risky, in view of the air attacks. It was eventually nine in the morning on January 20 that the three of us set out in a taxi—actually quite a luxurious car—over a billiard-like six-lane highway up to the border. There was Mike Kirsch of CBS News, through whose kindness we were able to make the journey, Chandran and I.

Kirsch had ordered the car for $ 3,000 and agreed to accept deferred payment from us for a share of costs. Baghdad was like a ghost town. There was very little traffic on the roads. We saw the top floors of a skyscraper under construction reduced to rubble. Along the way there were anti-aircraft batteries, hulks of bombed vehicles, a desert airfield strip by the roadside with three Iraqi fighters parked on it in full public view.

Across the border, after Iraqi customs had taken the film roll out of my camera in a meticulous search of the baggage, Kirsch hired another taxi, this time for $ 700 to take us to Amman. (Our hearts sank as we calculated the cost in rupees.) Jordanian passport formalities were cumbersome and time-consuming, and 140 km short of Amman, the taxi broke down in the middle of nowhere. Showing surprising consideration, cars and trucks stopped on being flagged, and one truck finally towed our taxi to the nearest township 20 kilometers away. There, after attempts quickly to charge the battery failed, our enter-prising driver produced some mechanics out of thin air, it seemed.

While we went to the nearest eatery whose menu ranged from soup to omelette—we ordered the latter which came inside a roti cut into two—the mechanics fiddled with the engine, and we were finally on the road again. It was 11.30 pm—three the following morning Indian time—when we reached our hotel in Amman. The good news at the end of the journey was that the CBS would foot the entire bill for the taxi rides.

War came to the Gulf suddenly, at 2.30 on the morning of January 17, seemingly taking the Iraqi authorities by surprise. President Bush had said that military action would come sooner, rather than later, but Baghdad was not prepared for an almost immediate reaction after the January 15 deadline for the withdrawal of Iraqi troops from Kuwait.

I was woken up at 2.30 in the morning by the stuttering of anti-aircraft batteries outside my hotel. Al Mansour Melia hotel was next door to two important targets, the Information Ministry and the television studios. In moments, the whole sky lit up and it was only after the first wave of precision bombing on selected targets that the siren sounded. After a pause came a second and subsequent waves, with the anti-aircraft fire and tracer bullets painting a pretty picture in the night sky.

The Defence Ministry headquarters was hit as were a refinery and the telecommunications tower. We huddled into the hotel's basement shelter, some of us in pyjamas, with a few foreign correspondents having succeeded in bringing in transistors. Many heads surrounded the tiny transistors as the BBC news and reports came on the air and President Bush's address placed the American action in perspective.

Peppy Music

On the local radio, there were incantations and, surprisingly, peppy music. But the biggest surprise of those early morning hours was the almost total lack of Iraqi response to the American and allied action. The anti-aircraft fire was largely ineffective, in view of the height of the bombing runs. Later in the morning, we tried to catch up on some sleep as it became clear at 5.30 that the bombing runs were over for a time.

In the morning, the city was being further denuded of its population as the spectre of war became more than a matter of rhetoric or diplomatic games. Private cars were piled high with essential belongings and taxis were packed like sardines to take people outside the city. There was no electricity and telephones went dead.

President Saddam, in a broadcast in the morning, was expectedly defiant and said the battle for liberating Palestinian lands had begun. He did not explain why he had not immediately carried out his threat of attacking Israel and Saudi Arabia.

It was not clear how crippled the Iraqi air force was after the pinpoint attacks on air and missile bases, but Iraqis were bracing themselves for a week or so of an increasing intensity of air attacks although the pattern suggested that American and allied forces would continue to be selective, concentrating on military and strategic targets, particularly in cities in Iraq.

The streets of Baghdad were empty, traffic lights did not work and taxis driving at a furious pace had a virtual run of the roads. Inevitably, taxi fares were raised ten-fold as the population became desperate to get out. The Indian chargé d'affaires and his skeleton diplomatic staff moved into the ambassador's residence, which had a basement.

After the surprise of the meagre Iraqi response to the initial American and allied bombing runs, the Saddam Hussein regime acted more to expectations on the morning of January 18 by launching somewhat symbolic missile attacks on Israel and Saudi Arabia.

This opened up the spectre of a wider conflagration, bringing in Israel into the conflict—an Iraqi aim—and shaking the Arab anti-Saddam coalition. But the Israeli response was measured and the American run of bombing raids on specific targets continued in Baghdad for the second day, causing civilian casualties, according to the Information Minister, Latif Nusayyef Jassim.

In a talk with correspondents that afternoon, Jassim expressed some satisfaction over the fact that by attacking Israel and Saudi Arabia, the initial American euphoria over the success of the first day's American raids had worn off. "We have demolished the legend of a short war", he declared. Declaring that "the computer has mistaken Iraq", the mustachioed Minister wearing a military cloak over his uniform, praised President Saddam by calling him twice "our hero, the great leader", rather modest praise in the Iraqi scheme of things.

One Week Later

The Iraqi claim of having destroyed the legend of a short war was obviously an exaggeration, but the first week's conflict in the Gulf War had demonstrated two things. The Iraqi capability to counterattack was far from destroyed and the aims of the two sides varied so greatly that there was a crucial link between the time-frame of the American-led operation and the political successes each side could achieve.

Apart from the massive air bombings that continued in Iraq and Kuwait by American-led forces, the war had been remarkable for the measured manner in which each side was conducting itself, despite the high level of rhetoric. The first victims of the war — two American and one British pilots — had been continuously shown on television screens in the Arab world. It proved the Iraqi point that notwithstanding the devastating fire power and accuracy of American and allied bombing raids, it was capable of bringing down American planes and capturing pilots.

Western strategists and experts had revised their assessments of how long the battle was likely to last. They are talking about months, rather than weeks. And much of the Iraqi diplomatic effort was concentrated on using this time it to try to convert the war into an Arab–Israeli confrontation. But Iraq was acting with deliberation as much as Israel because the consequences of a no-holds-barred war in the region were simply too horrible to contemplate.

A primary Iraqi aim was to bring Israel into the battle to break the Arab anti-Saddam coalition. But it was resisting the temptation of using chemical weapons even while lobbing missiles into Israel. In other words, even while trying to tempt Israel to get involved in the conflict directly, it was resisting turning the war into an Armageddon.

The horror of an Armageddon in the Arab world, as elsewhere, gave countries such as Jordan the opportunity to keep appealing for peace. As the battle was developing, there seemed little prospect of the main contestants immediately heeding Jordanian and other appeals. But Jordan was also a test case of how Arab opinion was evolving as the war took its toll. Peopled by a majority of Palestinians, Jordanians were passionately for President Saddam and equally passionately against President Bush. Indeed, the war had already produced the first legend in the Arab word, of 'Bush the Satan'.

Palestinians one met in Amman were too intelligent to believe that Saddam marched into Kuwait simply to help the Palestinian cause. They said that they were not "backing the winning horse" because no one knew the outcome. For the Palestinians, it was a question of using all available opportunities to place the issue of the continuing Israeli occupation of Palestinian land on the front burner. At the popular level, for many Palestinians, Israel was already engaged in the war and any number of Palestinians in Amman told me that Israeli planes were participating in the war with camouflaged American markings.

A Hero

On the political plane, President Saddam had already achieved some of his objectives. Saddam was a hero — more to the Arab world than to his own people. He had at the same time lit the fires of Arab nationalism which, in its new incarnation, had a strong and emotive religious element. This mix was powerful because it made it that much harder for those ranged against the Iraqi regime to maintain their positions. For instance, the semi-official *Jordan Times* said: "A great deal of our problem with the Americans, and to a lesser extent the Europeans, is that they have largely failed to understand us, and when they did not, their forces bombed some of us, only to hide the truth of what is happening from their people."

One worry of many Arab states, even those aligned against President Saddam, was that they did not want to see Iraq destroyed. The longer the war lasted, the more Americans would be tempted to try achieve their maximalist aims, to destroy the Iraqi military and industrial structure.

The Jordanian Tilt

As the Gulf War proceeded along a seemingly preordained course, Amman, the window on the war, waited tremulously for what the morrow might bring. The big question was whether Jordan would willy-nilly be sucked into a war whose dimension would change dramatically if Israel directly entered the fray.

The anti-American tinge to Jordanian views was unmistakable, but the official line, articulated by King Hussein and his administration, was to speak about American and allied actions more in sorrow than in anger. Crown Prince Hassan, the able spokesman for the regime, had warned of the great tragedy that might lie in store for the region and the world if the war took its logical course.

Of greater interest was the philosophical underpinning Jordanians were giving to justify Iraq's position in the Gulf War. For them, President Saddam's capture and annexation of Kuwait took second place because of the heavy American and Western involvement in the region. They suggested that Iraq was on the point of withdrawing from Kuwait after a few days but did not do so because of the arrival of American forces in Saudi Arabia. In their view, Saudi Arabia and Egypt panicked.

Intelligent Jordanians said that Saddam, whatever his deficiencies and the type of regime he had built in Iraq, had become the symbol of the Arab fight against the West. Jordanians traced the present events in the context of the rising wave of Arab nationalism, in alliance with Islamic fundamentalism, from the early eighties. For them, Saddam was mesmerising the Arab masses even more than Nasser was able to achieve in his heyday. Jordanians did not give up hope that Islamic fundamentalism, though essentially conservative in character, would eventually acquire progressive characteristics. Islam, in their view, had provided a nucleus for mounting protests against corruption and autocracy. Jordanians did not see any contradiction in seeking to assert Arab nationalism and evolve a form of pluralism and the repressive regime of Saddam Hussein.

Jordanian views were, in a sense, a throwback to the anti-colonial days of the fifties and sixties. They talked about the continued slavery of the Muslim Arab world and said that the Arabs were for Saddam because he had chosen to stand up and fight the West. In common with other Arabs, Jordanians talked about the Arab nation in the singular. To them, the concept was not a myth because there were underlying factors of unity.

The Regional Positioning

Turkey's decision to involve itself more directly in the Gulf War by allowing the use of its bases to the planes raiding Iraq and Kuwait had set alarm bells ringing in Greece, Cyprus and farther afield. Would Turkey now be assigned by the United States the role of the regional gendarme? it was asked. And what would happen to the Arab solidarity many were seeking to build on the wave of the new pan-Arab mood among the masses?

These were but two of the numerous questions that came to the fore as regional actors sought to reposition themselves while the Gulf War progressed. The contours of the future realignments were not entirely clear, dependent as they were upon how and when the war ended. But there were some indications of the form they would take.

The major countries in the region are Egypt, Iran, Syria, Iraq and Turkey, apart from Israel and the Palestinian movement that impinged on them all. Assuming that the war continued till the bitter end, Iraq would be out of the running for a considerable time as it rebuilt its sinews of industrial and military power.

The field in the short to medium term would thus be left to others. Turkey's interests seemed primarily to prove that it was a good North Atlantic Treaty Organisation member and deserved full membership and privileges of the European Economic Community. What concerned the Arab world more was whether it was hoping to revive a partial version of its imperial past—the famed Ottoman empire—by seeking to become a power of consequence.

Turkey remained on the periphery of the Arab heartland and future regional configurations would be decided in a larger measure by Egypt, Iran and Syria. Although Iran was not part of the Arab world, it remained an important player, and the fact that the new wave of pan-Arabism was riding on Islamic resurgence gave it the opportunity to deal itself into future configurations.

By the same token, the country of Ayatollah Khomeini could not take too kindly to Saddam Hussein's efforts to build himself up as the guardian of Islam.

Egypt was in a rather unhappy position, cast as it was in the role of the US's principal Arab supporter even as the Arab masses were being increasingly inflamed against the West by Saddam. In these circumstances, President Mubarak, who did a remarkable job in rehabilitating his country in the Arab world after Sadat's "heresy" of the Camp David accords, faced the ridicule and hostility of the Arab masses, if not their regimes.

Iraq's occupation and annexation of Kuwait had become a secondary question. Although Saddam's decision to couple his indefensible action with Israel's continued occupation of the West Bank and Gaza Strip was opportunistic, his motivation had receded in the Arab public mind because he had highlighted the fact that this cancer in West Asia had to be exorcised in order to resolve the region's problems.

Logical Decisions

Yasser Arafat's decision to desert Egypt, his favoured interlocutor until the Iraqi invasion of Kuwait, for Iraq and the anti-West coalition was logical. Any one who could place the Palestinian question on the front burner and use Islam and Arab nationalism against the West helped the cause of the Palestine Liberation Organisation.

The phase of moderation, symbolised by the close rapport between Arafat and Mubarak and the concessions made by the PLO, yielded poor returns. Whatever tragedies might befall Iraq in the coming weeks and months, Palestinians would be the gainers.

Israel came very much into the picture because the hardline approach of the Likud Government of Shamir frustrated all attempts to begin the process of peace. During my visit to Israel in 1990, I was struck by how the intefada movement had spurred an intense debate and divided the country down the middle. It was then the hope of many sober Israelis that changes in the leadership of the two main parties, Likud and Labour, by a new generation were imminent and would help begin the peace process.

Inevitably, a country unites behind the government at a time of peril, and the war was dramatically brought home to Israelis by an Iraqi Scud demolishing a neighbourhood in Tel Aviv causing many casualties and extensive damage. However, after the war, more Israelis than even before would question the wisdom of retaining the occupied territories at an enormous cost to Israel and the region.

This evolution would naturally take some time even as the short-term aim of the Israeli authorities was to gain more war material from the United States; thanks to the war, it had already acquired the Patriot missile interceptors.

Syria's President, Hafez Assad, was perhaps the best poker player in the region. He had chosen to join the anti-Iraq coalition to checkmate Saddam but had at the same time taken great care to distance himself politically from the Americans. Although he had already invited a swipe from Iraq on his Greater Syria ambitions in the guise of claiming a permanent overseeing role in Lebanon, he obtained the dividend of the US ceasing to support the Christian Lebanese general to give a chance to the Taif agreement on Lebanon to work.

Changing Mosaic

In this changing mosaic, the positions of Saudi Arabia and the Gulf states presented major problems because the further radicalisation of the Arab masses would trigger greater pressure for democratic change. How this change would come about would vary from one country to another and would be neutralised to an extent by the money power of these states. Partly, it would also depend upon the astuteness the ruling families demonstrated to give a measure of freedom to their citizens.

The irony was that, with his penchant for ruling autocratically with the support of an all-pervasive security apparatus, it was Saddam who should help bring about these portents for change. Indeed, the personality cult built up around him was in the class of Kim II Sung of North Korea.

Of greater import was the prospect of Arab unity, with two major regional players, Iran and Israel, being non-Arab, and Turkey seemingly more interested in securing its European moorings than to get too deeply involved in the divided Arab world. Pressures were likely to grow among the masses not only for greater democratisation but also for forcing their leaders to resolve inter-Arab differences.

The Nasser dream of building an Arab nation, which had fired the imagination of so many, proved to be ephemeral because of the all-too-apparent rivalries in the Arab world and because pan-Arabism was unable to fulfil the economic expectations of the people.

One argument of Saddam had struck a responsive chord in many countries, that rich Arab states should help out the less affluent. The rich rulers, particularly in the Gulf, would need to wind down their conspicuous consumption to avoid causing greater offence than they had caused.

President Saddam had set in train a whole chain of events he could have scarcely dreamt of when he decided to invade and annex Kuwait. That he was riding high in popular Arab consciousness was not in doubt. Most Arabs were convinced about the inequity of an international order which slapped a dozen United Nations resolutions to force Iraq out of Kuwait when the UN resolutions on Israeli occupation of the West Bank and Gaza Strip remained a dead letter.

Counting the Costs

So finally Kuwait was free, but the liberation of that country from Iraqi troops was but a small part of the story represented by the Gulf War. In the volatile region of West Asia an event such as the occupation of Kuwait by Iraq set off a chain reaction that ensured that things would not return to business as usual.

First, let us look at the international setting in August 1990. The world was congratulating itself on the end of the Cold War. The miracle of German unification was happening. The United States and the Soviet Union were set on a new course of friendly relations.

True, some of the revolutions in Eastern Europe were beginning to turn sour. Mikhail Gorbachev, the Nobel Peace Prize winner and the initiator of the momentous changes in the Soviet Union and the world, was running into a bad patch. His reforms, haltingly implemented, had brought about a grim economic crisis. And he had apparently not envisaged how the concepts of *glasnost* and *perestroika* would fuel separatist tendencies to threaten the integrity of the Soviet Union.

These were troubling events, but the euphoria of the great changes 1989 and 1990 represented had not quite worn off. After the long years of the Cold War and a world living by MAD (mutual assured destruction), the prospect of an era of peace and relaxation of tension was welcomed by all.

The world tended to forget that although the Cold War was dead, if not buried, the developed and the communist worlds had chosen to kiss and make up. Beyond these worlds lay the so-called Third World, with its myriad unresolved disputes, its poverty and historical tensions. As if to prove this point, President Saddam invaded Kuwait to begin a series of tragic mistakes and miscalculations that brought misery of Kuwait, to his own people and enveloped the region in the Gulf War.

The first major miscalculation Saddam made was to assume that the world would not take him to task for his indefensible act. The second was that he forgot that there was no countervailing Soviet force to the United States to help him tide over the crisis. The third mistake was in his misplaced confidence that by evoking the Arab–Israeli conflict and presenting it as one between Islam and Christianity, he would be able to split the anti-Iraqi coalition President Bush had assiduously built up.

Out of Touch

Having been in Baghdad during the first four days of American and allied bombing raids, the only explanation for President Saddam's miscalculations I could offer was that he was out of touch with reality. Democratic governance was not the rule in West Asia, but the kind of police state Saddam had built isolated him from the wider currents in the region and the world. He believed that after the eight-year war with Iran, a hefty debt to repay and a million-strong army with little to do, the solution to his problems lay in incorporating the oil-rich Kuwait to assert his hegemony in the region.

West Asia, sitting on much of the world's oil wealth, is no ordinary region. It had traditionally attracted the attention of the United States and the European powers. The Ottoman empire was cut up into states to be ruled by the European powers, and as the gushing oil wealth poured out, the United States, attaining unparalleled power after the end of the last world war, sought to secure its interests through a chain of pacts and arrangements.

The creation of Israel brought into being a new situation for the Arabs and Palestinians as wars were fought to settle scores. The United States made Israel its strategic ally, and although the Nasser era sent powerful waves of a pan-Arab movement, Arabs remained divided and Israel's acquisition and retention of occupied land on the West Bank and in the Gaza Strip, in addition to East Jerusalem and the Golan Heights, after the 1967 war became a new focus of Arab anger.

The Shah of Iran, who was beginning to play the role of a regional policeman with American blessing, was toppled by the hurricane winds of Ayatollah Khomeini's Islamic revolution. Indeed, it was the initial resulting confusion that tempted President Saddam to try to settle scores with Iran. Although Iraq, in the end, had the upper hand in the war, it took eight years for the war to end, and thanks to Saddam's misadventure in Kuwait, he was forced to give up all that he had won from Iran on a silver platter.

The sharpness of the American reaction to Iraq's invasion of Kuwait was principally because of Washington's perception that Saddam wanted to reorder regional relations against Western interests. For one thing, he would gain control of some 40 per cent of the region's oil wealth and with the military power he had been able to build up, he could threaten the network of relationships the US had assiduously built with such states as Saudi Arabia and, after the Camp David accords, with Egypt.

The United States chose to go through the UN Security Council route, rather than act unilaterally, because it wanted to buttress its threats with force. Given the state of relations with the Soviet Union and Moscow's preoccupations with domestic events and Western economic assistance, Washington was confident of securing its approval. Besides, with a China interested in rehabilitating itself in the West after the Tiananmen tragedy, Beijing's support could also be assumed.

The Americans, of course, had strong moral grounds to use force against the Iraqi occupation of Kuwait. One country cannot help itself to another in this day and age and cock a snook at the world. Indeed, the sense of shock over the Iraqi action was universal although assessments differed on how the goal of the liberation of Kuwait should be achieved.

As the merciless American and allied bombing raids pulverised Kuwait and Iraq, and President Saddam ultimately sued for peace in the hope of rescuing a part of his war machine and the basis of his own political support, the focus was increasingly on American war aims. It became obvious that in addition to freeing Kuwait, Washington was seeking to damage the Iraqi war machine to the maximum extent possible while attempting to create conditions for deposing Saddam.

American Aims

These larger American war aims made sense from the US perspective. A wounded Iraq, if its military senews remained largely undamaged, would continue to pose a threat to Kuwait and the so-called moderate Arab states such as Saudi Arabia and the other countries in the Gulf. Despite the kind of repressive regime Saddam ran at home, he had used subversive arguments such as sharing the oil wealth among all Arabs and people's rights and was attempting to marry his version of pan-Arabism to Islam.

With President Saddam having been humiliated and having failed to attain any of his major objectives, what were the prospects for the region? The United States had already come out with a tentative post-war scenario which sketched in broad terms the kind of security arrangements it would like to have. A key element in the plan presented by US Secretary of State James Baker was an underpinning by outside powers of a regional security system with such organisations as the Gulf Cooperation Council.

The Americans declared that they did not envisage the stationing of their ground troops on the Arabian peninsula on a long-term basis. But the obvious American goal would be to station naval and air forces sufficiently close to the area to protect its strategic interests and deter adventures of the Saddam variety.

Although Israel would remain a key American strategic ally in the region, it would have to remain outside the security arrangement. But the new system would have to reconcile the varying, and often conflicting, claims of the Arab powers and Iran and Turkey.

Iran took a high diplomatic posture in relation.to the post-war scenario. Indeed, Iran had been a major beneficiary of President Saddam's monumental errors. It had received full satisfaction on its claims, and the damage to Iraqi military and industrial power inflicted during the Gulf War was an insurance that it need not fear Iraq in the foreseeable future.

Turkey would expect some reward for permitting American and allied forces to use its bases while Syria would hope to increase its power and regional influence. Besides, it would be wrong to under-estimate Egypt, the traditional heart of the Arab world.

While the United States would seek to reconcile these rivalries and the place the Soviet Union should have in the region, two other issues would have an impact on the future. One was the all-important question of the Arab–Israel confrontation; the other the longevity of the new pan-Arabism Saddam had tried to build.

It was all very well to speak about the Arab nation in the singular, but one consequence of Saddam's invasion of Kuwait had been a deepening of fissures in the Arab world, with the Arab League split and some Arab countries fighting with American and allied forces, in however symbolic a fashion, to oust Iraq from Kuwait.

Beyond the region, the post-war scenario posed questions for India. In view of the dramatic assertion of American might, how strong would US presence be in the region? And assuming that the United States would be more, rather than less, visible in the area, how convergent or antagonistic would American and Indian aims be?

A New World Order

There was little euphoria in the Third World as the lessons of the Iraqi defeat were beginning to sink in. Each day brought new reminders of Iraq's continuing humiliation. This tragedy had two facets: the travails of the country and the wider consequences for the Third World.

It took the paranoia, cruelty and total miscalculation of President Saddam to get a coalition of some 30 countries, led by the United States, ranged against it. The Iraqi President not merely brought ruin to his country and Kuwait by invading and annexing the latter but also provided the US with an ideal opportunity to test its New World Order in relation to one country. With the exception of China, an American and European directorate in the shape of the permanent members of the UN Security Council is calling the shots. And Iraq had become a laboratory of experiments on the limits of sovereignty for a Third World nation.

The stiff cease-fire resolution on Iraq not merely specified that mass destruction weapons be taken out but ruled on permissible range of ballistic missiles. The terms of this resolution were being implemented, but beyond them Iraq had already been subjected to the concept of limited sovereignty. It had to swallow the bitter pill of the US and Britain providing a safe haven for Kurds in northern Iraq.

True, we live in an interdependent world, but abridged national sovereignty represented by such organisations as the European Economic Community was voluntarily arrived at for the common good, so were planned and hoped-for agreements on such issues as protection of the environment. In Iraq's case, not only was a rogue elephant sought to be disciplined but a new cosmology was being built to define the limits of sovereignty for a Third World country.

Draconian Resolution

Let us take a close look at the mammoth Resolution 687 under which the formal cease-fire came into effect. Iraq was required to "uncondi-tionally" accept "the destruction, removal, or rendering harmless, under international supervision" of all chemical and biological

weapons, all ballistic missiles of more than 150-km range, the destruction of all missiles capabilities, including launchers, and commit
itself not to acquire or develop nuclear weapons in the future.

These steps were justified not merely on account of Iraq's deplorable
record in the use of biological weapons and attempts to acquire nuclear
weapons as a lever of power but towards achieving two objectives:
establishing a nuclear weapons-free region in West Asia and "balanced
and comprehensive control of armaments" in the region.

Judging by the proposal put forward by the United States, both the
balanced and comprehensive nature of arms control were to be largely
determined by Washington, taking into account its security interests
and its strategic alliance with Israel. How a nuclear weapons-free zone
in the region could be created without bringing in Israel in more than
a symbolic fashion remained unexplained.

In a revealing testimony to the Senate Foreign Relations Committee,
a top State Department official had explained President George Bush's
arms control proposals. Apart from putting in place a regime of the
region's main arms suppliers, American arms sales were aimed at
stability, it was suggested, because they were "in the best interests of the
United States, the recipient states, and the cause of peace and stability".

A freeze was suggested on surface to surface missiles as also on the
production of nuclear weapon grade material, with all countries being
asked to subscribe to the Nuclear Non-Proliferation Treaty. This neatly
sidestepped the question of Israel's widely believed stockpile of nuclear
weapons but was in line with Washington's traditional policy of giving
its strategic ally in the region a superior military edge. Washington
was, of course, under no illusion that the process of arms control in
the region would be easy or quick. This would, in effect, mean that
Iraq would be one country that would be discriminated against for a
long time.

Some other aspects of Resolution 687 in dealing with a recalcitrant
Third World country were also worthy of note. For the first time, the
UN Security Council had directly decided to guarantee the inviolability
of an international boundary. This was, of course, related to the
agreement between Iraq and Kuwait signed in 1963, but nonetheless
was a path-breaker in its implications.

A number of consequences flowed from the experiment on Iraq.
The new rules applied only to the less powerful, perpetuating the
division between the Five (led by One) and the rest of the world. The
economically powerful countries such as Germany and Japan could
hope to graduate to honorary membership of the directorate, but not
others.

Besides, it was an open question whether a new Versailles Treaty
syndrome was being created in a part of the world already subject to
the historic Arab–Isreali confrontation. Unlike one defeated country

nursing its grievances, like in Germany's case in the past, Iraq's plight might find an echo in large parts of the Third World. If that were to happen, Saddam Hussein in defeat and amidst ruin would have the last laugh.

The Third World was, of course, in no position to respond to the new situation as it was shaping up. It was rudderless and disoriented, having lost the Soviet Union as a countervailing power to the United States. Besides, domestic crises had reached such proportions in many important Third World countries that they had little time or appetite to address wider questions of international polity.

India was in throes of a phase of transition that left it little time to grasp the nettle of problems flowing from a dramatically changing world. And we had seen the kinds of problems Algeria was beset with. Yugoslavia, the titular head of a Non-aligned Movement seemingly ready to bow out, was torn between its efforts to keep the country as it was and the growing irrelevance of NAM to its European orientation.

If the Third World were to acquire the feeling that the foolishness and paranoia of one leader in one country was being used to carve out a new world order to the disadvantage of the majority, the world would head for a new phase of instability. Frustration carries its own dangers, in a nation and in the international scheme of things.

Moving Towards Madrid

While the release of some Western hostages in Lebanon and hopes for the release of the rest had been in focus, events were gradually moving towards the proposed West Asian peace conference. There were compulsions on many sides to hold the conference and the active American involvement in the process was proof of the fact that its credibility was on the line.

In a sense, the Gulf War and the victory of US-led forces carried with them the moral obligation to address the continued Israeli occupation of Palestinian land. President Saddam made a vain effort to justify his invasion and annexation of Kuwait by linking his indefensible act with Israeli withdrawal from occupied land. But for the Arabs and much of the developing world, the United States could redeem its honour only by succeeding in getting Israel to accept the relevant United Nations resolutions.

Prospects for a new beginning in West Asia were more propitious than they had been for a long time because the end of the Cold War has meant that the major Arab countries had to evolve their future strategies without the countervailing power of the Soviet Union. The most dramatic change had been the Syrian position in accepting the American peace proposals while using Washington's benevolence to consolidate its position in Lebanon.

The Americans were careful in bringing the Soviets on board for the peace conference during the two powers' summit meeting in Moscow. The resumption of full diplomatic relations between the Soviet Union and Israel was on the cards, once the dates for the October conference had been agreed upon. Israelis had rightly argued that Moscow could not play an overseeing role without restoring diplomatic relations.

That said, some of the hurdles to convening the peace conference had still to be crossed. This was not surprising given the complexities of Arab policies, the deeper divisions in the Arab world caused by the Gulf War and the US strategic and military relationship with Israel. Besides, it was even open to question whether all the Arab states would want to see the emergence of an independent Palestinian state.

The two main hitches were the nature of the Palestinian representation and the defiant Israeli attitude in continuing to build Israeli settlements on the occupied West Bank. Israel objected to the direct participation of the Palestine Liberation Organisation and representation of Arabs from East Jerusalem, which it had annexed.

Some of these ambiguities remained to be cleared while others would be deliberately left undisturbed to get all the parties to the conference table. The issue of Palestinian representation, for instance, would have to be fudged, with the PLO approving a list without officially being participants. The agreed framework would, of course, be a joint Jordanian–Palestinian team.

The original concept of a United Nations-sponsored conference had already been considerably diluted, in view of Israeli objections. But it was still not clear what kind of a future role the conference would have. As far as the Israelis were concerned, the conference was a face-saving formula for the Arabs before they could get down to face to face talks with individual Arab countries and the Palestinians.

Opening Gambits

The peace conference would at best be the beginning of a long process. But its very convening would help defuse the Arab–Israeli confrontation up to a point. For a start, the Israelis were not even officially accepting the underlying concept of territory for peace and were giving their own unacceptable interpretations to the UN resolutions. What the Israelis had in mind was an autonomy package for the West Bank and the Gaza Strip, with a time-frame before further negotiations could be held with the Palestinians. Again, for the Israelis, East Jerusalem and the Golan Heights were non-negotiable.

At the talks these opening gambits would have to be tempered. It was, for instance, clear that Syria could not accept any arrangement which left the Golan Heights with Israel. In all likelihood, Israel would have to surrender the Heights, with cast-iron guarantees for its demilitarisation.

The East Jerusalem problem was more complex, striking as it did the religious chord on both sides and the fact that Israel had integrated it with West Jerusalem. Some special status for Jerusalem would have to be evolved. As far as the West Bank and the Gaza Strip were concerned, the time-frame for moving from autonomy to independence, with delimitarisation and possible confederation with Jordan, would have to be credible.

Hardline Israelis were, of course, totally opposed to the peace conference idea because they believed, with some justification, that once the process started, it could have only one end: the giving up of almost all, if not all, occupied territory. And they had convinced themselves that the interests of the Jewish state, living in a hostile neighbourhood, demanded the retention of all occupied land. By the same token, it was the hope of the United States and many others that once the process of individual talks between the Israelis on the one hand and the Arabs and Palestinians on the other started, the sharp edges of each side's proposals would begin to be rounded. There was, besides, an element of desperation on the part of Palestinians because the longer the process took, the stronger would be the Israelis' position since they were continuing to change the situation on the ground.

In essence, the United States was seeking to conduct an orchestra where individual musicians were playing discordant tunes. The central issue of the Arab–Israeli confrontation was overlaid with inter-Arab rivalries, the trauma of the Gulf War, the lack of enthusiasm of some Arab states for an independent Palestine and the overriding American strategic interests.

The United States was still trying to cobble together a security arrangement for the Gulf states whose precise contours remained to be defined. An American commitment to the security of these states was not in doubt but it had to determine how the presence of its ground troops would sit with Arab and Iranian susceptibilities. Despite the recent agreement among Egypt, Syria and the Gulf Cooperation Council, the Arab component in the security system was likely to be merely the icing on the cake.

Partly, the future scenario would be determined by the shape of things in Iraq. Washington was waiting for the fall of Saddam even as it continued to de-fang Iraq under United Nations auspices. While thus far defying all predictions about his impending fall, Saddam had brought misery to his people and helped Washington to emasculate his country's sovereignty.

Egypt and Syria had their own regional ambitions as they adjusted to a new world in which Iraq was out of the running as a major player for some time and the Soviet Union had opted out of playing an interventionist role. Besides, the question of integrating Iran in the West Asian equation remained an open one.

Indeed, Iran, for its part, was seeking to readjust its sights in the post-Khomeini period. Its helpful attitude to facilitating the release of Western hostages was only the latest indication of its efforts to come to terms with Washington and the West in general. Iran believed that given its size, location and potential, it should have its place in the new scheme of things. And it could only be inhibited in playing such a role if it continued to project the United States as the Great Satan.

The end of the Gulf War and the increased clout of the United States offered an opportunity that came rarely. West Asian shuttle diplomacy had until recently been associated with Henry Kissinger, but if James Baker succeeded in his shuttle diplomacy, he would score over the high-profile Kissinger and make West Asia a less dangerous place.

Two Cheers for the US

There was a lot riding on the West Asian peace conference in Madrid because it represented a unique chance to begin the end of the Arab-Israeli confrontation, which had led to several wars and continuing periods of high tension for decades. No one believed that it would be an easy task to unentangle a skein of relationships that had become synonymous with wars, abductions and terror.

But United States Secretary of State James Baker deserved credit for having got the protagonists to the point of a ceremonial conference leading to what were called two-track negotiations: Israel's talks with each of its Arab neighbours and separately with a Palestinian–Jordanian delegation. Looming in the background was the Palestine Liberation Organisation Israelis said they would not talk to and the powerful American presence.

These projected talks were crucial primarily for the Palestinians but also for the region and the world. Over the decades, West Asia had passed through many phases and Israel, with the strong backing of the United States, had destroyed many Arab illusions. At the receiving end had been the Palestinians whose homelands were conquered by Israel in the 1967 war. The West Bank and the Gaza Strip had retained the status of occupied territories while Israel had annexed Arab East Jerusalem and the Syrian Golan Heights.

Over the decades, Israel had been seeking to change the demography of the occupied territories by settling Jewish communities, merely to invite polite disapproval from the United States. The PLO, the legitimate representative of the Palestinians, had itself been involved in factional fights and had been fighting with Israel and some of the Arab States such as Jordan, with little success. The factional quarrels among the PLO spawned terrorist movements while the main Fatah movement had been under the charge of a remarkable leader, Yasser Arafat.

Egypt's decision to make a separate peace with Israel through the Camp David agreements, with US prompting and monetary inducements, represented an important signal that one phase of Arab bluster and war moves was over. Egypt had invited the opprobrium of the Arab world but it received back its lost territory (it was happy not to receive the Gaza Strip which it had administered) although with strict demilitarisation provisions. Basically, Egypt decided to sit out its isolation until it was invited back into the Arab fold.

Egypt's "betrayal", as some of the Arab states and the bulk of Arab people viewed it, rankled. Israel had no doubt won a great strategic victory in ensuring that with Egypt out of the reckoning, the prospect of a combination of Arab states launching an attack on it became remote.

Syrians Flexibility

The Iraqi defeat in the Gulf War served further to divide the Arabs and gave the PLO the liability of having supported the losing side of President Saddam. But the equations among the Arabs were changing, the most dramatic being the siding of Syria with the US even as the Arab masses rooted for Saddam, despite his inexcusable and foolish conduct in invading and annexing Kuwait.

The change in the Syrian position was an indication of the impact on the region of the cataclysmic events happening in the world. There were the revolutions in East and Central Europe, the dramatic changes in the Soviet Union whose "new thinking" in foreign policy came in the shape of dumping its ideology and seeking cooperation with the United States and the West. Power was inevitably tilting towards the US, particularly after its victory in the Second Gulf War, and the failed abortive coup in Moscow leading to the disintegration of the Soviet Union meant that as things stood, there was only one world power to reckon with.

Saddam, while facing inevitable defeat, had cleverly linked his indefensible occupation of Kuwait with the continuing Israeli occupation of Palestinian lands. The United Nations had pronounced on the subject and had asked Israel to withdraw from the occupied territories on the condition that its Arab neighbours recognised Israel's existence within the pre-1967 borders. But the Israelis, with US backing, simply chose to ignore these resolutions.

For the United States, with its new power and prestige, tackling the Arab-Israeli conflict presented a moral imperative; even more than that, its ability to seek legitimacy in West Asia over and above the defence and other deals it had and would arrange with the Arab rulers, depended upon a less partisan attitude towards Israel. In the United

States, where lobbies are accepted as legitimate instruments of influencing policy, the Jewish lobby remained a formidable force.

While the Arab states had generally been appreciative of the new reality—the collapse of the Soviet Union as an effective superpower had meant that there was no strong countervailing force to the United States—the Israelis had been somewhat complacent in their close strategic and economic and political relationship with Washington. They were shocked by President Bush linking a $ 10 billion loan guarantee for housing with the West Asian peace process and getting away with it, despite the strong Jewish lobby.

The Arabs and Palestinians had moved further from their known positions than Israelis in making the Madrid peace conference possible. It had required eight trips to the area by James Baker to fudge contentious issues such as Palestinian representation and twist arms and offer blandishments to move the conference proposal forward. Although the Soviet Union was co-sponsoring the peace conference, it was primarily an American show. And Moscow had restored full diplomatic relations with Israel to be able to play this somewhat symbolic role.

Apart from the official stances of the contending parties, the real questions boiled down to Israeli agreement to exchange territories for peace, with inevitable border adjustments. This presented dilemmas for Israel and the Arab states. Israelis were split down the middle over the question, with perhaps the majority opting for peace (Israel had never known real peace since its turbulent birth).

Arab Reservation

The Arab states, which paid routine lip-service to an independent Palestinian state, had their reservations. The truth was that the Palestinians and Israeli were the two most vital elements in West Asia. Among the Arabs, Palestinians tended to be better educated and they had helped administer many of the smaller countries. Their suffering over the decades also gave them a burning pride in their identity.

All that could be hoped for out of this new opportunity for peace was that an agreement could ultimately be arrived at for the autonomy of the West Bank and Gaza Strip with the binding provision that their future status would be determined after a fixed period. That future status, to be acceptable, would probably be in the shape of a demilitarised independent Palestine in a federation with Jordan.

But an early test of the peace process would be a freeze on the building of Israeli settlements in the occupied territories. There would be little point in launching this exercise if Israel were to continue to change the demography of the West Bank and Gaza while the central point of the parleys was the exchange of territories for peace.

A Benchmark

Two conclusions flowed from the historic West Asian peace conference in Madrid. It was a singular achievement of American diplomacy to get Israel and all its immediate Arab neighbours to face and listen to one another at one table after some 40 years. At the same time, the slanging match between Israel and Syria and the hiccups over the next phase—bilateral talks between Israel and the Arabs— were indications of the long road to peace.

The conference itself revealed that the participants were very conscious of the American diplomatic capital invested in it. They were appealing both to their domestic constituencies and world public opinion to make their points. In other words, as each party sought to make its pitch, it was very conscious of the fact that it should not be accused of breaking the conference.

The three elements of the individual presentations, as Baker pointed out in an impressive concluding speech, concerned peace, land and security. But he was, in a sense, begging the question because the essential point was how you arrived at the correct mix. For the Palestinians and Arabs, it was primarily a question of Israel vacating Palestinian and Arab land conquered in the 1967 war.

For the Israelis, any surrender of land was connected to security and peace. In any case, the Israelis had not accepted the contention that they should give up any of the conquered territory for peace although they had said that everything was on the table for discussion. But surely they sought to put the cart before the horse by initially insisting that bilateral talks with the Arab countries and Palestinians should take place in the region; in effect forcing the Arabs to recognise Israel by going there or inviting Israelis to an Arab country before a compromise package was in place.

These were early days for the peace process. Although the Americans might have been surprised by the intensity of name-calling between the Israelis and the Syrians, Baker publicly chose to take it in his stride by dismissing it as "maximalist" positions understandable at this stage of the peace-making game. At the same time, Baker warned the participants that they, not the co-sponsors (the Soviet Union's role was largely supportive), had to make peace although Washington would continue to pursue its diplomacy privately and in public.

The broad scenario for a peace settlement was already sketched out. It was to give Palestinians on the West Bank and in the Gaza Strip autonomy even as discussions had to be held in a time-frame to decide the future of the territories. Such a future dispensation, in all probability, would involve a federation or confederation of the Palestinian entity with Jordan. Also a matter for future negotiation would be the question of border adjustments to the pre-1967 boundaries.

Deep Suspicions

The main hurdle was how to reach the point of real discussions and negotiations. Suspicions between the Israelis and Arabs were so deep, underlined by the turbulence and blood-letting of more than four decades, that there was at this stage little give and take. It was, in a sense, an acknowledgement of American clout and power that the participants had got as far as they had.

The participants were zealously guarding their known negotiating positions. The fact of American diplomatic dominance in the world precluded precipitate action, but the parties involved were loath to give up their trump cards: territories, as far as the Israelis were concerned, and full diplomatic recognition of and dealings with Israel for the Arabs.

But the three-day Madrid conference had thrown up interesting patterns. The Palestinians, for one, had been striking a moderate pose, despite the fact that the chief Palestinian delegate made all the traditional points in his speech. As was to be expected, the Syrians had been striking up the most strident postures, with the Israelis giving as good as they got, and the Syrian Foreign Minister reverting to attack Israel, this time in rediscovering the terrorist antecedents of the Israeli Prime Minister, Shamir. It suited the latter to declare that nothing in the conference surprised him.

Indeed, the Arab–Israeli diplomatic confrontation was taking place on two levels: posturing to safeguard their interests and to seek to influence American public opinion about their efforts for peace. It was, therefore, logical that Shamir, who made a point of leaving Madrid after making his rebuttal on the morning of the last day of the conference, should stress his efforts for peace while insisting on holding bilateral talks in the region after an initial round in Madrid. It was also part of the Israeli tactic to suggest that the Arabs had still not recognised Israel's existence and that at least some of the Arab countries sought its annihilation. In other words, the Israelis were saying that there were no takers for the peace Jerusalem was offering. That it was a flawed peace, subject to negotiation, was not being stressed in Jerusalem.

The answer lay with Washington, rather than with the Arab and Israeli protagonists. Baker had given his country the role of a catalyst and although he continued to protest that neither the US nor the Soviet Union sought to impose a solution, the contours of a final compromise would very much be an American plan.

Baker's stress on his disappointment over the lack of confidence-building measures by the participants was a pointer to an essential prerequisite for a forward movement in the peace process. It was clear to the meanest intelligence that once the peace process got going in the second stage, Israel could not continue to build new settlements on the occupied territories because it would make nonsense of a search for peace. At the same time, Israel wanted an Arab concession before quietly forswearing new settlements.

The Americans had grasped one central point to underpin the peace process. President George Bush's inaugural address to the conference suggesting the necessity of "territorial compromise" for peace raised Arab hackles, but Baker in his concluding address and otherwise stressed the sanctity of United Nations resolution 242 and the American understanding that it stood for land for peace.

A Peace Framework

Without this basis, there could be no Arab incentive for making peace with Israel. In fact, President Bush went further to detail the peace framework. He said: "Negotiations will be conducted in phases, beginning with talks on interim self-government agreements. We aim to reach agreement within one year. And once agreed, interim self-government agreement will last for five years; beginning the third year, negotiations will commence on permanent status".

Baker was right in saying that despite the many hurdles that lay ahead, the Madrid conference represented a new benchmark in efforts for a West Asian peace. Both he and the Americans generally had not underrated the nature of the difficulties that would be encountered. And it was obviously in the interest of the Bush administration that the main hurdles in the long obstacle race were crossed before the start of the American Presidential election season, vulnerable to the influence of the Jewish lobby in the US.

But the ironies and the hypocrisies of the arrangements for the Madrid conference would not be lost on the American public or the world. Jerusalem's reservations on not talking to Palestinians from East Jerusalem or with the Palestine Liberation Organisation were respected in letter while the chief Palestinian spokesman was in the "objectionable" category and the chief Palestinian delegate made it clear at the conference that his allegiance, as that of other Palestinians, was to the PLO.

And despite the hot words exchanged between Israel and Syria, no delegate walked out of the Madrid conference, with Shamir describing Syria as one of the most tyrannical states in the world and the Syrian Foreign Minister holding aloft a picture of a 32-year-old Shamir on the wanted terrorist list. Yes, Madrid did represent a benchmark.

The Hiccups

No one with an understanding of West Asia had anticipated that the American-sponsored peace process would run a smooth or even course. But events were placing unbearable strains on it, which could derail—or greatly delay—the long journey to peace.

It was the juxtaposition of events that had set alarm bells ringing in world capitals. The elections in Israel imposed their own logic and rhetoric. Just during this sensitive period, the smouldering Palestinian resentment in the occupied territories led to stabbing incidents and Jewish retaliation. And in line with Israel's tooth for a tooth policy, their warplanes had been pounding targets in Lebanon.

In short, the Arab–Israeli confrontation was alive and kicking. None of the parties involved in the peace process had repudiated it, but even making allowances for the extravagance of rhetoric in the region, it would be more difficult for the participants to get to the nub of the issue that needed to be resolved: a satisfaction of Palestinian aspirations while ensuring Israeli security.

The wider regional backdrop of these events was hardly encouraging. President Saddam remained in saddle in Baghdad while his country continued to be subjected to a United Nations imposed embargo in a situation that was at best a stalemate. The milder sanction imposed on Libya remained suspended in mid-air, as it were, as Washington ruminated over its next step.

Other regional actors were trying to position themselves advantageously. Up to a point, Syria's hands seemed to be full with troubles in Lebanon and renewed Israeli warnings. Turkey and Iran were paying much attention to Central Asia, with the latter more than willing to assume the leadership role in the Gulf. The Gulf states themselves were trying to emerge out of the economic and security consequences of the Gulf War.

The central message of these developments was that the Arab–Israeli peace process would be long and the incipient leadership rivalry among the regional players portended friction. Indeed, the two sets of problems would interact as the United States and its principal Western allies remained the guarantors of security of the Gulf in particular.

The centrality of Washington's strategic alliance with Israel was not in doubt. But the United States' ability to influence events, in particular an Arab–Israeli rapprochement, would depend upon Arab perceptions. The building of Jewish settlements in the occupied territories was at the very least a bargaining chip for Israel and the United States had done well to distance itself from this activity. But the continuing embargo on Iraq—despite President Saddam's measures—were creating an anti-American mood in the Arab world.

Washington's dilemma was that its strategic interests required a special relationship with Israel as also the cultivation of defence links with Saudi Arabia and Egypt. The Gulf states had, of course, gratefully accepted the United States' umbrella because they considered it their most durable form of defence. But the United States' effectiveness in the Arab world was dependent upon the people's acceptance of an American role.

And such an acceptance was crucially dependent upon the people's perceptions. Some American analysts suggested that "the Arab street" did not count; it was the rulers or leaders who laid down the law. But there were limits beyond which the leadership, however archaic the form, could not prevail. Ironically, the Gulf War was a trigger for greater political activity in the region, leading to demands for opening up closed systems.

Sober Assessment

The Palestine Liberation Organisation had remained largely quiescent, mindful as it was of America's prevailing clout. In the PLO's sober assessment, the United States was the only country that could deliver an autonomous Palestine, leading to independent statehood. But if the process towards the first stage dragged on interminably, the organisation could become largely irrelevant as the Palestinians in the occupied territories set their own pace of confrontation with Israel.

It could be argued that conflict was endemic to West Asia, given the explosive potential of the Arab–Israeli confrontation on the one hand and the great disparities of immense oil wealth and poorer Arab countries on the other. But that was cold comfort to the United States' strategic calculations.

The problem with the United States' single-minded resolve to defang Iraq, with Israel's blessing, was that others in the region—primarily Iran—wanted to assume the leadership role. Washington's game plan to have a reasonably strong Iraq without Saddam's extravagant ambitions to balance Iran did not work. It was now left with frustrating Iranian ambitions while continuing to humiliate Iraq.

Egypt, in many ways the region's leader, was suffering the handicap of its great dependence on American largesse and its economic problems. Symbolically, President Mubarak flexed his muscles on occasion to refurbish his Arab credentials, but such demonstrations were taken with a pinch of salt by his neighbours and the wider Arab world.

West Asia had, indeed, arrived at a crucial fork in its tempestuous history. Could the regional ambitions of individual countries be kept in some check while the arduous process of an Arab–Israeli reconciliation was maintained?

Despite its power, Washington was as susceptible to regional factors as it was before the disappearance of the Soviet Union as a power factor. What had changed in the region was the recognition that with no other countervailing power, countries had to accommodate themselves to the fact of a one-power equation or face penalties.

This could be a double-edged sword because Arab frustrations could lead to desperation and the United States bore the additional responsibility of being seen to be even-handed while safeguarding its strategic alliance with Israel. Given the compulsions of a presidential election year, its task was doubly difficult.

One hope was that after the Israeli elections, Jewish compulsions to strike up heroic postures would subside. Ultimately, Israel's compromise with Palestinian nationalism would be made on the basis of *realpolitik* and an assurance of its security interests. The United States was an essential component in the process, but it would require a high degree of statesmanship on Washington's part to remain undeflected by regional storms in pursuing its central purpose.

The consequences of the Second Gulf War, however, would continue to work themselves out. Washington had to strike a balance between Saddam Hussein's defiance through the very fact of retaining power and the need for a reasonably strong Iraq to balance Iranian ambitions. It would also remain Washington's purpose to get the Gulf states to arrive at a regional equilibrium not so heavily dependent upon external Western support. The fiasco of the Damascus Declaration revealed the suspicions of the Gulf states towards ambitious Arab neighbours.

The objective of the exercise was to give an Arab underpinning— by Egypt and Syria—to the security of the Gulf. But the Gulf states felt more inclined to rely on American and Western protection.

Kuwait, 1992

As Kuwaitis picked up their lives since the Iraqi invasion nearly a year earlier, one thing was clear. Life could never be the same again, and it was the Kuwaitis who reminded the world that they had a long way to go before they could return to their original affluent lifestyle. It was doubtful that they could ever regain their former carefree existence.

The invasion and occupation of Kuwait had seared the Kuwaiti psyche. The Kuwaitis, and others, who remained prisoners in Iraq, according to officials, still numbered 2,000-odd and through stickers and posters and an intense public campaign, Kuwaitis were reminding themselves and the world that they had not forgotten their less fortunate brethren.

Americans were heroes in Kuwait. Those countries that supported the Iraqi invasion were still viewed with different degrees of disfavour and the Kuwaiti ruling establishment had decided that, instead of relying on the empty rhetoric of the Arab nation, they would seek security where they could obtain it. Hence the Kuwaiti decision to sign a defence agreement with the United States and plans to sign similar agreements with Britain and France.

Kuwaitis were emphasising the role of the six-nation Gulf Co-operation Council (GCC) for two reasons. It gave them psychological support and since most of the Gulf states were sailing in the same boat, they had common problems to discuss in facing the future. The GCC proved a broken reed at the time of the Iraqi invasion, and, despite the brave words about forming a joint Gulf army, there were few illusions in Kuwait about the ability of such a force to safeguard the security of their states.

Kuwaitis were raising loans abroad to be able to finance the immense reconstruction effort. Losses from the oil fires, mercifully put out, were put at $ 120 million a day. The borrowings were against future oil exports, and Kuwait could hope to reach the export target of the pre-war days only in 1993. Kuwait still had a tidy sum in reserves and had investments in multinational companies. But in relative terms, it was a time for belt-tightening.

Political Compulsions

As against the new demands of reconstruction were the political compulsions. Elections to a national assembly had been promised for October 1992. The ruling establishment seemed to feel that it needed to restore the people's standard of living to the pre-war level. The occupation of Kuwait and the war had disturbed the relative even tenor of the old days. Apart from the trauma of the occupation, the younger generation was in a more rebellious mood, family ties had loosened and women in particular were demanding their rights after their participation in the resistance movement.

Kuwait had the unique institution of *diwaniya*, discussion and recreation groups that met regularly around a known personality to discuss problems and let off steam. Few themes are barred and, in West Asian terms, the institution represented a radical departure from the traditional themes of conformism. One *diwaniya* I attended in Kuwait city was presided over by a woman, a rare occurrence in itself, although she belonged to the ruling family.

Dr Rosha Al-Sabah was vice-rector of the university and taught comparative literature. She presided over a mixed group of men and women, poets, university men and others interested in expounding their views. Dr Rosha herself was forthright in demanding that a mere 9 per cent out of a population of 800,000 Kuwaiti citizens should not form the ruling elite. The remaining 91 per cent was composed of women and naturalised citizens. Dr Rosha, of course, was for giving women the right of vote.

Questioned on the fate of Palestinians in Kuwait, the gathering was of the unanimous view that a people who had been given a state and all welfare benefits had "stabbed Kuwait in the back" during the occupation. And the intensity of feelings on the humiliation and worse Kuwaitis suffered during the occupation was to be heard to be believed. Groups had been formed, some of them around Islamic ideas, but the dissidents were not a cohesive group. According to Dr Rosha, funda-mentalism was growing, particularly in the university. Girl students voted for fundamentalists and the students' union was challenging a ruling by the dean of the medical school banning the wearing of the strict Islamic dress for women in laboratories for hygienic and practical reasons.

Kuwait city still wore the scars of the occupation. Along the sea front, windows in houses were still bricked up with openings for slits, house fronts were daubed with red circles crowned by the names of Iraqi commanding officers occupying each house. The Iraqis expected an American attack from the sea and hence made their preparations, a feint that served the United States and its allies well. Overall, damage to the buildings in the city had not been as extensive as it could have been although Iraqis stripped homes and officers of all they could carry.

In the oilfield areas, the work of bringing the resource-earning oil back into play was continuing and Kuwaitis were already demanding an increase in their quota of oil production, once they had restored normal supplies, to make up for their immense losses. One oilfield area I visited was in Ahmadi. The sand was drenched in oil, there were vast lakes of oil as workmen sought to restore normalcy. Kuwaitis were talking no chances and elaborate security rings were in place to guard oil production against sabotage.

While waiting for the day when oil revenues would start flowing again in abundance, the Kuwaiti establishment was seeking to build a new nationalism on the basis of the shared tragedy of seven months of Iraqi occupation. "Help POWs", "We have not forgotten you" and other such stickers and posters were constant reminders of the unaccounted missing, still believed to be in Iraq. And Kuwaitis wore their humi-liation during the occupation days on their sleeves to emphasise their common resolve to resist the invader.

One of the problems was that Kuwaitis were a minority in their own country. The expatriate worker, from the Indian subcontinent and the Philippines, was a common sight. Although Kuwaitis were plan-ning to reduce their dependence on expatriates and were imposing restrictions on their employment and length of stay, the very task of reconstruction meant that the demand for foreign labour would, in immediate terms, grow, rather than diminish.

Gulf Seeks Security

The three days of deliberations of the six-nation Gulf Cooperation Council held in December 1991 in Kuwait, which bound the Gulf States with Saudi Arabia, was rich in rhetoric and ceremony. The rulers of the six states—Qatar, Bahrain, the United Arab Emirates, Oman,

Kuwait and Saudi Arabia—sat at a round table in a lavish tent in a complex built for the conference in the damaged Bayan palace compound to signify the conclusion of their conference.

But the GCC left the vital questions unanswered. How could the Gulf states ensure their security? What role could Iran play in the new dispensation? Could the lip-service being paid to a future role for Egypt and Syria under the rubric of the Damascus Declaration ever be translated into a vital security underpinning? Could the goal of evolving a joint army of the Gulf states be more than a symbolic expression of their desire jointly to face a dangerous world?

The Gulf War and the Iraqi invasion of Kuwait and its liberation under the leadership of the United States had traumatised the Gulf states because they had underlined their vulnerability. Here were countries sitting on 40 per cent of the world's oil wealth. They had small indigenous populations and relied in varying degrees on the expatriate worker. And there were predators in the area jealous of their wealth and desirous of helping themselves to dollops of them if they could, as Iraq demonstrated.

The Gulf War had not merely deepened the divisions in the Arab world but had also made the Gulf states deeply suspicious of the motives of the other Arab states. They were wary of Egyptian and Syrian motives, and even more wary of Iran's regional ambitions. At the same time, they realised these countries' capacity to make life difficult for rulers with immense wealth without the population base that could give them strength.

In view of their traumatic experience of Iraqi occupation, Kuwaitis decided to cut through the anti-American rhetoric, a staple diet in West Asia, publicly to embrace the United States to safeguard their security. But the others were hesitating about how far and how publicly to follow Kuwait's example.

Appropriate Noises

True, Kuwaitis had sought to balance the choice they have made by making appropriate noises about unifying the Gulf states, the virtues of the Damascus Declaration and the brotherhood of the Arab nation. But the contradictions involved in this exercise were apparent.

For the Gulf states, the Palestinian question evoked more ambivalent reactions because of Kuwait's experience during the occupation. Kuwaitis could never forgive the Palestine Liberation Organisation chairman, Yasser Arafat, for his support of Iraq, and accused "quite a few" Palestinians of collaborating with Iraqis during their occupation of Kuwait. From a total of over 400,000 Palestinians in the pre-invasion era, only some 40,000 remained in Kuwait, and they were on sufferance.

There was little let-up in public in the anti-Israeli rhetoric, but for the Gulf states Palestinians, who had provided the backbone in administration, health services and other fields in many countries of the region, had become unwelcome guests and were generally regarded with suspicion. And the Gulf states, in particular Kuwait and the United Arab Emirates, were making efforts to refine their polices on the expatriate worker in order to limit the numbers and they were encouraging the indigenous people to have more children.

On the domestic front, the Gulf states were painfully aware of the appeal radicalism could have for their populations. These countries were governed in the traditional manner, with more, or less, popular potentates exercising absolute power.

The Gulf states were chary of giving Iran a direct security role in the region. They had supported Iraq in the Iran-Iraq war, but Iran's neutrality in the second Gulf War won it some marks. Iran's hopes of cashing in on a measure of goodwill its approach to the Gulf War created had, however, been belied.

Iran's Opposition

One problem was that Iran's opposition to outside powers overseeing the region's security collided with the new mood in the Gulf of ensuring their security by a tie-up with a power that had demonstrated its will to come to Kuwait's assistance. The other was that although Iranian revolutionary rhetoric has been suitably tempered, it symbolised a threat to the traditional rulers.

Thus the search for seeking security for the Gulf states continued as they tried to balance their needs with the temper of their peoples and their efforts to dampen radical demands.

The dilemma of the Gulf states could not be resolved in a hurry. After all, they were not the major players in the region and were dependent as much on the activities and national interests of the United States and countries such as Iran, Egypt and Syria and the meandering process of an Israeli–Arab reconciliation as on their own wisdom to influence the outcome.

In Kuwait, for instance, one met individuals who were highly critical of the shape of the government that ruled the country. It was the same mixture as before the invasion, they said, despairing of the ruling family striking out on a bold new path. Such critics did not always have a political axe to grind; rather, their concerns stemmed from the realisation that the prevailing order could not last unless the ruling families were prepared to move with the times.

The Arab–Israeli confrontation struck at the heart of the problem because unless the Americans could be seen to be moving Israel towards the goal of a fair peace, anti-American sentiment could only grow. Beyond a point, the Gulf states could not ignore this sentiment. It made their task of seeking security by obtaining an American guarantee that much more difficult.

The Gulf states had yet to arrive at a *modus vivendi* with Iran. It was all very well to suggest, as Kuwait did, that the Iranians could have a maritime security role, a proposition that seemed unacceptable to Iranians. How far Iran and the Gulf states could come to a compromise settlement remained a question mark.

Egyptian and Syrian roles were more ambivalent. Egypt was seen as being within the American sphere of influence and hence not an independent actor. Syrian efforts to trim its sails to the prevailing Western winds were viewed as a tactical exercise. It was seeking to make gains in the region in its new incarnation. Its precise goals, outside the influence it wanted to continue to exercise in Lebanon, were somewhat imprecise.

The longer term American goals in the region were clear, but the precise instruments through which it would seek to achieve them were not defined. Partly, it would depend upon how far it could succeed in influencing the Arab–Israeli reconciliation process; partly, it would be determined by the regional balance that took shape.

The Gulf region remained in a state of flux, but unless the rulers of these states could inspire confidence in their people about the future, they were skating on thin ice.

A Testing Ground

However one looked at them, the alarm bells over Iraq were a true picture of the uncertainties that plagued West Asia two years after Iraq's invasion of Kuwait. Iraq was a symbol of the new world disorder in more senses than one. It had become a testing ground for the limits of UN power and the might of the United States and its special Western allies. And despite all the humiliations meted out to President Saddam, he continued to thumb his nose at his prosecutors.

The United States was hampered not merely by President George Bush's uphill struggle to win re-election—he was vulnerable to the charge of playing domestic politics in Iraq—but also by the fact that the coalition he had built up two years ago would disintegrate if the US took war again to Iraq. The decision, ostensibly led by Britain, to exclude Iraqi aircraft from the southern Shi'ite zone under pain of their being shot down was a kind of half-measure that had characterised the Western response to a country defeated in a war refusing to lie down.

The UN Security Council had passed a whole range of resolutions which could be taken as justification for much of what the West wanted to do in Iraq. The difficulty arose from the West's, particularly the United States', strategic perceptions and the sympathy Saddam continued to evoke at the popular level in much of the Arab world.

Strategically, American concerns were governed by the need to retain Iraq's integrity, both as a check on Iran and out of fear that any unravelling of the country would lead to chaos that would be detrimental to its interests. Official American reiteration of seeing Iraq survive as one country was an indication of US consistency on this point.

The zone carved out for the Kurds in the north was an unhappy Western compromise because while it naturally encouraged long-held Kurdish aspirations for an independent state, the West could not be a handmaiden for the achievement of this goal. It would spell the break up of Iraq and would set alarm bells ringing in the capital of the US ally, Turkey, saddled with its own—often acute—Kurdish problem.

By the same token, any encouragement of Shi'ites in southern Iraq would mean an acquisition of strength for Iran. Washington was already wary of Iran's potential and ambitions and had no desire to gift a part of Iraq to it. Yet the West had to make a symbolic point to try to discipline a truculent Saddam.

Apart from performing the miracle of surviving in power two long years after his country's defeat, President Saddam was playing a game of attrition with the US and its chief allies, in this instance France in addition to the unfailingly loyal Britain. And he seemed to be succeeding in the cat and mouse game he was playing.

Long Stand-off

Take the long stand-off between the UN inspectors and the Iraqi government outside the agriculture ministry building. In the ultimate compromise reached, Baghdad won several points against the backdrop of the rising crescendo of American threats by having a Russian, rather than an American, lead inspector. And the UN venture was made to look rather foolish because if there were any compromising documents in the ministry, they would not have been left undisturbed for weeks.

Saddam seemed to have learnt a few lessons from his foolishness in refusing to accept a last-minute compromise to stave off the attack of the US and its allies by retreating from Kuwait. In a tactic he had now perfected, he stopped just short of the brink by giving in while continuing to make his propaganda points. For instance, Iraqis dismissed the United Nations as an advertisement front for the United States.

But President Saddam, in his own impish way, seemed to be making a larger point. The United States wished to make an example of Iraq, after the latter's totally indefensible attack on and annexation of Kuwait, for its own reasons. With the demise of the Soviet Union as a competing power, the US had the ability and means to enforce its agenda on any recalcitrant power, particularly a country which had outraged the world by invading and annexing an independent nation and a member of the UN, threatening American strategic interests in the bargain.

The result was what had been described as the mother of all UN resolutions that sought to subject Iraq to the most obtrusive inspections and draconian conditions ever imposed on a member state. The US and its allies went further in carving out a no-go Kurdish zone. A set of subsequent Security Council resolutions strengthened the noose around Iraq's neck. And a resolution permitting Iraq to sell oil was hemmed in by such conditions and projected monitoring mechanisms that Baghdad contemptuously rejected it.

UN Unfairness

Although the rest of the world chose to go along with the American agenda on Iraq despite misgivings among non-permanent members of the Security Council, President Saddam was demonstrating that, whatever his sins, the UN had been unfair to Iraq and he had the power to embroil the world organisation in an endless series of contests in which even a stand-off was a victory for him, given his country's present patent weakness.

President Saddam was, therefore, pointing up the lop-sided nature of a world organisation in which the majority had no real say and had now been placed outside the pale of decision-making by the end of the two-power mechanism which had enabled the developing countries to exert some influence through a competing Soviet Union. The former Soviet Union was foolish enough to boycott the Security Council for a time to enable the US to fight the Korea war under the UN flag; it had been co-opted by Washington to follow its agenda.

This symbolic contest between Iraq and a UN under Washington's wings was taking place in an area which was as potentially unstable as it was rich. The Iraqi rhetoric, matched by Western threats, had made Kuwaitis feel insecure, comforted though they were to an extent by their country's military alignment with the United States. And the border demarcation between Iraq and Kuwait, made under UN aegis, was likely to remain a bone of contention far into the future.

Traditionally, the American decision-making ability in the heat of a presidential election campaign gets impared. Fighting as he was with his back to the wall, President Bush's options were reduced because whatever decisions he took would be interpreted as motivated by his desire to improve his re-election prospects. President Saddam, of course, had no such problems.

Perhaps Saddam was banking upon the American predicament to conduct a more vigorous phase of his propaganda campaign, driving UN inspectors up the wall and combining defiant rhetoric with adaptability in order to ward off actual strikes. Many nervous countries in the Gulf in particular were waiting.

A new elected President or a re-elected President Bush would, however, continue to face the legacy of the Gulf War. President Saddam was as much a symbol of West Asian instability as he was of America's unfinished business in the region. The point was whether and on what terms the US would be able to come to grips with the many ramifications of a war won on the battlefield turning murky in its aftermath.

Hebron Massacre, 1994

The world was facing its moment of truth in West Asia. For the massacre in Hebron in February 1994 went far beyond the unspeakable murders of Palestinians praying in the mosque during the holy month of Ramadan. They revealed the depth of Jewish–Arab hostility and called into question the basis on which the secret Oslo agreement between Israelis and the Palestine Liberation Organisation was arrived at and the tortuous incomplete negotiations conducted to implement it.

This basis was that in bridging the Arab–Israeli divide, the world had to adopt a step by step approach. The first step was Palestinian self-government in the Gaza Strip and the Jericho enclave with the future shape of the Palestinian entity being left for subsequent talks. The assumption was that during this phase Palestinians and Israelis would learn to live with one another and help to evolve a future settlement.

The PLO's agreement to the scheme was less than enthusiastic, but Arafat accepted it because, however unsatisfactory the plan, it provided an opening to a future Palestinian state. Second, this was the only agreement on offer and, with the end of the Cold War and the disintegration of the Soviet Union, there was no countervailing power to the United States to help the Palestinians.

Arafat bore the criticism he faced from Palestinians outside the Fatah and even from his mainstream wing with fortitude because he believed that he was leading his people to freedom, deferred as it was. But he was to meet with bitter disappointment as the process of negotiations dragged on. Even more ominously, Israeli negotiators insisted on and obtained the right of screening all persons entering or leaving the Palestinian autonomous areas.

The agreement Arafat signed with the Israelis in Cairo with a heavy heart in a sense represented a turning point for many Palestinians. They felt that their initial suspicious were perhaps justified and that instead of the process leading to independence, Israelis wished to build a golden cage for Palestinians. So keen were the Israeli negotiators to deny the Palestinians any symbol of statehood that they looked askance at moves for a Palestinian currency or even a postage stamp. The Israeli settlements on the occupied land were outside the ken of the discussions inasmuch as they were to be protected by Israeli troops and were to enjoy a special status.

Rabin's Miscalculation

Where the Rabin government went wrong was in assuming that it had all the time in the world to score its points and bring the PLO into line. Arafat's warnings were clear enough, that delay would create complications and disillusion more Palestinians. Further, he berated President Bill Clinton for his laid-back position and pleaded with Washington to be more directly involved. But the Clinton administration, focused as it was on the domestic economy or unavoidable fire-fighting jobs abroad, was content to let the Israeli–PLO talks proceed at the leisurely pace set by Tel Aviv.

Washington could not have foreseen the nature of the crime committed at Hebron and sought to repair the damage by asking Israelis and the PLO to come to Washington for "talks till agreement". The Rabin government, while rejecting demands for disarming the settlers and for an international presence in the occupied territories, promised to ensure that such crimes would not be repeated. This offered scant comfort to the Arab world as the PLO deliberated and the enormity of the crime against Palestinians sank in.

While the United States picked up the pieces of a peace process begun in Madrid, hammered out in Oslo and discussed in Washington and many other world capitals, it would be idle to pretend that the chain remained unbroken. PLO negotiators could not return to talks with Israelis as if nothing had happened. The first question that would have to be discussed was what to do with the Israeli settlements on occupied land. How could the embryonic Palestinian entity live with areas bristling with guns outside the control of a future Palestinian police force? The measures announced by the Israelis did not provide the answer.

It was not merely a question of blaming a lone insane gunman out to sabotage the Israeli–PLO agreement, as the Israeli tended to do. The crime, committed by one or many, had revealed in a flash the weakness of the assumption that once the first phase of the autonomy deal went through, it would inevitably lead to an independent Palestinian entity. Had the Israeli negotiators been more understanding of and generous to Palestinians, the Hebron massacre could have been treated as an aberration. But each round of negotiators had seen haggling over legal technicalities, an effort by the Israelis to give the PLO as little as possible. PLO declarations on a time-frame for the conclusion of negotiation had repeatedly and immediately been amended by the Israelis. To the outside world, it seemed, the PLO was the supplicant.

The Israelis seemed to have been living in the dangerous world of illusion that led them to believe that the PLO was the weaker party and they could take the fullest advantage of the reality of the post-Cold War world. They should have known that peace was a give and take process and not a one-way street, that an irreparable disruption of the peace process would not mean a mere return to the old hostility but its escalation, with unpredictable consequences for Israel and the region. In other words, the alternative to peace was war.

Men of goodwill in the region and the wider world still hoped that the Hebron massacre would shock the Israelis and the United States into the realisation that dilatory methods of negotiations and the Israeli propensity to score points were not paths to peace or success. First, Washington had to work out with the Israelis how the latter could satisfy the PLO on armed Israeli settlements in their midst being free to target any Palestinian of their choice. An anachronism that could have been overlooked in the first phase of the autonomy plan had now assumed a central role and could not be resolved by old methods.

The question, in essence, boiled down to the Rabin government's willingness and ability to face the reality of a future independent Palestinian entity. This was the basis on which the PLO accepted the half-way house represented by the Oslo agreement enshrined in a declaration of principles symbolised by the Washington handshake of Arafat and Rabin. There could be no place in the future for Israeli enclaves. It was a question of how and when these should be dismantled, rather than whether they should exist.

Death of Oslo, 1996

If there was an air of normality in the Palestinian autonomous territory of Bethlehem in March 1996, with Palestinian police handing out parking tickets to errant drivers, the calm was deceptive. In the main market, second hand goods changed hands and the vegetable and fruit stalls drew crowds. In Assad's textile shop carrying an assortment of frilly children's clothing and piles of leather jackets, the tenth applicant of the day came in search of a job—any job.

"The Israelis have imprisoned us", Assad told me. "They have not even left a window open." He was, of course, referring to the blockade imposed by the Israeli authorities after the series of bombing raids in Israel. Palestinians could not go to work in Israel and there was no prospect of the reopening of borders until after the Israeli election at the end of May 1996, if then. "All Palestinians who can try to find a way to get out and go away", he said.

In the Manger Square, the few tourist coaches looked incongruous in the hustle and bustle of Palestinian life. Farid Azizeh, a Bethlehem town councillor, ran a neat restaurant. He was 65, a Christian, and was angry. "We were better off before Oslo," he said, referring to the Israeli–PLO agreement. "Why, I have an Israeli friend, an officer, of 28 years' acquaintanceship. And now he won't even take my telephone calls. Where is Hamas? Find me a Hamas. The Israelis are just depriving us of our livelihood. I have a Honduran passport. I'll just sell my flat and leave."

The desire to escape the difficult situation too many Palestinians find themselves in was understandable. And for too many, Oslo had meant sorrow and pain after the brief bursts of joy that greeted the inauguration of the Palestinian autonomous areas whose entrances and exits were guarded by Israeli soldiers. Assad and Azizeh did not plan to leave their homes but they were among a growing army of Palestinians turning against the Oslo agreement although there was little criticism of Arafat from the people I met, except to commiserate with his lot.

The Israelis, on their part, had graduated to demanding "separation" from the Palestinians and suggested that the economic deprivation and hardships caused by the closure of the autonomous areas should be addressed by the mythical international community. "Fine," says Ashrawi. "Let us discuss borders and the formation of two states." That is precisely what the Israeli did not want to discuss.

Barak's Bluntness

The annual conference of the International Press Institute met in Jerusalem, in itself a foolish decision, because the plan to hold a parallel meeting in Jericho never materialised. The Palestinian leadership rebelled at the IPI choosing West Jerusalem. But in an effort to appear non-partisan, the IPI approached Ashrawi, and she came to address the gathering in her personal capacity to demolish the theories Israeli leaders had built up so carefully. Fighting a tough election as Prime Minister Shimon Peres was, he was very much on the defensive, all security-conscious. But it was his foreign minister, the former chief of staff, Ehud Barak, who called a spade a spade.

It was a frightening picture, frightening for the cause of peace. Barak made it plain that the peace process was made possible because of Israel's position of political and strategic strength. He listed the following assets for Israel: the collapse of the Soviet Union, Israel's unique relationship with the United States, the only superpower, Iraq's defeat in the Gulf War and the Arabs' "perception" of Israel being a nuclear power. He believed that Israel and the Palestinians were heading towards separation, which would be better for the future relationship. He said the basic difference between the Labour Party and the Likud was that the former believed that to exercise full control over the occupied area, Israel would either have to be a bi-national state or a non-democratic one, neither of which was a desirable idea.

Others, such as the former long-time head of the Israeli foreign office, David Kimche, filled in the blanks. He expected at least 100,000 Israeli settlers to be regrouped and remain on the West Bank, Jerusalem would stay under full Israel control with the Palestinians allowed "complete municipal autonomy". The Palestinian headquarters could be in Ramallah. But Kimche conceded that the Palestinian authority was "a state in the making" although his hope was that it would have at least an association with Jordan and have a kind of Benelux arrangement to include Israel.

It was easy for Ashrawi to pick holes in the Israeli arguments. The transition process, she said, had faced tremendous difficulties because new settlements had been built on occupied land, agreements such as the release of Palestinian prisoners had been defied, there was a continued siege of Jerusalem and attempts at dictating terms had not stopped. Israel had been pre-empting issues: Jerusalem, land, settlements, while the corridor between Gaza and the West Bank had not been built. There was a context to the problem of violence and security—"let's discuss the roots". She said an outside neutral sponsorship was needed to rescue peace. "Let's rescue peace, not merely the peace process," in her words.

The objective of detailing these views at some length, as they were propounded for the benefit of the world's editors and publishers, is to underline a stark fact. The peace process, as envisaged at Oslo, was dead. The problem was how to revive it before failure overwhelmed the Israelis and Palestinians. Even the so-called softer Israeli view of the future encompassed an undivided Jerusalem as the Israeli capital, usurpation of some 11 per cent of the area of the West Bank to be joined to the Jerusalem area and the continued presence of 100,000 Israeli settlers on the West Bank under Israeli jurisdiction.

Given this scenario and the known and publicly announced American bias towards Israel, how could any Palestinian leader accept such a future? In Ashrawi's view, Hamas was not a monolithic organisation. It should be brought into the peace process while seeking to isolate the extremists in Hamas. The closure of territories was not the answer. Palestinians, she suggested, were a very volatile constituency.

Flawed Democracy

In the old quarter of Jerusalem, a shopkeeper gave me his interpretation of Israeli democracy. There were four categories of democracy, in his view, and the four were treated differently. Category one: white Israelis; two, Arab Israelis; three, Arabs in Israel; four, Palestinians in Gaza and the West Bank. He, as an Arab living in Israel, could go to the West Bank but a Palestinian living in the West Bank could not come to

Jerusalem. The shopkeeper told me of a new point that hurt all Palestinians. Rabin's assassin was sentenced to life imprisonment, but his house remained undemolished even as Israelis systematically blew up the homes of Hamas bombers. Palestinians might have learnt to live with discriminatory Israeli policies but they had not reconciled themselves to double standards.

The conventional wisdom was that the peace process had to remain in suspension until the Israeli elections were over. The reality was that the closer the two parties moved towards the final status negotiations, the clearer it was becoming that the solution Israel was willing to offer would be unacceptable to any self-respecting Palestinian. Israelis were prepared to give Palestinians a chequerboard of a state as part of a federation with Jordan, keeping to themselves Jerusalem and large slices of occupied land.

According to Binyamin Begin, son of the late prime minister and a prominent member of Likud, the Oslo agreement had nothing to do with genuine peace and was "dead on arrival" on the lawns of the White House. Begin might have been pre-empting the result, but there could be no doubt that it was dead.

Getting at Truth

What was the Arab perspective of the West Asian peace process? Was there, indeed, an Arab prospective or only one correct perspective? Which objective was more difficult to achieve: Peace between Israel and Syria and Lebanon or between Israelis and Palestinians? Did Benjamin (Bibi) Netanyahu represent a small group of ideologues like himself or a larger phenomenon in Israel? Was the United States playing a helpful role in promoting the peace process?

These were some of the questions that were raised, and tentative answers given, at a brainstorming session organised by the International Press Institute in Amman. Among those participating, in addition to a bevy of editors and publishers, were King Hussein, Prince Hassan, President Hosni Mubarak's adviser Osama El-Baz, former Jordanian prime minister Abdel-Salaam Majali, former Jordanian foreign minister Kamal Abu-Jaber, and the deputy minister of economy and commerce of the Palestinian Authority, Samir Hleileh.

It was glorious weather in Amman—sunny and balmy—but the prognostications of the peace process, as they were made in a hotel conference room and in the Royal Palace, were not as bright. Indeed, those who analysed the situation were divided between those who believed in a happy ending and others who could not see a silver lining to the dark clouds enveloping West Asia. There was, of course, a compulsion to believe that peace would ultimately break out, or else the arduous labours to bring about a *modus vivendi* between Arabs and the state of Israel would be futile.

Perhaps the most interesting assessment made was that the Arab world and the wider world beyond it were not merely fighting Bibi Netanyahu but a wider Israeli phenomenon of ideologues who considered the entirety of Palestine to be Israeli holy land. Hence, in Abu-Jaber's view, it would be easier for Syria and Lebanon to make peace with Israel than for Palestinians to do so. It was recognised that Bibi would have to, and would, make compromises but other Israelis who held the same views would not. Bibi and the hardliners of his inclination represented a powerful component of Israeli opinion. What was left unsaid was that there would be eternal strife between Israelis and Palestinians.

El-Baz, being in a singular position to know the inside story of negotiations in view of President Mubarak's key role, pleaded that it was important not to tar all Israelis with the same brush. Opposed to Bibi and other ideologues were the Labour Party and the Peace Now movement, and the Jewish diaspora was unhappy with Bibi's handling of the peace process. El-Baz believed, despite all evidence to the contrary, that the Likud prime minister would have to change his views on the formation of a Palestinian state because although he was an "absolutist", he was also a politician who wanted to succeed. And the Palestinians had gained legitimacy in the peace process.

Bibi's Lament

El-Baz thought there was a point to Bibi's lament over the Hebron negotiations that the delay in reaching an agreement was due to Arafat's desire to wait for the end of the US presidential election in the hope that a re-elected President Bill Clinton could exert greater pressure on Israel. If Bibi gave the impression of twisting in the wind on a stake, it was because of Arab suspicions that once he was taken off the hook, he would quickly revert to dragging his feet on implementing the other agreements such as Israeli withdrawal from the rural areas of the West Bank, the release of Palestinian prisoners and beginning serious negotiations in the "final status" talks. Palestinians realised that Bibi remained under intense pressure from the world on implementing agreements Israelis had already signed.

It was again El-Baz who sounded the warning note that it was unrealistic to expect the United States to exert crude pressure on Israel, but he and other Arab participants spoke of the "American silence"— the need for the American position "to be declared" to persuade Israelis to follow the path of peace, in El-Baz's words. In a felicitous turn of phrase, Abu-Jaber, who had reverted to his professional duties, suggested that Bibi was more interested in the process than in peace. And it was he who propounded the theory that it would be more difficult to make peace between Palestinians and Israelis than between the Jewish state on the one hand and Syria and Lebanon on the other.

The red herring Netanyahu had thrown in suggesting a subsidiary Puerto Rico model for the future Palestinian entity was laughed out of court, El-Baz describing it as ridiculous, suggesting that Bibi was day-dreaming. Mejali, on his part, pointed to the trend towards the right in Israel since the seventies but for a short break represented by Rabin and Peres. Peres had tried and failed to integrate Israel into West Asia whereas Bibi believed that his country had to depend upon military might and, Mejali believed, was not keen on integration in West Asia at all but was seeking integration into Europe. Bibi's grandfather was a rabbi in Lithuania of the exclusivity school, came to West Asia in the twenties, had nine children and changed the family name to Netanyahu, meaning "the gift of God".

Majali, together with the other participants, asked a question which did not need an answer. If Israel continued swallowing Palestinian land, what was the point of talking? And there were the shades of the apocalyptical vision, that if Bibi continued to pursue his policies, he would be releasing tremendous forces lying dormant. Let us, Majali pleaded, agree on a definition of peace. The seeds of conflict would remain in the soil if Bibi pursued his policies and the question for the former Jordanian prime minister was Israeli mentality, conscious as he was of the fact that pan-Arab security had collapsed totally in 1967.

Pressing Issues

For Samir Hleileh of the Palestinian Authority, the daily issues were pressing even as priorities were chalked up—infrastructure, start-up costs of ministries, etc. and the problem of covering the deficit. It was, he confessed, a shaky Palestinian Authority and a shaky economy, the Palestinians reduced to make-work schemes employing between 20,000 and 25,000 persons in order to contain dissatisfaction. International investors, he said, had looked askance at the Palestinian plan for an airport and a sea port, but the Palestinian territories were closed for seven months in 1996 and "without direct access [to the outside world] we cannot survive". The Palestinian territories lost a quarter of the gross domestic product (GDP) in per capita terms due to Israeli-imposed closures and Hleileh suggested that although there was conflict of ideas and beliefs in the Palestinian Authority, donor intermediaries were not sensitive to the "empowerment" of the PA.

The new port would take two to three years to complete, according to Hleileh, but the airport was ready. However, the Israelis were insisting on every detail being agreed upon before allowing the airport to function, with Palestinians refusing to allow double checks on incoming traffic. There were such important but mundane problems as collecting taxes (primarily VAT), the collections in Gaza being less than half of what they were under direct Israeli rule while the West Bank collections exceeded 140 per cent of the old figure. Hleileh reckoned that tax leakage to Israel was in the region of $ 180 million a year. The figure for security and police staff and bureaucrats for Gaza and the West Bank were 36,000 and 66,000 respectively; it was, the Palestinian minister added wryly, "one method of providing employment".

The unique brainstorming session ended in the royal palace in Amman over high tea, and the last word belonged to Prince Hassan. Asked whether he was happy with the treaty Jordan had signed with Israel, he answered, "Normalisation has not prevented us from speaking the truth".

America in the Dock

On the face of it, Iraq was on the wrong side of the law by imposing its own ban on American inspectors in the United Nations teams overseeing Iraqi disarmament for more than six years in the autumn of 1997. But Baghdad had chosen its moment carefully to make a telling and just point. How long must a country remain under sanctions imposed by an American-dominated UN Security Council? And how long can one country, however powerful, use the veto mechanism to pursue its own foreign-policy objectives under the cloak of the United Nations?

By all accounts, the Iraqi leadership was waiting for an opportunity to challenge the United States. Although the resolution that was finally passed over Russian, French and Chinese abstentions, threatening a travel ban on categories of Iraqi officials, was a pale shadow of what the Americans wanted, Baghdad saw its opportunity to cross swords with Washington yet again. Instead of giving relief from the crippling UN-imposed sanctions, the Security Council, under the baton of the United States, was threatening tougher action on the ground that Iraq was withholding information from UN inspectors, led by Richard Butler who had earned praise from the Clinton administration for relieving them of the chore of getting around Indian objections to the CTBT, the Comprehensive Test Ban Treaty. And Butler was suitably belligerent.

Rising to the bait, the United States had held out the possibility of military action under the recognised euphemism of "no option being ruled out" even while activating its diplomacy to try not to use force. Russia and France had jointly spoken against the use of force (with China earlier making the same point) while calling upon Iraq to back down. And Jordan had added its voice to plead for a peaceful resolution of the new crisis.

Unlike during President Saddam Hussein's fateful misjudgement of US and Arab governments' reaction to his invasion and annexation of Kuwait, he was using his present tactic against the US for a studied political purpose—to raise the whole issue of UN-imposed sanctions and their political motives and to present the United States with the unpalatable choice of another round of military action that would serve to alienate the Arab world further—after the partisanship of the US on the Palestinian–Israeli confrontation had made what is called Arab street opinion increasingly anti-American. At the same time, President Saddam was challenging Russia, France and China to come out from under the American shadow in the UN—no one expected Britain to do anything other than follow the American lead.

There were thus two plays being staged in the world theatre—a formal Iraqi challenge to the US in the UN ambit and a second, more subtle, play-within-a-play in which Baghdad was seeking to bare the real American motives for continuing UN sanctions. In the latter sub-plot, Saddam Hussein was a necessary prop for a continuing major American military presence in the region as also for the arms sales the US could achieve. And there was the strength of the weak when driven against the wall: they had little to lose in courting a further fight with Goliath. Even after paying a tremendous price for President Saddam's unforgivable action in invading Kuwait, the US-inspired UN sanctions had devastated and pauperised a whole nation, and there was no end in sight.

In Baghdad's view, a continuing stalemate was the worst of its opinions. A whole army of UN inspectors of various nationalities, leavened by discreetly placed US personnel, went up and down the country trying to discover forbidden munitions. When discovered, these were dutifully destroyed. At other times, some spot investigations were prevented raising an orchestrated US cry, and the UN was again brought into the picture. Iraq was lying and hiding forbidden arms, said the UN inspectors. But despite the obvious power and clout of the United States, the other permanent Security Council members barring Britain were beginning to register their mild protests while the people of Iraq continued to groan under their growing privations. The oil-for-food deal had done less than was hoped for, with the US having been tempted to use it for its political purposes.

Veto Hammerlock

There was something terribly wrong with a veto system that could give any one of the permanent members the right to leave a whole nation out in the wind twisting in the hot sun to die a slow death at the altar of US strategic interests. How could a UN mechanism be made an instrument of oppression, whatever the justifications offered? Could one country run the United Nations as a fiefdom (ironically without paying its obligatory dues)?

These were uncomfortable questions to answer even though no one disputed America's unique power and position in the post-Cold War world. The conventional wisdom was that the US would not agree to have the sanctions lifted until the Saddam regime went. On the other hand, America would seem to have a vested interest in the continuation of the regime. One way out of the dilemma of interminable sanctions would be to have "smart" sanctions which would become invalid after a time unless renewed afresh by the Security Council.

The Iraqi regime's immediate objective in taking on the US at this stage was to highlight the contradictions in the American position on West Asia. There were few Arabs in West Asia, if any, who would call the US an "honest broker" in the Palestinian–Israeli confrontation. While this crisis was being exacerbated every day by the actions of Israeli Prime Minister Benjamin Netanyahu, who was more honest than his Labour opponents in stating the Israeli objectives, the impoverishment of an entire people was gaining the US more opponents in the Arab world. America might rule the waves, as Britain once did, and the skies as well, but it could not succeed in achieving its goal by might alone.

America Upstaged, 1998

Amidst a sense of relief in the Arab world over the agreement signed by the UN secretary-general, Kofi Annan, and the Iraqi government in February 1998, averting imminent US–British air strikes on Iraq, was a matrix of reactions that highlighted the complexities of the issues involved and the main actors taking part.

The reactions to the deal, brokered after days of long and arduous discussions, ranged from the obvious delight of the Gulf and wider Arab world to the caution, if not scepticism, of the United States. The Clinton administration seemed to be unsure of how distrustful it should be of the deal and how much credit to take for forcing President Saddam Hussein's hand by an ostentatious display of fire power.

Russia and France, on their part, were claiming credit for Annan's success for their insistence on a diplomatic solution. Indeed, a Russian deputy foreign minister had set up camp in Baghdad for weeks to pursue his country's mediation efforts. Britain's Tony Blair, as the main backer of the American hard line, was content to sound tough, to the unhappiness of many in the European Union for his failure to evolve a common policy during his country's rotating presidency.

And even as officials in Washington talked about waiting to see the fine print, Americans were facing the obvious problem of pulling back from a military confrontation at the last minute after the high-tech war machine was in place for giving Iraq "significant" knocks. A day earlier, Albright had introduced a very undiplomatic and jarring note by publicly proclaiming that American "national interests" would take precedence over the United Nations and what it chose to agree upon.

We had it on the authority of the UN Secretary-General that the essential and main features of the UN Security Council resolutions, particularly on free access to all sites without setting deadlines, had been accepted by Iraq and there was a signed document to prove it. Amman's suggestion at the post-signing ceremony that the inspections should be completed in "reasonable time" would imply that the Iraqis did make the point that these inspections could not be continued indefinitely—seven years was long enough to punish a people.

The Iraqi leadership decided not to insist on written time limits because it was persuaded that instead of blocking an agreement, it would be best to leave the time-table to work on the basis of political compulsions favouring Iraq.

American Problem

Judging by the Israeli reaction to the UN–Iraq deal in terms of the assertion that Iraq would continue to pose a threat, American disappointment over the last-minute understanding reached in Baghdad would perhaps acquire a sharper edge. For in the American policy-making establishment, the protection and arming of Israel were a central consideration, together with protecting the oil resources and their access to the West. But being deprived of launching air strikes on Iraq—Washington could hardly go ahead unilaterally to bomb Iraq after the agreement—posed a major problem for the Clinton administration precisely because it was pursuing a "dual containment" policy in relation to Iraq and Iran, without much thought or foresight.

With Iran, "wrestling diplomacy" might lead to a gradual thaw in relations, particularly after the assumption of the presidency by Khatami, but America's dilemmas would not go away. As a holding operation, the US was likely to retain the beefed-up forces it had in the Gulf region—there were some suggestions to make the enhanced force semi-permanent—but there would be opposition from several Gulf states if they were required to pay for it, apart from the political objections that would be raised by at least some of the states in West Asia.

The American approach to Tel Aviv's insolent building of a Greater Israel by reducing Palestinians to serfdom in virtual Bantustans had merely added fuel to the fire, the perception being that the US had first deprived the Iraqi people of food and medicines for seven long years and then gathered an armada to bomb the once-prosperous country back to the Stone Age.

It should be clear to American policy-makers that their attempts at justifying their starkly different approaches to Iraq and Israel struck no chord in Arab hearts. For much as people in the Arab world might dislike some attributes of President Saddam Hussein, American policies were serving to present him as one who dared to defy the world's bully who was aligned with, and protected, Israel.

There were compelling domestic reasons for American administrations to support Israel's policies, however wrong-headed and disastrous they might be for American interests, but unless Washington could control Israel's behaviour and approach to Palestinians, it had to steel itself to continue losing influence in West Asia.

A Pebble in a Pond

The old aphorism of things getting worse before they get better seemed to be coming true in West Asia in early March 2002. Just as Arabs and the wider world were despairing of the levels of violence escalating each day, with Palestinian suicide bombers being answered by Israel with bombs from modern fighter jets and missiles from helicopter gunships, a pebble had been thrown into the pool of blood. And that pebble had been making bigger and bigger circles.

The pebble was, of course, thrown by Saudi Arabia's Crown Prince Abdullah bin Abdul Aziz Al-Saud most discreetly through a *New York Times* columnist. And it consisted of an old formula, land for peace, taken to its logical conclusion of full recognition of Israel with full withdrawal to the pre-1967 borders. But both its timing and the weight of the Saudis had made the world's chancelleries sit up.

The Bush administration, largely disengaged as it had been from the worsening confrontation, first dismissed the idea as a "minor development" only to undertake a somersault, with the President calling Prince Abdullah and sending two senior officials to Riyadh. In a sense, Vice-President Dick Cheney's much publicised planned tour of the Arab world to promote the concept of an American air war taking Iraq's President Saddam out had been upstaged by the proposal to make peace in the orgy of violence between Israelis and Palestinians.

What Prince Abdullah proposed to Thomas Friedman of the *New York Times*, published in his column on February 17, was "full withdrawal from all occupied territories in accordance with UN resolutions for full normalisation of relations". Further, he suggested that he had pigeonholed his plan to make the proposal public at an Arab League summit in Beirut scheduled towards the end of March because of the levels of Israeli oppression of Palestinians.

Senior Saudi officials had amplified the plan as "more a vision than a plan or initiative". Indeed, apart from the restoration of occupied land on the West Bank and in Gaza to the pre-1967 borders, the evocative issue of the return of Arab East Jerusalem was mentioned although the other prickly issue of the right of refugees' return to Israel had not been broached.

Next only to the American views, Israeli Prime Minister Ariel Sharon's reaction was significant because although the plan contained elements that were anathema to him, he had described it to a European interlocutor as "an interesting idea". He had been unable to provide either peace or security to his people in his year in office and he could not openly rebuff the only glimmer of hope that had appeared on the horizon. Nor could he afford to alienate a world that had looked askance at the manner in which he had been making his point through the use of a modern fighting machine on a civilian population and undertaking military incursions into Palestinian refugee camps and habitations.

The plan had taken on a life of its own. The Saudis were traditionally coy in taking the political centrestage on controversial issues. And with the Oslo peace process in tatters and an uncompromising hardliner at the helm in Israel, there had seemed no way out of the 17-month-long intefada. The American and Israeli mantra of demanding peace first before substantive discussions was a barren path because it let the extremist Palestinian factions set the agenda. Nor was it helpful to humiliate Arafat by confining and grounding him and destroying his means of transport.

The American-led war against Iraq to force it to reverse its invasion of Kuwait led to the Madrid conference on West Asia because the Arab world had shamed Washington by drawing a parallel between its approach to Iraq and Israel. The beginning of the process led to the Oslo accords that now lie buried. Similarly, the September 11 events and their impact on America and the world had particularly shaken up West Asia with Washington, for instance, questioning Saudi policies.

Camp David Formula

The spotlight had turned back to the Camp David formula towards the end of the Clinton presidency under which some 95 per cent of the West Bank and the whole of the Gaza Strip were to be returned to a Palestinian state, with Palestinians enjoying conditional sovereignty over Muslim holy sites in Jerusalem. Although Americans were quick to blame Arafat for rejecting the formula, the Jerusalem proposal was unacceptable and the issue of the return of refugees was unresolved.

Some American comment suggested that they construed the Saudi ideas as a fence-mending exercise with the US because of the level of hostile attention the Saudi nationality of most of the hijackers had attracted. In real terms, the search for a motive was irrelevant because they provided a new opening which could only be firmed up at the Arab League summit.

Arafat welcomed the Saudi proposal and had sought prompt American support for it, realising as he did that only if President Bush were to abandon his not so benign neglect of the Israeli–Palestinian confrontation could Israel be brought to the negotiating table. And it was an indication of European interest in the new Saudi initiative that the European Union's foreign and security policy chief, Javier Solana, paid a quick visit to Sharon and Arafat before going on to Riyadh. Collectively, the Europeans did not bear the stigma of being biased in favour of Israel.

The hurdles before setting the stage for a substantive dialogue were formidable and there were few who would bet on a more helpful era in West Asia in the short term. But peace between Israelis and Palestinians could only come about if the United States abandoned its foolish ventures in taking President Saddam out and instead concentrated on helping to take Palestinians and Israelis out of the cauldron of death and despair.

Facts of Life

Events were swirling at such breakneck speed that yesterday's big initiative became a non-event; military coercion reached new, previously unimaginable, levels; suicide bombers found holes in a supposedly impregnable fortress and the world tut-tutted and watched the horror of suicide bombings and the incongruity and cruelty of an army shooting its way into civilian areas in an almost farcically unequal battle.

Two images stood out in the welter of events. One was the new halo bestowed by Israel on Yasser Arafat, smiling and defiant as he talked to the world's leaders over the telephone and granted television interviews by candlelight. The Israelis said they have "isolated" him, confining him to two rooms in his headquarters that lay in ruins, with water and electricity connections cut off. The second image was of a Bush administration totally out of its depth, symbolised as much by the impotence of the mediator, General Anthony Zinni, as by the breezy manner of President George W. Bush's commentary on events from his holiday ranch.

The UN Security Council was also brought into the picture, with the United States choosing not to veto a resolution seeking a cease-fire and the withdrawal of Israeli forces from Palestinian cities. Earlier, the US had permitted the Security Council to speak about a Palestinian state. Everyone understood that the United Nations was a bit player in the deadly West Asian drama, and Israel immediately made clear it had no intention of acting on the resolution.

It was tragic that the macabre dance of death should have to be enacted when everyone knew the ending. No one could doubt that there would be an independent Palestinian state comprising at least 95 per cent of the present occupied territories on the West Bank and in the Gaza Strip, with the bulk of East Jerusalem as its capital. What remained to be worked out was to define the Palestinian refugees' right of return to Israel in practical terms and the mechanism for the stewardship of Jewish holy places in East Jerusalem.

So much had been compressed in days that the public espousal of the land for peace deal by Saudi Arabia's Prince Abdullah, made at the Arab League summit in Beirut, was almost forgotten. Yet this was the first time than an important Arab state, the guardian of the two holiest sites for Muslims, had offered full normalisation of relations in exchange for the occupied territories and the return of the refugees. Now that the Oslo peace process lay buried, here was the promise of Arab acceptance of Israel in their region.

It was singularly unfortunate that at a time the United States, as the protector and mentor of Israel, could have wrapped up a deal that could have ensured Israel's existence in peace and security should be in a bind of its own making. Ariel Sharon's rise was due to the failure of Ehud Barak to bring peace and security, despite his brave, if eccentric, attempts. In sharp contrast to President Bill Clinton's hands-on policy, President George W. Bush took an arm's length approach, understandably interpreted by Sharon as a licence to act as he would wish to.

The nature of Israeli actions in Palestinian areas — comprising the use of F-16 fighters, helicopter gunships and battle tanks and targeted killings of Palestinians — came to be counter-productive, with the response coming in the rising tide of suicide bombings. Sharon viewed the post-September 11 mood in America as being particularly auspicious for his penchant for using military force to seek political solutions.

Setting Scores

Apart from the thrust on Afghanistan, the Bush administration had devised its own set of priorities in West Asia, and it consisted of settling scores with Iraq's President Saddam Hussein. Belatedly, Washington realised that Vice-President Dick Cheney's planned West Asian safari to win friends and influence people in relation to a future American military intervention in Iraq became an occasion for his hosts to unveil their agenda: America's approach to the Israeli–Palestinian conflict. And to drive home the point, Iraq used the Arab League summit to proclaim its acceptance of Kuwait as a nation state and made an ostentatious reconciliation with Saudi Arabia.

How long the deadly contest between Israelis and Palestinians would last in this phase remained to be seen. It was clear as daylight that a mere cease-fire held little attraction for Palestinians unless it was linked to a political process that would follow. True, the Saudi land-for-peace formula was a vision, rather than a detailed road map, but the process should begin soon. And the longer the Bush administration took to get to grips with the problem while reading homilies on the evil of suicide bombings, the less would be the agony of Palestinians and Israelis alike.

For their part, Israelis should face up to the difficult decisions they had to make. Neither Barak nor Sharon had been able to live up to his promise of providing peace and security. The Israelis were divided down the middle on seeking peace with Palestinians, with the moderates enjoying something of a majority in calmer times when feelings were not as inflamed. Barak's road was more promising because it would eventually open up the prospect of a Jewish and a Palestinian state living in peace side by side.

It would be foolish to underestimate the complexities of the situation. The US was trying to cope with fighting a "war on terror", with its pronounced West Asian links even outside the central figure of Osama bin Laden. Much as the Bush administration would wish otherwise, the Israeli–Palestinian confrontation played a central part in fuelling the anti-American rage in the Arab world. Those who have lived in the region or studied its problems knew that the basic Palestinian cause was just. It was for the Bush administration to reconcile its strategic alliance with Israel and the domestic compulsions that guided American policy with doing justice to the Palestinians.

Nothing short of a viable and sovereign Palestinian state would bring peace to West Asia, despite the undoubted hyperpower status the United States enjoyed in the world.

Bush's Learning Curve

President George W. Bush should have been forewarned. Even as his Secretary of State Colin Powell was trying to square the circle in West Asia, Israel struck back, as it always did when it wanted to achieve an objective in Washington. The political battle had been effectively moved from the region of conflict to the corridors of power in the United States.

Only twice before in the history of Israel's interaction with the United States had US presidents aced Tel Aviv — for a limited period and a limited objective. One was during President Eisenhower's time over the Suez Canal; the other during the presidency of W's father, Bush Senior, when he withheld guarantees of a $10 billion loan to discipline Israel on its expansion of settlements on occupied land.

Israel had traditionally maintained a well-oiled set of lobbies in Washington around the nucleus of the American Jewish elite. For much of the time, Israel reigned supreme on Capitol Hill as the fortunes and electoral prospects of many Congressmen and Senators were dependent upon Jewish bounty.

So it was hardly surprising that even as the voice of the Eastern establishment, the *New York Times*, was lecturing Israel on having "insulted" the President of the United States of America for contemptuously flouting his public demand that Israel withdraw troops from Palestinian cities, Ariel Sharon released his secret weapon. He despatched the former prime minister, Benjamin Netanyahu, to pump hands on Capitol Hill, telling sympathetic, if not fawning, legislators with the help of a map that Palestinians wanted the whole of Israel and the occupied territories. For many Israelis, facts were not a hindrance to presenting their case.

American Double-Speak

Despite W's reiteration of his message and his amplification that "without delay" meant "now", Israeli incursions into Palestinian areas continued and expanded. And it was not lost upon the Arab world that Powell's West Asian safari, which won a public rebuke from the King of Morocco, made its unhurried way to Jerusalem giving Sharon ample time to finish his bloody job. Along the way, the secretary of state softened his President's demand because the Israeli prime minister, primed by opinion polls, was in no mood to listen.

The web of Israeli interaction with the US policy-making establishment was deep. Any US president, always perilously close to an election of one kind or another in the American scheme of things, needed rare courage, if not foolhardiness, to go against Israel's interests, as perceived by Tel Aviv.

W's initial mistake was to assume that taking a hands-off approach to a region in which Israel had been nurtured and brought to adulthood by the power and money of the United States would mean anything but giving a licence to a man of Sharon's track record to do his irresponsible worst. When events began to cascade out of control, W periodically sent the luckless General Zinni to the region. It was like sending a single fire engine to douse the flames of a whole city. Israel's iron fist—the full scale of the carnage in Jenin had still to be revealed— was answered by suicide bombers.

It was the arrogance and foolishness of Sharon that he not merely smashed the infrastructure of the laboriously built and European-financed Palestinian Authority but condemned Arafat to the status of "an enemy", finally confining him to two rooms in his shattered headquarters in Ramallah after cutting off water and electricity supplies. He thus had no Palestinian interlocutor to talk to. Learning a painful lesson from Vice-President Dick Cheney, who had set preconditions to meeting Arafat, Powell demanded merely the

Palestinian leadership's condemnation of suicide bombings before eventually granting him an audience.

Self-Inflicted Wound

If W now found himself between a rock and a hard place, it was his own fault, compounded by his lack of experience in international diplomacy. As even the likes of Henry Kissinger had documented mournfully, Israelis were the toughest negotiators and never tougher than in crossing swords with American presidents. The Bush administration was trying to cover up its embarrassment for having been rudely disobeyed. The stakes were particularly high in the conflict.

Given the scale of Israeli operations and the rage among Palestinians and in the wider Arab world, the US policy-making establishment was mulling the options. The former Labour prime minister Ehud Barak was helping the process in his own fashion. He had proposed a fenced-in Israel initially taking in 25 per cent of the occupied West Bank and the two parties returning to the Camp David negotiations of Bill Clinton's presidency. This formula should be implemented unilaterally if necessary, in his view.

American policy-makers, on the other hand, were also looking at an imposed solution on the premise that animosities between the two sides had reached a stage when only an American diktat could work. Traditionally chary of peace-keeping assignments for American forces, the Bush administration would baulk at such an outcome.

The moral of the story was that all the world's problems could not be folded into an American-led "war on terror". Whatever the shape of the future Israeli leadership, a country that sought peace and security could have neither unless it gave Palestinians a viable independent state of Palestine. And that state had to comprise annexed Arab East Jerusalem. Further, the state of Israel had to atone for the injustice done to the Palestinians, driven out of their homes in what is Israel, by symbolically accepting some of them even as they have, over the decades, demanded atonement from the world for the persecution they suffered in Europe.

History in Aid of State

Histoy is many things. It is a lesson for the future. Sometimes, it repeats itself as a farce, but it is almost universally used as a myth for nation-building. It is equally often employed as an instrument of state policy. Nowhere is the last aspect used more effectively than by the state of Israel because its very rationale, even for those who accept it, lies in the distant past and less distant European events.

Any visitor to Israel is brought face to face with history in the museums and other reminders sponsored by the state, with busloads of young schoolchildren being brought to these institutions almost every day to inculcate in them a sense of their unhappy past. Israelis traditionally wear their history on their sleeves. Why the people of West Asia should pay for the persecution suffered by Jews in Europe is a matter that has been lost in the politics played by Britain and the United States and by "the facts of the ground".

Israel was by no means alone in using Nazi Germany's treatment of Jews to gain political advantage in the post-war era. Britain and France employed this unsavoury history to keep West Germany down, despite its economic weight and population, and it was in rather recent times that Germany regained its full sovereignty as the last vestiges of World War II occupation were dismantled. But an older generation of German leaders was willing to suffer the consequences of the past in governing their country while setting their sights on bringing prosperity.

Two events happened to change this putting down of Germany: the reunification of the two Germanies, despite British opposition and French unhappiness, and the coming to power of a new generation untainted by the past, symbolised by Gerhard Schröder. The reunification gave the Germans political weight and Schröder's chancellorship spelled out in no uncertain terms that Germans had done enough penance for their past and would not allow its evocation as a stick to beat the new Berlin Republic with. If only reluctantly, Germany's European neighbours accepted the new reality.

But the battle over Germany's past was being fought anew, this time between Europe and the United States. The provocation was Israel's treatment of and conduct towards Palestinians and the level of America's pro-Israel sympathies and the nature of its policies. There were well-known domestic factors, in addition to Washington's strategic needs, that influenced US policies whose blatant pro-Israel nature could be gauged by the kind of resolutions routinely passed the Congress and the Senate. Election prospects of Congressmen and Senators were often dependent upon their equation with American Jewry and Bush Senior's defeat in his last election bid was laid at the door of his one act of delaying a $ 10 billion loan guarantee to pressure Israel on its policy of expanding illegal settlements on occupied land.

Prime Minister Ariel Sharon's decision to send his troops on a military adventure in Palestinian towns and territories with the full force of American-supplied weapons of war—F-16s, tanks and helicopter gunships—in response to suicide bombings killing Israeli civilians created an outrage in Europe. The reaction in the United States was different. An indulgent George W Bush administration had given Sharon much room for manoeuvre even while publicly calling on him to withdraw troops "without delay". And in perhaps the most ironic twist, W called Sharon "a man of peace" even while taking to task Arafat, confined to his battered headquarters, his Palestinian Authority destroyed and his civilian infrastructure in ruins.

European Response

Europe, being closer to the scene of tragedy and without an all-powerful Jewish lobby to contend with, responded differently. Europeans, including officials of the European Union and governments, questioned Sharon's methods, the brutality of the force used against Palestinian civilians, the destruction of the Palestinian Authority's civilian infrastructure (including files of the heath and education ministries) and routine Israeli assassinations of Palestinians. There was also a greater resonance in Europe of Israel's actions because of the large Muslim minorities — from North Africa in France and Turks in Germany. There were also, regrettably, acts of vandalism of Israeli cemeteries and monuments, particularly in France.

The devastation and deaths in the Jenin refugee camp in particular brought about an almost universal outcry, and Israel hastily agreed to receive a United Nations fact-finding team to limit the damage. After the UN Security Council agreed to send a team appointed by Secretary-General Kofi Annan, Israel successfully sabotaged the project while members of the team cooled their heels in Geneva. And Tel Aviv rode out of the crisis scot-free, riding as usual on the copious American shoulders. It was the United States against the United Nations and the UN lost, again.

However, Europe was not prepared for the avalanche of American criticism on the alleged pro-Arab sympathies of the old continent. And the unkindest cut of all was the suggestion that Europe was being anti-Semitic in the attitude it had adopted towards the Israeli-Palestinian problem. True, these charges were being made by wide segments of the American media, rather than by the US ruling establishment, but they reflected official opinion.

Europe's sharp reaction, in particular the European Union's blunt response by Javier Solana, the foreign policy and security chief, was an indication of the anger in European capitals. It was also perhaps intended to demolish the long-held myth that by criticising Israel and its conduct towards Palestinians, an individual or a nation became anti-Semitic. Europe was now saying collectively what Germany had said earlier as a nation state.

Solana called to account "those who want to give the impression that Europe has been transformed into a xenophobic, racist and anti-Semitic territory". The American theme song often is that Europe is burdened with its past and hence takes a more pro-Arab and anti-Israeli stance. This was an ostentatious American display of the uses Israel has been making of history. The extreme right was presenting problems in Europe but it remained a fringe movement and was motivated by a complex set of factors.

There was, however, a silver lining to the new crisis in cross-Atlantic relations. Like Germany, the European continent might have emancipated itself by refusing to let others use the tyranny of history for ulterior motives. It was not the end of history, but it could mark the end of the exploitation of a doubtless tragic chapter of history for selfish ends.

The Imperial Power

Oil Weapon, 1973

President Nixon's year of Europe in 1973 was ending on a note of bitterness never before experienced between West Europe and the United States. The West Asian war and its consequences had left their mark on Nato and the concept of the Atlantic alliance. West Europeans felt frustrated and the Americans appeared to be keen on creating the impression that they wanted their allies to be penalised for their policies. The Arabs had succeeded in dividing West Europe and the US by using their oil resources as a political weapon.

But oil was only one factor, however important, in the difficulties between West Europe and the US. Essentially, it had served to aggravate their differences over the future shape of their relationship, in particular over sharing the defence burden and making concessions on trade and monetary issues.

Henry Kissinger's initial call for a new Atlantic Charter was met with scepticism in West European capitals. The basic American premise he disclosed was that with an emergence of an affluent West Europe and the achievement of a Soviet–US power parity there was need to redefine the Atlantic relationship. What the Americans wanted was that West Europe had to pay more for its defence, both in money and men, and make significant concessions in trade and monetary policies. The predictable European response was to assume that the Americans were using their defence role to force the European Economic Community to make major concessions.

France led the European defiance for two reasons. Traditionally, General de Gaulle and his successor, President Pompidou, had sought to use the Common Market to build up an independent European personality. Besides, in the French view, if the EEC was collectively to be a new power centre, how could it have a one-sided relationship with one of the two superpowers? Second, the French insisted—and most of their partners agreed—that defence, trade and monetary issues could not be lumped together. There were different forums and time scales for discussing and resolving them.

Europe's main problem was that, since the Americans were insisting on a collective EEC reply and they had the military and economic strength to create greater problems for Europe, they had to be placated. A somewhat vague and general statement on future relations followed and agreement was reached to issue three separate statements to coincide with President Nixon's visit to Europe. The French tactic in the negotiations with their EEC partners was not unexpected. Having taken an extreme position, they made last-minute minor concessions which were greeted with relief by the other members who declared that the final compromise was a triumph of the community's ability to act together.

The Americans were far from satisfied, as Kissinger made clear, but the consultations were continued to define the new Atlantic relationship and to make the declarations more substantial. But the West Asia conflict overtook these consultations and helped to aggravate mutual suspicious. For the Europeans, the last straw was the state of alert of US forces all over the world without consulting Nato. For the Americans, the crisis point was reached when West Germany publicly asked them not to ship arms to Israel through their sea ports.

European Shock

France blamed the superpowers for fuelling the war machine in West Asia. The Americans rebuked the allies for refusing to support their position and, in the case of West Germany, for hindering the supply of arms to Israel. It was the US Defence Secretary, Schlesinger, who made the first critical reference but this was later repeated by the State Department and President Nixon. West Europe was shocked and, though the governments outwardly remained calm, there was no mistaking their indignation.

The issues posed by the Americans were clear. Were the Nato alliance and the American commitment to defend Europe to serve only Europe or were they able to serve the US's strategic interests? If the US was unable to move its troops to an area of vital interest in an emergency, it would have to review its commitment. The European answer, though not yet publicly stated, was equally clear. The Americans could not unilaterally commit Europeans to one side in a conflict in another part of the world although, in the event of a general war, West Europe's sympathy and support would go to the US. Secondly, the Americans could not violate national sovereignty, as they had done in West Germany's case.

These charges and counter-charges increased differences among the Atlantic partners as the war continued. While the two superpowers continued to supply arms, they were also trying to evolve a cease-fire formula. The US was primarily interested in keeping Soviet troops out of West Asia; but in the process it also kept out British and French troops. Before the shock of the US alert hit Europe, the position of the major countries in the EEC had already crystallised. President Pompidou was following the policy of "pro-Arab neutrality" laid down by General de Gaulle in 1967. Italy quickly sided with the French, in view of its almost total dependence on West Asian oil. Britain too adopted a similar posture.

West Germany was placed in a difficult position. A majority of the people was sympathetic to Israel but the Brandt Government had been trying to adopt a neutral position for some time; besides, the threat of an Arab oil boycott was real. In the event, the Germans decided to remain neutral—as far as official policy was concerned. The Dutch, with their emotional attachment to Israel, were not able to restrain themselves. The result was that the Netherlands became the only EEC member to be blacklisted by Arab oil producers.

The Bonn Foreign Ministry's protest to the US against shipping arms to Israel from Bremerhaven port reportedly followed a warning by the Arabs. Bonn was in any event offended by the US bid to ship arms to Israel from West Germany. It might have ignored the air-lifting of arms from American bases but resented the loading of Israeli ships in a German port, especially without prior permission.

Bonn's Misfortune

It was ironical that Bonn should have been singled out by the Americans for their rebuke. It had been the most faithful and consistent supporter of Nato; besides, most of the US troops committed to Europe were in Germany. It was, therefore, embarrassing for Brandt to be cast in the role of the ringleader of dissidents. The irony of this situation was not lost on France, which had been more critical of US policies than others. One French comment was that Nato had to be facing a crisis if the Americans had to rebuke West Germany, Turkey and Greece.

While West European governments were trying to play down the crisis, the consequences of the war and the American response to it marked a new turn in the Atlantic relationship. It was recognised in many EEC capitals that their inability to play a role in the war and in peace-making sprang from their inability to agree to act together.

The EEC was facing many problems in reaching the goal of economic and monetary union by the end of the decade, as decided as the summit of the Nine in Paris. Their differences arose from their differing national interests and they did not have the same approach to the EEC. The economic and monetary problems, however, were not as important as the obstacles to a common European defence. The French, committed to an independent nuclear capability, were convinced that in the last analysis each country had to look after its own defence.

Even if the French were persuaded to agree to an Anglo-French European nuclear deterrent, American agreement would be essential because Britain was dependent on the US. If agreement was reached on a European nuclear capability, what would happen to West Germany? Would it agree to an inferior position decades after the end of World War II? On the other hand, the prospect of a German finger on the nuclear trigger would immediately produce reactions from the Soviet Union and its East European allies.

Post-Victory Scenario

The West Asian drama was being enacted at two levels. The United States was in the process of reordering its relations in the region after its victory in the Second Gulf War and the collapse of the Soviet Union. Both these developments had strengthened American hands vis-à-vis Israel. At the other level, the business of calling a peace conference to begin an end to the Arab–Israeli confrontation was engaging US diplomacy.

The two issues were inter-connected because the new American clout in relation to the Israelis and the Arabs gave it a rather unique window of opportunity. One result had been a conscious US effort to correct somewhat its traditional tilt towards Israel by President George Bush successfully rebuffing the Jewish lobby in the US on the Israeli demand for loan guarantees of $ 10 billion. More than the amount involved, the symbolism of an American President saying 'no' to Israel had not been lost on Jerusalem or the Arab world.

In an astute counter-move, the Palestinians on their part had given a positive reaction to the US peace proposals. Many loose ends were still to be tied and the question of Palestinian representation through a joint Palestinian–Jordanian delegation would have to be fudged. The words of disapproval from Israel were not interpreted as a final answer.

The Israeli problem was that the nation was split down the middle on the question of making peace with the Arabs. On the Palestinian question, the territories for peace proposal, which formed the basis of the relevant United Nations resolutions, perhaps a majority of Israelis would favour it, depending upon how the question was posed. But the turbulent history of the region and the Israelis' own role in it caused fear in Jerusalem. Having learnt to live with the gun and on the strength of the gun, Israelis found it psychologically difficult to adapt to the possibility of living in peace.

Israel remained an important strategic ally of the United States, but the terms of the relationship between the two countries were undergoing a subtle change. Washington was telling Israel that it could no longer enjoy a veto over perceived American interests in the region and that the US administration had now the gumption to take on the Jewish lobby.

President Bush chose to go to the heart of the Israeli–Palestinian tangle by deferring the loan guarantee request for settling Soviet Jews. For the record, the US had always opposed the building of new settlements on the occupied territories, but turned a blind eye to them. The Israelis had continued to build new settlements and as if to snub the US, a new settlement had gone up almost every time US Secretary of State James Baker made a trip to the region.

Once the question of Palestinian representation was resolved, the peace conference was to serve as a curtainraiser to individual talks between the Arab states and the Palestinian–Jordanian delegation on the one hand and the Israelis on the other. Logically, the conference should have a referral role in being able to assess the progress of the talks after a time although for Jerusalem, it was a mere fig-leaf for the Arabs in order to be able to hold one on one talks.

American Plan

The American plan envisaged a two-stage operation: a period of autonomy for the West Bank and Gaza Strip followed, after a specified period, by talks on the future of these areas. The emotive question of restoring East Jerusalem to the Palestinians was not being tackled immediately nor was the question of returning the Golan Heights to Syria, although both these issues were bound to be raised in future discussions.

It was the American hope that once the peace process got going and Arabs and Israelis could discuss their problem at a table, the rough edges on either side would begin to wear out. The question of an independent state of Palestine was left for the future. It was, for instance, open to question whether many Arab states would want to see a separate independent state of Palestine; most would prefer to see it in a confederation with Jordan.

It was, of course, clear to everyone that the peace conference was an American show, despite the somewhat symbolic co-sponsoring of the Soviet Union. It was equally clear that the question of American credibility in the region was on test, in view of the role played by it in the Second Gulf War. The Palestinians, for one, had accepted the American argument that they had the most to gain from a peace conference; even from the tactical point of view, the decision of the Palestine National Council, the Palestine Liberation Organisation's parliament in exile, made sense.

No one familiar with West Asia would have illusions about the difficulties involved in ending the Arab–Israeli confrontation. But the post-Cold War era had brought in its wake challenges as well as opportunities and the certainty that the process of building new equations was taking shape. Any reordering of relations had to be a two-track affair, from the American point of view.

American efforts to begin the Arab–Israeli peace process was a necessary psychological prop to the future role the US was seeking to carve out for itself. The contours of such a role were still being mulled over but they consisted of two elements: a new security set-up and the equations to be worked out among the major countries of the region: Egypt, Syria, Saudi Arabia and Iran.

The new Syrian flexibility was a result of the collapse of the Soviet Union as a world power while both for Egypt and Saudi Arabia, their close links with the US had to be tempered by their peoples' perceptions of America. Iran, as a major power in the region, was in the process of ending its isolation from the West; the fact that Teheran had tentatively chosen to oppose the peace conference meant that it wished to use the issue as a bargaining chip with the US.

In immediate terms, the security arrangements consisted of a link-up between Egypt, Syria and the six-nation Gulf Cooperation Council and a defence agreement between the US and Kuwait. But a more permanent security arrangement had still to be worked out. Here Iraq in its defeat cast a long shadow.

President Saddam Hussein was still in place in Iraq and the game he was playing with the US, wearing the UN hat, over free inspection of nuclear and other sites was serving a propaganda purpose for him in the Arab world. The strong American reaction was making Washington's Arab allies distinctly uncomfortable; for another, Iraq was spreading the word that the US was bent on persecuting Iraqis.

In any event, the end of the Iraqi drama was not in sight. And until there was a definitive end to UN sanctions and the political demise of President Saddam—the two were inter-connected—the shape of the future West Asian power equations would remain hazy. Indeed, President Saddam could derive some vicarious satisfaction from muddying the West Asian waters for the US.

The crux of the matter was that while most Arabs had been quick to make a change in the light of the new realities, Israel had yet to adapt itself to America's increased weight in the region and the world. The manner in which the Israeli Prime Minister, Shamir, handled the loan guarantee question showed that he was still relying on the old technique of influencing American policy through the Jewish lobby in the US.

It had taken the Israeli establishment some time to readjust its sights and play down what had been a humiliating showdown. It would be foolish to underrate the influence of the Jewish lobby on American policy-making, particularly as presidential elections approached, but Bush had shown that a President who felt secure could afford to take on Israel on issues viewed as vital to US foreign policy interests.

End of History?

The United States was groping for an answer to the future. While the precise contours of that future were still uncertain and beset with dangers, an agonising debate was in progress on how the United States could safeguard its own and broader Western interests. The debate was proceeding on two planes—the philosophical, and at the political level, with Democrats charging the Bush administration with harbouring a nostalgia for the Cold War.

The debate flowed from a central phenomenon of our times: the demise of the messianic creed of communism as a world phenomenon. Mikhail Gorbachev's attempt to refashion his country more in tune with modern times and accepted freedoms had transformed the world scene. And the resulting debate in the US was swirling round two theses presented by Francis Fukuyama of the State Department's policy planning staff and Lawrence Eagleburger, deputy assistant secretary of state.

Writing a provocative essay in *The National Interest* journal in his personal capacity, Fukuyama used a selective interpretation of the German philosopher Hegel to suggest that the world might be witnessing the end of history, "the end point of mankind's ideological evolution and the universalisation of Western liberal democracy as the final form of human government". This followed from the defeat of the two major challenges to liberalism, those of fascism and communism.

For Fukuyama, "the death of this ideology (Marxism-Leninism) means the growing 'common marketisation' of international relations, and the diminution of the likelihood of large-scale conflict between states". And, doubtless to provoke debate, he ended his thesis on the following controversial note:

"I can feel in myself, and see in others around me, a powerful nostalgia for the time when history existed. Such nostalgia, in fact, will continue to fuel competition and conflict even in the post-historical world for some time to come.... Perhaps this very prospect of centuries of boredom at the end of history will serve to get history started once again".

Eagleburger's thesis, propounded in a lecture at Georgetown University in Washington, was on the hard-nosed theme of protecting American interests in the future. But it gave expression to an echo of Fukuyama's nostalgia theme in the words: "For all its risks and uncertainties, the Cold War was characterised by a remarkably stable and predictable set of relations among the great powers".

Eagleburger consoled himself with the thought that the US would remain "for long into the next century the only power able—or at least willing—to think in global terms and to fashion policies in the overall political, economic and security interest of the West".

But Eagleburger's recipe for managing the future followed a predictable course. He pleaded for retention of the Western consensus, in the North Atlantic Treaty Organisation and otherwise, and cast doubts on the irreversible nature of the changes in the communist world. What had served the West for 40 years still provided Eagleburger the beacon for the future.

There was an inherent contradiction in Eagleburger's thesis. On the one hand, he suggested that the "uncharted waters" America was entering required a new compass. On the other hand, he pleaded: "...The positive and indeed revolutionary changes which are sweeping the world today are reversible, and they could not be sustained by the efforts of the United States alone. They can, however, be sustained, and the dangers which exist turned into opportunities, if the Western democracies renewed their commitment to a collective and cooperative approach to the major issues which confront them".

Future Dangers

What had added piquancy to the American debate was the widespread feeling that President George Bush's cautious brand of international diplomacy, particularly in dealing with the other superpower, was not quite the answer to the breathtaking changes taking place in the world. In Washington's view, the future held two major dangers, in addition to transnational issues and the possibility of the poor countries' problems spilling over into the North. They were the trade and economic tensions symbolised by the unification of the European Economic Community and by Japan and the fear that the disintegration of the European communist world would lead to the disintegration of the Nato edifice.

The Americans' major political worries were, indeed, Euro-centred. And Eagleburger's thesis contained an almost plaintive plea to the West Europeans, telling them that "It is the Europeans themselves who have the principal political stake in making the transition to a new and undivided Europe a peaceful and orderly one". And he said, "Already, we are hearing it said that we need to take measures to ensure the success of Gorbachev's reforms. This, however, is not the task of American foreign policy, nor should it be that of our Western partners".

The American debate increasingly tended to turn to the adequacies or otherwise of President Bush because he had thus far shown that he was singularly lacking the grand vision that could be the only answer to the exciting present and a pregnant future. He began his presidency with a long foreign policy review, and although he was able to surmount the last crisis in Nato by his proposals on conventional arms cuts, he had done little to fire the imagination of his people with new foreign policy goals. The new momentum in superpower relations was due mainly to Soviet nagging and concessions, rather than to new thinking in Washington.

In his reaction to Fukuyama's essay, Senator Daniel Patrick Moynihan had tartly suggested: "It would be small consolation to find at the end of history, or at least at the end of the twentieth century, 'the basic principles of the liberal democratic state could not be improved upon' if in the process the principal liberal democratic state finds itself exhausted from the struggle, depleted, demoralised...He (President Bush) is free to change American policy toward the Soviets as much as he wishes, without risk of being said to have subverted it".

Perhaps President Bush had assumed the American presidency at the wrong time in world history. His caution—his critics called it timidity—was more suited to the predictable nature of the Cold War phase of world politics, rather than the uncharted waters Eagleburger had talked about.

Merely to preserve the Nato edifice and to extract trade concessions from the European Community and Japan were an inadequate answer to the changing world. Eangleburger might well warn West Europe of the danger of competition in expanding relations with the East, but the dynamic of the disintegration of the communist state, being dramatically revealed in Poland and Hungary, would inevitably draw West Europe closer to the East.

Washington acknowledged that the German question was back on the international agenda—but had not suggested an answer, except to talk of the value of continued Western strategic consensus. Admittedly, Washington had to be careful in publicly revealing future plans, but all indications suggested that the Bush administration was not thinking in terms of an imaginative conceptual answer to the extraordinary ferment in Europe.

Nato and the Warsaw Pact might become increasingly irrelevant to the issues that would excite Europeans in the future. At the centre of changes in Europe was, of course, West Germany. Its future was now delicately poised between a stronger European Community and the appeal of reunification and asserting its economic primacy in East Europe.

Eagleburger's lecture at Georgetown University ended with the thought that managing the future would require "American leadership of the highest order". President Bush's leadership qualities had, indeed, become the central subject of debate. Americans were asking the right question.

Second Thoughts

Rather soon, the New World Order of President George Bush's description was becoming old-fashioned. The end of bipolarity had led to the military pre-eminence of the United States, but its efforts to impose an order of its liking had run into a host of problems.

Nothing illustrated this better than developments in West Asia, although the uncertainties raised by the disintegration of the Soviet

Union and the break-up of Yugoslavia underlined the ferment the world was passing through. Indeed, West Asia had the seeds of a North-South confrontation and highlighted the very different perspectives of the West, principally the US, and the Arab world.

The United States led an alliance to win the Second Gulf War, but the victory became flawed by President Saddam Hussein's refusal to bow out. And over Libya, the American success in getting the UN Security Council to pass a sanctions resolution with a dealine if Tripoli refused to oblige was at the cost of five abstention votes, including China's and India's.

In both cases, the United States was right on the substance of the issues involved. Saddam Hussein violated all canons of international justice by marching into and annexing Kuwait. The Libyans had the duty of coming clean on surrendering the two men accused of planting bombs on planes which led to a large number of deaths.

However, the problems arose out of the United Nations' inability to be the world's policeman and Arab—and the Third World's—perceptions of American, and Western, double standards. The United Nations cover for American and Western actions in Iraq illustrated US resolve and its ability to muster enough votes in the Security Council. The Western view outside Washington had been that since the UN was in no position to mount a military operation on the scale required, it was in order that the United States and its allies accomplished the task of righting a wrong.

In the Libyan case, the United States was on less secure ground although the underlying theme of punishing the perpetrators of the crime of terrorism enjoyed near-universal support. Even more than over Iraq, the Security Council resolution raised several questions. Had mediation been given a fair chance before resolving to enforce mandatory sanctions? How long would the United Nations remain susceptible to succumbing to American wishes? Why were only some countries disciplined while others went scot-free?

It was clear that the United States was using its military dominance in the world after the collapse of the Soviet Union to seek strategic and political advantages for itself. President Bush had publicly proclaimed the goal of his country remaining the world leader. Washington was able to secure a Western consensus on Iraq and Libya to fashion UN action along its desires—avoiding the divisive strategic issues with West Europe.

Inevitably, the US had to sacrifice morality and justice on occasion in pursuit of its strategic and political objectives. Its selective policy of arming the countries of West Asia was only one example. It was also using the Western consensus effectively on such issues as nuclear and missile proliferation while employing its political clout to seek a better deal for itself on the trade and economic fronts.

Two Problems

The United States had two major problems in refashioning the world after its interests. It window of opportunity was limited by the emerging power status of the European Economic Community, Japan and, ultimately, Russia. Second, American plans could succeed in the medium term only if it could build a durable consensus to include the countries that counted in the world.

On the first score, the US could only try to speed up the process of refashioning the world in line with its present and future interests. Its dilemmas were greater in respect of the Third World, the events in West Asia being a piquant pointer.

The Bush administration has had the sagacity of grasping the opportunity presented by the end of the Second Gulf War to begin the long process of getting to grips with the Arab–Israeli confrontation. As the $10 billion loan guarantee dispute with Israel had demonstrated, Washington was keen to maintain a semblance of even-handedness between the Arabs and Israel.

However extravagant and unjustified Arab feelings might be in relation to Iraq and Libya, the bulk of the Arab masses reacted instinctively and felt that US actions were vindictive and partisan. The anti-Iraq coalition the US was able to build had fallen apart, as far as its Arab members were concerned. Statements out of Washington suggesting the need for another series of bombing raids on Iraq to take out its alleged remaining nuclear facilities merely added fuel to the fire.

Admittedly, the world was sought to be refashioned along American and, up to a point, Western lines. When developed countries had felt compelled to support the United States for their own interests, the Third World was in no position to cock a snook at the United States. But such a coercive acquiescence could not provide a stable basis for a new world polity. Growing anti-American feelings in the Arab world, however questionable the actions of a Saddam Hussein or a Gaddafi, were an expression of people's frustrations with the prevailing tenets of US policy.

West Asia had been a traditional powder keg, with its oil wealth, its anachronistic structures of governance and the frustrations of the poor in the non-oil-producing countries. US efforts to form an effective security environment to protect its strategic and geopolitical interests in the region have had some success. But relationships with governments whose base was being eroded by swelling anti-American feelings could at best be tenuous.

Unlike Israel, which set its own rules to protect its security, the United States, as the world's pre-eminent military power, could not for long enjoy such freedom of action. West Asia presented a major challenge to American policies because regional and personal ambitions against a backdrop of instability and Arab-Israel enmity collided with US interests.

The concept of an Arab nation, fashioned by Nasser, failed to work in any realistic or geopolitical sense many years ago. Psychologically, the idea still had an appeal and Arabs were willing to applaud any Arab ruler, however wrong-headed he might be, seen to be standing up against mighty America.

US administrations were no strangers to bouts of anti-Americanism in different parts of the world. What distinguished the mood in the Arab world from a recurrent phenomenon was its intensity and that it was happening at a time of great uncertainties around the world.

Washington saw its compulsions in West Asia in clear terms. Apart from securing its strategic and political interests, the US viewed the region as the crucial area to make its other policy objectives stick. They concerned the non-proliferation of biological, chemical and nuclear weapons and of medium- and long-range missiles.

American efforts had run into trouble. Many countries in the Third World did not buy the Western concepts of enforcing non-proliferation goals and the fact was that Israel, with a widely believed nuclear arsenal, remained outside the net. In this area, *realpolitik* entered American calculations. As the main strategic US ally in West Asia, Israel enjoyed a dispensation not applicable to any of the Arab friends or allies.

The short point was not Libya's unreasonableness in refusing to hand over the two accused but the symbolism involved in the attitudes of Tripoli and Washington. As the Arabs reactions to the UN Security Council resolution revealed, Gaddafi was the new Arab hero defying the US. For Washington, Libya was a rogue elephant who had to be disciplined and taught a lesson.

The freedom of American action was circumscribed by Bush's election campaign to retain the presidency. Thus far, President Bush had resisted giving in to the powerful Israeli lobby in the US on the loan guarantee, but the situation could change if his re-election chances dimmed. In any event, an election year in the U.S. distorted American policy.

The larger issues would remain beyond U.S. Election Day. They concerned questions of war and peace in West Asia and America's ability to pursue its policies without provoking a revolt in the Arab world. The prospect of a New World Order was at best a mirage; at worst, it was self-delusion.

World View, 1993

With the advent of 1993, the world's agenda was so overloaded with prickly problems that, instead of President Bush's New World Order, we were destined to face disorder. The end of the Soviet

Union and the fall of communism had changed the parameters of debate and relationships so drastically that a period of instability and readjustment of political and military alignments was inevitable.

Two facts stood out in the emerging world. The United States remained the world's pre-eminent military power and the United Nations had entered the most effective phase in its history under American tutelage. It was equally clear that rival centres of power were growing in Europe and Japan to challenge American dominance against the setting of increasing ethnic and religious clashes mixed with large doses of regional nationalism.

There were numerous crisis areas around the world, but the future would be largely determined by how the new American President, Bill Clinton, handled the relationship with Russia, how the constituents of the former Soviet Union made the transition to an ordered life and how Europe managed its own contradictions in taking the process of integration forward while helping find solutions to such tragedies as Yugoslavia.

Despite the break-up of the Soviet Union and Russia's reduced status in the world, the Moscow–Washington relationship held the key to the future because upon it would depend the stability of Europe and in such areas as West Asia and the Indian subcontinent. And the mainspring of Russian success would flow from its ability to begin to surmount its mind-boggling problems in transforming the economy.

While Germany and Japan were surely but slowly emerging out of the shadows of the last World War to take their rightful place, the continuing tragedy in Bosnia-Herzegovina and the American foray into Somalia indicated that they had some way to go. Nothing illustrated this point as clearly as the United States virtually running the United Nations in its key areas of peace-keeping and peace-making. It was the only power with the capability and will to intervene in regional conflicts and crisis situations.

The United States and the West in general could help Russia with money and moral and political support, but they could not solve Russian problems for President Boris Yeltsin. The latter was fighting with his back to the wall even as economic privations and chaos impinged on the country's politics. Thus far, the Russian President had proved to be a shrewd political operator but his skills would be severely tested in the year ahead.

A second major problem for President Yeltsin was his country's relations with the former Soviet constituents. The Commonwealth of Independent States experiment was doomed from the start; it was in any case a device to get Mikhail Gorbachev out. However the conflicts in and among the new republics were resolved, they would continue to impinge on the 25 million ethnic Russians living in what had become foreign lands.

American Dominance

The United Nations had an activist secretary-general in Boutros Boutros-Ghali, but his efforts to give the organisation a measure of autonomy in coping with the growing number of crises around the world had met with a dusty answer. The truth was that the United States was loath to give up its privilege of orchestrating how the UN system should cope with a crisis, and any substantial military help offered came with an American commander, whatever the composition of the multinational forces.

The UN could not remain merely an arm of American foreign and security policies, but there was no country or group that could effectively challenge Washington's sway in 1993. Europe was not quite ready nor was Japan in a position to fill American shoes. A restructuring of the UN was still years away.

Europe had discovered that its march towards a European Economic Community that could rival the United States in a common market and political clout had run into problems of local nationalism and economic woes. The EEC had inaugurated its single market leaving out some areas and although the Maastrict Treaty was back on track, concessions had to be offered to Denmark, in addition to the initial concessions given to Britain.

The engine of the EEC, a reunified Germany, had slowed down as a result of the inevitable problems arising out of integrating the former German Democratic Republic in the Federation. Apart from the financial drain this had meant for Bonn's exchequer, it had sprouted the ugly problems of an underclass which was seeking salvation through neo-Nazism. The anti-foreigner feeling was not restricted to Germany; in most EEC countries, recession and the psychological problems of adjusting to a new world had made foreigners scapegoats.

West Asia still loomed large as a world crisis area and after a moderately promising start in Madrid, the new Israeli–Arab peace process brokered by the US had run into heavy weather. The ingredients of an Arab-Israeli reconciliation remained the main stumbling block, and the new US President would have to commit his administration to a major effort to move the peace process forward.

In the short term, the more vulnerable countries of the region, particularly in the Persian Gulf, had chosen to seek safety in American protection. But for many countries, their immense oil wealth and archaic forms of government remained combustible sources of instability. The Arab–Israeli confrontation helped accentuate national problems in West Asia.

The African continent had more than its share of troubles and conflicts. Not unexpectedly, the promising beginning to a new South

Africa had yielded place to killings, political crises and painful read-justment. Essentially, the two main sides to the conflict remained committed to creating a new, more democratic country, a process that should move forward in 1993.

African Disorder

But a rash of civil wars and conflicts in many African countries had brought home to the world the continent's instability. Nature's ravages and man-made hunger had combined to bring misery and death to vast populations. As the American-led international effort in Somalia indicated, the process of stability and economic well-being would be out of reach for many in Africa.

On the other hand, China was devoting its energies single-mindedly to its economic well-being even as it modernised its forces. Beijing was looking upon its relationship with the new American adminis-tration with some foreboding. But being pragmatists, the Chinese leaders were already making soothing noises for Washington's benefit. The US relationship was key to the Chinese goal of becoming an economic and military power in world terms. China needed US investment and trade and technology and the chances were that Beijing would make peace with President-elect Clinton, despite problems.

Where did the so-called Third World fit into this picture? The non-aligned countries made a bid to re-attune themselves to the new world at their summit in Jakarta the previous year. Even as the creed had lost much steam in the changing world, most belonging to the Non-aligned Movement (NAM) felt there was the political necessity of using it to demand a place in the sun. With major countries in NAM immersed in domestic problems and turmoil, the movement failed to make its mark in the new configurations.

Nearer home, the South Asian Association for Regional Cooperation was facing a crisis. Coupled with the economic necessity of a regional grouping was the handicap of Indo-Pakistani enmity. And the Ayodhya temple crisis in India and the reactions it evoked in Pakistan and Bangladesh had set back hopes for the slow progress of an idea whose time had come.

The reality was that there was little prospect of the Third World counting for much in shaping the world after the end of the Cold War. India's ability had been considerably hampered by the process of redefining its national identity and philosophy, but most other members had their own problems to contend with. Some Third World countries had chosen to subsume politics in achieving economic success. But there was little cause for cheer.

The CNN Effect

When the world's media were ordered out of Baghdad four days after the beginning of the Second Gulf War, there was one exception. The Cable News Network (CNN) was allowed to stay in solitary splendour. Peter Arnett stayed in Baghdad for the duration of the war, much to the envy of the rest of us, raising controversies in the United States over being "used" by the Iraqi authorities.

I was reminded of those early days of the war over Baghdad on seeing CNN score another scoop. It was the only international television or news organisation allowed to accompany Jimmy Carter, the former US president, to North Korea. Other news organisations and the world listened to and watched CNN.

CNN was the pioneer in worldwide satellite television news reporting, and the Second Gulf War pitchforked it into hundreds of millions of living rooms. It represented a quantum jump in the power and reach of media, a phenomenon no one could ignore. *Time* magazine gave Ted Turner the accolade of the Man of the Year, and he and his organisation certainly deserved the praise they won.

While CNN had become an accepted fact of life, its very success raised questions. Wonderful as it was for a journalist or political analyst to watch a major news event take place as it took place, didn't it distort reality by giving the "literal truth" to the layman? Second, had CNN crossed the dividing line between an observer and a participant?

To an extent, journalism had become more personalised over the decades. In the print media, personal bylines—once a scarce commodity—had been proliferating. But personalised journalism came into its own with the advent of television, with news anchors becoming international celebrities, demanding and receiving a commensurate price. Walter Cronkite was perhaps the most famous television news journalist of the pre-satellite era. But his forte remained presentation and interpretation, despite the film clips shown on the programme. Instead of the traditional journalist's felicity in writing an in-depth analysis, the television journalist had to have the ability of talking coherently and instant interpretation. The element of superficiality the latter method lent the subject was unavoidable.

But the television journalist, despite his greater prominence, was above all a reporter interpreting events. Although political journalists around the world were often tempted to don the mantle of the statesman, rather than the reporter, advising their country's, or the world's, leaders what to do, they remained on the periphery of decision-making. Their words or revelations could influence events or, on occasion, the fate of individual leaders, but they stayed on the sidelines. The most striking instance of television's ability to influence public opinion was in turning large numbers of Americans against the Vietnam War.

Satellite journalism, symbolised above all by CNN, was taking the journalist away from his mooring. He was in danger of becoming a participant in the political drama. Baghdad had shrewdly assessed the benefit it would derive by having one agency transmitting pictures instantly around the world because its movements could be controlled. CNN, therefore, became a factor for decision-makers in Washington and elsewhere around the world. The importance of CNN had thus grown even as it was blurring the distinction between an observer and a participant.

CNN Reality

The emergence of this phenomenon posed problems not only for the profession of journalism but also for decision-makers. The instant telecast of pictures of an event or a misfortune imposed pressures on decision-makers to act instantly. It remained to be determined, for instance, what contribution was made by satellite television to President Bill Clinton's unfortunate foray into Somalia. As an American official had quipped, there was reality and there was "CNN reality". The two could be in collision, and it required steel nerves and prudent judgement to withstand public pressures to do something instantly.

Which brings us to the other problem CNN's success spawned. A layman, in the developed world as in developing countries, had neither the time nor the inclination to master intricate matters of international diplomacy. For instance, only a minority in the West read the so-called quality newspapers; the majority relied on television to find out what was happening in the world. For those without the background or knowledge about a major world crisis, satellite television, by its very nature and the demands of the clock, was a poor teacher. The ubiquitous common man was, therefore, likely to get a distorted picture of a fast-moving development and, when aroused, could be wrongly impassioned.

Those at CNN and in other satellite organisations said they were trying to do an honest job and instant coverage of events was leavened with more deliberate comment, often by experts, in "talk shows". Ironically, the latter programmes were often skipped by the majority and catered to a narrower audience which read serious newspapers in the first place. Television's power had been traditionally acknowledged by governments around the world; the authorities, even in the West, were more restrictive in dealing with television than they were with the print media.

What had changed was the reach of television, with the mushrooming of satellites around the world. It was this reach which was tempting governments on the local and international planes to coopt satellite television, in particular its most powerful exponent, in promoting their interests. Iraq and North Korea were not the first states, nor would they be the last, to use media to their advantage. During my time in the former Soviet Union, I discovered that the communist authorities had mastered the art of using the dictates of deadlines for news agencies to promote their cause. And it had become a matter of routine for White House staff in Washington to time important announcements with an eye on the main television news bulletins.

With 24-hour television spanning the globe, the old deadlines were gone, and CNN's credo of staying with the news as long as it took was encouraging governments simply to adopt it as a participant in all but name in staging an event. The more CNN became the sole international witness to some news event, the more it would have to ponder over the price of its "scoops".

Clinton's Tasks

President Bill Clinton was relishing his unusual role as the choreographer of a peace extravaganza, for the laser beam he had promised to focus on domestic issues had faltered, and there was no better cure for a bruised presidency than pirouetting on the world stage. After the disaster in Somalia, the botched intervention in Bosnia, things had gone right for Clinton. And he rattled them off at his White House press conference: Haiti, North Korea, Iraq, and West Asia.

There was a palpable fear among some that he might be pushing his luck. What was conceived as a glittering ceremony to witness the signing of a peace treaty between Israel and a second Arab state had been transformed into President Clinton's odyssey to West Asia, with the focal point being his visit to Damascus. For the imperfect peace that had come about between Israel and some of its Arab neighbours could get nowhere without bringing Syria on board. President Assad was willing, provided Israel committed itself to a full withdrawal from the Golan Heights

The irony was that without the Israeli–PLO agreement, the perceptible changes that were taking place in West Asia would not have occurred. And this agreement and the autonomy experiment on the Gaza Strip and Jericho were being buffeted by the anti-peace activists on the two sides as Israel reverted to its traditional medicine of closing the autonomous areas and raining bombs on southern Lebanon. And Israeli ministers were talking about the "separation" of Jews and Palestinians, as if such as absurd thesis could form the basis of reconciliation in the region.

President Saddam Hussein demonstrated that he was capable of stirring the pot. The American response was swift, and, unlike the last time, the Iraqi president thought that discretion was the better part of valour. But the new crisis was a reminder that there was unfinished business in Iraq, triggering a debate in the United States on whether the US-led forces should not have toppled President Saddam more than three years earlier. Yet out of the Second Gulf war came the Madrid peace process.

Given the history of Arabs' confrontation with Israel, it was not surprising that the movement towards peace should be halting and interspersed with blood. But as President Clinton sought to make peace between Syria and Israel, he would do well to remember that the PLO–Israel agreement that spurred negotiations on other tracks could also come to haunt the peace process. There could be no peace short of Palestinians getting their due. And increasingly Israeli methods of retaliating against extremist acts were coming to mock the concept of peace.

Yasser Arafat had indicated that he would seek US help in getting nations to deliver on their promises of financial assistance. Even more important than money would be Clinton's ability to convince the Israeli leaders that they should not make the Palestinian Authority's task more difficult than it was by piling on economic miseries on Palestinians and expecting Arafat to wave a magic wand to make such opposition groups as Hamas disappear.

Palestinian Doubts

There was a sharp division among Palestinians on the merits of the autonomy agreement with Israel between those who saw it as a necessary route to an independent state and others who believed that Palestinians had been short-changed. The majority was inclined to give the experiment a chance, and now this majority was assailed by fresh doubts as the autonomy process sputtered. To believe that a guerrilla movement could suddenly transform itself into a government that worked like clockwork would be unrealistic, nor should anyone have illusions about the Herculean nature of the task of the Palestinian Authority in building the Gaza Strip practically from scratch, woefully inadequate as it is in infrastructure while a high proportion of the young remained without jobs.

Arafat was trying to coopt elements of the Hamas movement into the system. His chances of success would become increasingly bleak if Israel continued to follow its traditional policy of immediate and disproportionate retribution for any attack on Israelis by Hamas extremists. The Israeli Prime minister. Yitzak Rabin, perhaps felt that he had to demonstrate resolve in the face of the shock caused by the suicide bombing of a bus is the heart of Tel Aviv. But he was in danger of seriously undermining the basis of the new thrust for peace in convincing more Palestinians that they took the wrong path through the autonomy agreement.

Any possible breakthrough in the stalemated indirect negotiations between Syria and Israel would bring President Clinton kudos, and his popularity ratings would go up. But the whole peace process would rest on shifting sands if the PLO–Israeli experiment failed. The dispute over Israel pointedly giving Jordan's king a continuing role in East Jerusalem's holy sites without an agreement on its future with the Palestinians had been interpreted by Arafat as a deliberate provocation, further muddying the waters.

A Panting Tour

After the dust had settled on President Bill Clinton's panting tour of West Asia, it was time to examine the vital question on bringing peace to the region. In terms of "photo opportunities" and symbolism, the Jordan–Israel peace treaty was the centrepiece of the President's trip. But the more important questions related to breaking the Israeli impasse with Syria and revitalising the Jericho-Gaza First autonomy experiment. President Clinton's stop-overs in Kuwait and Saudi Arabia were happy events inasmuch as the American leader was basking in the Gulf states' gratitude for the promptitude with which US forces came to the region to cope with threatening Iraqi troop movements.

For all the media attention President Clinton attracted, the outcome of the visit was disappointing. It would seem that he yielded to the temptation of trying to overwhelm President Assad with the symbolism of a US presidential visit to win an agreement without giving him an unequivocal Israeli commitment to a full withdrawal from the Golan Heights. The result was that he was left claiming "progress" on the Syria–Israel track, but little more.

On the equally, if not more, important question of giving a push to the Israeli-PLO peace process, President Clinton publicly gave precedence to Yasser Arafat's task of suppressing terrorism and the need for accountability before release of aid than to helping sort out the political impasse that had overtaken the implementation of the autonomy experiment. Even more ominously, the US secretary of state, Warren Christopher, suggested that Arafat should choose between Hamas on one hand and Israel and the US on the other. The Clinton administration was in effect undercutting Arafat's efforts at coopting elements of Hamas even while fighting extremists in the organisation.

On the plus side, the peace extravaganza did build up a hopeful atmosphere in the region, with old walls falling away and revealed the striking changes that had come about since the Madrid peace process began. Minefields were cleared for the Jordan–Israel peace treaty signing ceremony, and even more dramatically, some 2,500 leaders and businessmen from the Arab states, Israel and other regions were holding a three-day meeting in Casablanca to consider and debate a new economic blueprint for the region. A reminder of unfinished business was the refusal of Syria and Lebanon to attend. And pointedly left out were Iraq and Iran, apart from Libya.

There were rumblings in the background. Apart from those opposing the partial peace process, the Hezbollah in South Lebanon made their point by continuing barrages on Israel's self-declared security zone even as President Clinton flitted from one Arab capital to another. Hamas, which had claimed responsibility for the devastating bomb in the heart of Tel Aviv, vowed that it would continue to oppose the peace deal and target Israelis.

Diplomacy was conducted at two levels—the public and the private. When Clinton chose to invest the prestige of the US presidency in breaking the Syrian-Israeli impasse, he would have hoped that the two parties were close enough to an agreement to permit him to bring about a diplomatic coup. This did not happen and Clinton was left with little option but to give hints through his officials that he would return to Damascus soon—when it did happen. The plodding Christopher would, in the meantime, return to his shuttle diplomacy.

No Breakthrough

What happened in private between Clinton and Assad was not revealed. Presumably, the latter was willing to make tactical concessions once his central point—an Israeli commitment to withdraw from the whole of the Golan—was accepted. Indeed, earlier Syrian comment had suggested that the US president's visit to Damascus would have been more useful had it preceded a stop in Israel, reversing the schedule. In the event, President Clinton arrived without the key to a solution, and while the Syrians made him welcome and reiterated their commitment to a just and comprehensive peace, there was no breakthrough.

President Clinton's meeting with Arafat in Cairo was, by all accounts, a hurried encounter and the president was perhaps under a compulsion to emphasise the issue of security for Israel after the Tel Aviv tragedy. Neither he nor his secretary of state gave any indication that they were conscious of the complexity of the situation Arafat faced nor of the formidable economic and political problems he had to surmount even without the closure of the autonomous areas ordered by Israel, depriving some 70,000 Palestinians of their livelihood.

The impression Palestinians gained from the Clinton trip was that they got nothing out of it, and as the US had choreographed it, the race for peace would be run without them. There was the all-important problem of bringing Syria on board and concomitantly resolving the South Lebanon issue; there was the question of ending the Arab economic boycott of Israel. Substantive discussions between Israel and the PLO on the future Palestinian entity would not begin for some two years by which time the momentum for peace would be unstoppable and the PLO would have to make the best of a bad bargain. With pardonable hyperbole, Clinton had decreed that the peace process was already unstoppable.

This was a dangerous feeling for Palestinians to nurture and for the US to give them cause for nurturing. The PLO gave the critical push to the peace process and it simply could not be left on the shelf and forgotten. The critical question was not how Arafat dealt with Hamas but how he could give his people tangible evidence that they were leading a better life and there was hope for them to attain genuine independence and statehood.

Tangling with Iraq

Would Iraq's Saddam Hussein have the last laugh? The Kurdistan Democratic Party, temporarily allied with Baghdad, was trumpeting its seizure of the last important town in northern Iraq and President Clinton had started talking about the limits in influencing events inside Iraq. He was talking not merely of the widely reported Central Intelligence Agency-funded plot to murder Saddam, which had gone awry, but of the unwelcome set of options he had in a dicey situation driven by the compulsions of the US presidential election campaign.

President Clinton's Republican opponent, Bob Dole, was already sharpening his knife to take the re-election seeker to task for declaring success for his air strikes on Iraq when the winner seemed to be President Saddam, who could have gained more in reasserting control over the North than he lost out in the damage inflicted on his military installations in the South. The American strategy of retaliating in the South to punish Saddam for going to the help of a Kurdish faction in the North was determined by the Arab states' and Turkey's reluctance to become staging posts for the attacks and the extremely low American tolerance levels to deaths of their troops.

On the diplomatic front, the White House would have been surprised by the vehement reaction of most of the region and even of some of its Western allies to the cruise missile strikes on Iraq. Not since the Second Gulf War had so many in West Asia opposed an American action so strongly although governments, many of them needing US protection for their own security, had been more diplomatic in their reactions. Perhaps the objections were best articulated by France, which called the action unauthorised by any UN Security Council resolution and said the attacks were uncalled for because President Saddam had moved troops inside his own country and went to the aid of the major Kurdish faction in the North at its invitation. Having made their point, the French quietly went back to policing the "no-fly zone" in the South with the US and Britain, in itself illegal, although not over the extended portion notified from one day to the next by an American fiat.

The Americans were not the only ones surprised by the intensity of the Arab reaction to external involvement in Iraq. The Turkish government learnt to its cost that its foolish plan to appropriate a slice of Iraqi territory in northern Iraq had no takers, except for the Americans and perhaps the Israelis. Ankara was apparently having second thoughts on the wisdom of such a step and was mending its plan, if not scrapping it altogether. There was much concern in the Arab world over threats to the territorial integrity of Iraq because it could spark off a new acute phase of instability in the region, bound hand and foot as Iraq already was by surveillance aircraft policing the better part of Iraqi skies. No one was surprised by CIA-assisted and funded efforts to help assassinate President Saddam, which was part of the agency's hoary tradition of eliminating "inconvenient" foreign leaders, efforts that had singularly failed in getting rid of Cuba's Fidel Castro.

The US, of course, was seldom inhibited by "legalities"—Warren Christopher's definition of the French objection to the air strikes on Iraq—in pursuing its policies. The inhibitions stemmed from Clinton's re-election bid, and the minefields he had to avoid to retain his lead over his Republican rival. The Democrat had many things working for him: an economy that was looking up, low unemployment, the Republican excesses after their congressional triumph in 1994 and some modest successes in the foreign policy field, including the domestically popular Saddam-bashing air strikes. But one wrong move in Iraq and Clinton's popularity ratings could go into a tailspin to the benefit of Dole. Indeed, President Saddam had the power to see another President after George Bush lose his election.

No Soft Options

Even assuming that President Clinton's next action would be determined by his own electoral compulsions, as was his original decision on air strikes, there were no soft options. The Kurds, particularly the losing faction, the PUK temporarily aligned with Iran, felt betrayed by Washington which knew from the beginning that a Kurdish state carved out of Iraq, Iran, Turkey and Syria was not on the cards nor was the dismantlement of Iraq. American efforts to bring and keep the two main and traditionally fractious Kurdish factions together to seek a wide measure of autonomy from Baghdad had been half-hearted. The victorious KDP faction had been begging for American help before deciding to sup with the devil.

One option, of getting directly involved in the Kurdish North in Iraq, had been ruled out by the Clinton administration as being too dangerous, given the risk of getting bogged down in the morass. The other options would range from further air strikes on Iraq from a safe distance or from the Gulf waters or get a regional power such as Turkey to undertake massive military operations along Iraq's northern borders. The first would multiply the protests from the Arab world and it was by no means clear that, despite Ankara's ill-judged security zone idea, it would be willing to court collective Arab opprobrium to do Washington's dirty work.

Despite the wishes of Washington and the countries of the Arab Gulf Cooperation Council to keep the old anti-Iraq coalition of the Second Gulf War, it had disintegrated. France, for one, could retain some influence in West Asia only if it sought to detach itself from the US in critical areas of policy. In the Arab world, leaving aside the personality of President Saddam, it was becoming increasingly unacceptable to the people that Iraq should be bashed for what it chose to do within its own borders, with the US imposing unilateral measures. And there were strong feelings on American moves to deny the long-suffering Iraqi people even the limited monitored oil-for-food sale agreed upon earlier.

Predictably, the Israeli prime minister, Benjamin Netanyahu, had backed Washington's air strike on Iraq, using the crisis further to underline his country's usefulness as the primary US ally in the turbulent region. On the other hand, his ostensible commitment to peace made in Washington was far from convincing. The Likud government was, indeed, a stark reminder to the Arab world of the partisan nature of US administrations, in particular the present one, on any question relating to Israel vis-à-vis the Palestinians and Arabs.

Israel's Prisoner

The United Nations resolution on the explosion in Jerusalem and on the West Bank and Gaza strip in September 1996 was full of symbolism. It positioned the world against Israel and the United States as the latter reneged on its agreement for the compromise resolution to abstain. It represented a defeat for the US inasmuch as Washington did not want a debate at all and no resolution. And, despite its diplomatic language, the thrust of the resolution was criticism of Israel and a call for closing the offensive tunnel that opened up on to the Arab side in Jerusalem.

The reverse for the United States was as striking as it was for Israel. Because the way Washington had been conducting world affairs in the post-Cold War era was to demarcate the areas it wanted to keep the United Nations out, seek the UN umbrella when it suited its interests and, on occasion, involve the UN in a problem to bury it or wash its hands of it. Of course, when things did not quite work out as they should—in Somalia or in Bosnia—there was always the UN to blame.

The world, therefore, was faced with the prospect of being a mute witness to the horrendous events in the occupied territories if it were to follow the American prescription. The UN Security Council, the primary world organ for keeping the peace, however inadequately, would have passed over days of bloodshed in silence. But the ultimate vote—14–0 with one abstention—spoke for itself. It also signalled the end of the era in which Washington could always have everything its own in the Security Council. The drama of the UN vote apart, the Israel-PLO confrontation was now centrestage and, in Hannan Ashrawi's colourful language, the Palestinians and Israelis were fighting over Jerusalem's soul. It used to be said that both Rabin and Arafat were prisoners of the Oslo accords and the orchestrated handshakes on the White House lawn and of each other. After Shimon Peres' defeat, Benjamin Netanyahu was seeking to break out of the prison with tragic results. All American efforts were directed towards putting him back in, but Netanyahu was using the levers Israelis have so masterfully employed for so long in influencing US politicians and administrations. Netanyahu was, in effect, saying that Bill Clinton, seeking re-election, was Israel's prisoner and had to side with it even with the world ranged against Israel in the UN Security Council.

There were, of course, limits to how far Netanyahu could go. Europeans were a factor because of their benign trade dispensation towards Israel and, without a dominant Jewry influencing government decisions, they were in a better position to discipline Israel if they wanted to. Further, Europe had to keep an eye on its flourishing trade with the Arab world. But with Britain rarely marching out of step with the United States and Germany still under American political tutelage, only France made rhetorical gestures of independence. The tragedy was that if Europeans had greater self-confidence and agreement on the kind of Europe they wanted, they could have been a major factor in promoting peace in West Asia.

Band-Aid Effort

Bound by the compulsions of the presidential election and the powerful Jewish lobby, President Clinton was largely restricted to mending the broken pieces of the vase of Oslo. And the obvious beginning was a meeting between Netanyahu and Arafat, a symbolism meant to signal a return to negotiations. The problem was that since he was swept to power, he had refused to negotiate and the charade of his first meeting with the PLO leader was just that. The outlook did not look promising.

The compact between Israel and the Palestinians, propelled by the Second Gulf War, was there would be a trade-off between land and peace and the building of a measure of trust between the two sides after decades of bloody conflict. Despite the many heartbreaks, delays and false starts, the peace process was reaching somewhere. Although the most difficult questions remained to be tackled, for once the American faith in CBMs (confidence-building measures) seemed worthwhile. The Labour government was officially expecting the formation of a future Palestinian state and Rabin had made the decision in principle to trade off the Golan Heights for peace with Syria.

The sharp division in Israel on the peace process was clear enough, and the opposition Likud's rhetoric logically led to the Prime Minister's assassination. On the Palestinian side, the opponents of the Madrid process did their bit through a run of suicide bombings to reverse the sympathy wave for Rabin's successor, Shimon Peres, in favour of a narrow victory for the fire-breathing Netanyahu. The suicide bombers became inactive after Peres' defeat. Netanyahu was doing such a splendid job of demolishing the Madrid edifice that any help from the Palestinian opponents of the peace process was unnecessary.

Netanyahu and Arafat planned to meet in Washington under President Clinton's auspices together with the leaders of Egypt and Jordan, but the dissonance between the two sides was so great that it seemed difficult to envisage a minimum of trust that had to precede a compromise. Rather, the Likud Prime Minister was giving the impression of suffering from a siege mentality, interpreting anything not to his liking as a form of blackmail to extract concessions from him. It would indeed appear that Netanyahu had boxed himself into a corner of his own making. The only choice left for him was either to stick to his hardline policies casting Palestinians as little more than serfs or lose face and perhaps the support of the extreme conservative parties in the government.

It was, of course, clear that a continuing impasse in a peace process gasping for breath could only lead to another explosion. And as the level of killings indicated, the count of the dead and the injured could only grow. Some Israelis were threatening to station troops again in the so-called Palestinian autonomous areas, which would be the last nail in the coffin of the Madrid peace process. Some Palestinians were talking about the need to revive the intefada.

Beating the Drum

One had become accustomed to the Americans' hyperbole and apparent belief in their uniqueness and greatness, never before achieved by any nation on Planet Earth. In a rather routine way, President Clinton and other officials declaimed that the United States of America was "the greatest", rather in the manner of the newly-humbled American boxer had used the phrase as his signature tune.

There was, indeed, a lot Americans could be proud of. Theirs was a dynamic country, ever experimenting, ever thrusting forward, ever innovative, an always "can do" nation. The competitive spirit was inculcated at a young age and was apparent even in the placid world of think tanks, as I discovered during a two-year stint with the Carnegie Endowment of International Peace in New York. The shower of Nobel Prizes Americans carried off almost while doing their daily shopping was impressive. And Americans had achieved excellence in the military field.

Set against these attributes were the less endearing qualities of Americans. Their lack of interest in the rest of the world, their propensity for teaching children the virtues of making money at a very young age, their view of government — all government — as evil, the built-in selfishness that comes with riches and prosperity, their arbitrary unselfish acts, often breathtaking in scope, their belief that American democracy was the best in the world. These are traits one observes in the collective American psyche.

Deep down, the Americans had always believed in their exceptionalism, but their post-Cold War incarnation as the sole surviving superpower had disturbed the American balance in some ways. Arrogance—a quality one did not usually associate with them as a people—had come to the fore. So had the streak of isolationism that had never quite left the US since the founding of the republic. And a world which had largely left behind the strident era of what was the most compelling ideology of the present century confronted the phenomenon of the sole surviving superpower also becoming the world's most ideologically-inclined nation.

The stage was set by Ronald Reagan, who successfully combined his conservative inclinations with a simple and intense hatred of communism best summed up in his description of the Soviet Union as the "evil empire". There was nothing cerebral about Reagan's ideology; it was a gut feeling and hence eminently suited to populist treatment. No doubt this gut feeling mixed well with the desires of the infamous military-industrial complex—so called first by a successful US general and later president—and the persistent theme of all disclosures of American estimates of the might of the Soviet Union was of their gross exaggeration. According to conventional American wisdom, the disintegration of the Soviet Union and the diminution of its successor state seemed to have increased, rather than diminished, the need to enhance American military strength.

Rogue States

There are of course, the "rogue" states, duly announced by Washington, and the need to maintain forces to fight two regional wars at the same time. Besides, there was need to continue Reagan's discredited "Star

Wars" programme to meet a Russia turning malevolent, and, of course, taking care of the odd missile that might come the American way, fired by a "rogue" country or group. The former Soviet president, Mikhail Gorbachev, made the wry comment that it was strange that Republican Congressmen and Senators had insisted on a *larger* military budget than proposed by the Clinton administration.

As the first country at the cutting edge of modern technology, the United States has had problems in coping with the socio-economic consequences of this technology. There is little doubt that while ingenious machines can accomplish wonderful tasks, the human mind takes infinitely longer to use these machines wisely, and the stress machines and their influence on life-style causes has some unwelcome consequences. Americans had a tendency to experiment with, if not embrace, extreme solutions, as was apparent from such phenomena as the Christian Right and a worship of cults.

Among the alienated were white, less well-off males who had been left on the shelf by the demands of the Information Age. Their resentments reduced them to psychological specimens who hated government, "liberalism", foreigners and the United Nations. The irony was that there was little liberalism, as understood in the rest of the world, left in the US, and the Clinton administration had got the best deal ever out of the United Nations by co-opting it as an arm of US foreign policy while refusing to pay the bills.

The tragedy for America, and the world, was that given its present unique status in the world, it did not have the inclination or time to resolve these problems at a natural pace. The US was too busy running the world in its fashion and the true perception of problems was often hidden by a new belief in American infallibility. With the world to command, the US had produced its own brand of arrogant men and women—US spokesman Nicholas Burns and Ambassador to the UN Madeleine Albright, to name two in the government, or columnists such as William Safire. The leitmotif of these persons was that they had the answers to all problems and if the world did not like it, it could lump it.

This long prelude is an attempt to divine the reasons for the extraordinary gung-ho performance of US Defense Secretary William Perry. The manner in which he had been telling the world, in particular the "rogue" states such as Iran and Iraq, that he was spoiling for a fight was unprecedented for a country possessing real military power although it would come naturally to a tinpot dictator. In Kuwait, Perry thundered while explaining the "dual commitment" policy towards Iran and Iraq: "We are prepared to fight a war". And as an aside he warned President Saddam Hussein, "Don't think of coming back to Kuwait again". And before he returned to Washington, he mourned the podium at the Naval post-graduate school at Monterey, California, to declare, "Any country which would use chemical, biological weapons against the US, its troops, its allies, we would respond with overwhelming force".

On the eve of retiring as defence secretary, Perry perhaps wanted to project the great things he had done to the American military to make it the fighting force it was— echoes of Vietnam seemed to have receded. And there was also the American tradition of freewheeling public diplomacy. However, while agencies such as the Central Intelligence Agency were known to have pursued their own policies, often contrary to the government's, a US defence secretary did not have that privilege. In other words, if the policies being projected by Perry were those of President Clinton in his second term, the world better take cover.

Facts on the Ground

The Clinton administration's reluctance to engage itself in West Asia, except on Israel's behalf, was finally having the salutary effect of showing the world, including Americans, the wages of its skewered policy. For the well-worn formula adopted by President Clinton and his senior officials of not offering their own solution was one way to favour the Israelis as they merrily went on colonising more and more Palestinian land could only encourage an escalating level of violence. The reaction of the Netanyahu government was Pavlovian: no deal without security, a concept always endorsed by Washington.

And, after a time and much humming and hawing, another reluctant attempt was made by Washington to pretend to mediate by sending a man viewed as an Israeli partisan by Palestinians. The result was either failure or a patchwork truce that was blown sky-high by the next explosion caused either by suicide bombers or the unwise buffer zone, carved out of Lebanese territory by Israel, which it was seeking to hold on to by sending planes to bomb Lebanese targets. And West Asia continued to lurch from crisis to crisis.

Yet it should be plain to the dimmest wit that harping on security while colonising more Palestinian land and making a mockery of the entire basis of the Oslo agreements could not ensure security for Israel. And the issue of war and peace in West Asia was for a change beginning to be debated in the United States for what it was, rather than in the context of President Clinton's love for Israel, the power and money of the influential American Jewish lobby and the deep American suspicion of Arabs that made US administrations rely on Israelis as their strategic partners in the region.

Regrettably, the post-Cold War world had given the United States the luxury of making mistakes because there was no other power or combination of powers that could force Washington to abandon its foolish policies. A change in American policy had, therefore, to come from within, despite the besotted nature of Capitol Hill's relationship with Israel. And it was a hopeful sign that Americans were beginning to ask real questions such as the correlation between justice and peace and the reluctance of President Clinton to risk annoying Israelis to the slightest extent.

It is not lost upon the American policy-making elite that the feisty new secretary of state, Madeleine Albright, had not dared to go to West Asia during the first six months, preferring to conduct diplomacy at long distance. She knew that given her president's deep attachment to Israel and unwillingness to take any risk in displeasing Jews, her foray into West Asia could only lead to a failed mission, whatever the gloss placed on it. Perhaps she herself was not averse to Clinton's policy, having only recently discovered her Jewish roots. Indeed, the bulk of senior Americans dealing with the region had no doubts about their own Jewish roots. The dominance of Jews in senior American policy-making positions on West Asia was easily explained in that other competent men and women would ordinarily prefer specialisation in the "sexier" regions of the world.

Palestinian Reality

Yet the lessons of Israeli–Palestinian turbulence should have been clear to Americans as to the more thoughtful Israelis. "Security" was not manna from heaven to be plucked and enjoyed, and, in the circumstances of West Asia in the closing years of the twentieth century, it could never be achieved by Israel remaining a colonial power policing Palestinian areas, bottling up entire populations at will, making access to and from Palestinian territories a nightmare for the Palestinians themselves and the world and generally telling the Palestinians that they were little better than serfs and must live on bits and pieces of territory that must not be armed. This was the reality anyone who had been to the so-called Palestinian territories would bear witness to.

Terrorism against innocent civilians for any cause is abhorrent and must be condemned, but it was time Americans paused to consider what options they were leaving Palestinians. Under the guise of the peace process, Israelis were carving up much of the occupied West Bank and Gaza Strip while reciting the mantra of security. And in her first substantive remarks on West Asia since assuming office, Albright was content to harp on Israeli security while giving no hope to Palestinians about tomorrow, hiding behind the argument that the two parties should sort out the problems themselves after heavily tipping the scales in favour of Israelis.

Israelis, including the leader of the Labour Party, made no secret of their policy of exploiting the unique position of their protector and supporter in the post-Cold War world as the sole surviving superpower to secure gains they could not have dreamed of achieving in the era of two superpowers. But they as well as the Americans were being short-sighted in shackling Palestinians hand and foot while the benign Clinton administration looked on. Because the American-supported Israeli policies were laying millions of landmines that would splinter peace in the region for generations.

It is arguable whether the Israelis and Americans were serious in expecting Arafat to give Israel "security" while they were doing everything in their power to humiliate him and the mainstream Fatah faction. If Arafat chose to make more concessions than he had made thus far — remember the tunnel skirting the Al Aqsa mosque that stayed open despite the many Palestinians killed protesting against it and the continuing building work on the so-called Har Homa Jewish settlement in the heart of occupied Arab East Jerusalem—he would be handing over his people to the Hamas movement.

Every day the actions of the Israeli authorities were driving Palestinians into the arms of Hamas whose words had a greater resonance among the people against the backdrop of Israeli actions. And we had Netanyahu and President Clinton and his administration asking Arafat to provide Israelis security. Given their actions, the only way Israelis could achieve security was by using one of the atom bombs they were reputed to possess, but then it would be a security of the graveyard, for Palestinians and Israelis, and others as well. Short of such medicine, it was doubtful that Israelis could see through the first decade of the twenty-first century in the master–servant relationship they were prepetuating with Palestinians.

Baghdad's Signal

However the high-wire act between Iraq and the United States ended—the scripted return from the brink of another bloody confrontation—the United States' ability to hijack the United Nations for its ends would undergo a change. For by challenging the impartiality of American inspectors in UN teams in Iraq, Baghdad had highlighted a situation increasingly upsetting the rest of the world. If the United Nations was becoming an American fiefdom, there was not much point in having a world organisation.

In technical terms, Iraq was in breach of the law because a country's officials wearing the UN hat became international civil servants. Reality, as we know, was quite different, as the scramble for senior posts (not merely for the perks involved) showed. The Americans could use proxies such as the Australian Richard Butler to head the UN Iraq commission and any number of obliging Brits, but the Iraqis were

unerringly targeting the US in saying that the UN sanctions exercise—
the most draconian in UN history—had been maintained for close to
seven years to serve the Clinton administration's political and strategic
objectives. Looking at the decades-long US sanctions against Cuba,
Baghdad was seeking a time-frame for terminating them.

A world grown weary of American arrogance in the post-Cold War
era was looking at the crisis through different eyes. While Washington's
European allies were following the Clinton administration's lead in
the eastward expansion of Nato and in slapping sanctions on some
countries even though disagreeing on bread and butter trade issues,
they were restless. If the post-Cold War world meant the hegemony of
one power, they wished to change it. The much-heralded multipolar
world had still to arrive, but the Iraq crisis was something of an
opportunity to stake out a different vision of the future.

Against this backdrop, it was disingenuous of UN Secretary-General
Kofi Annan to suggest that the UN mission to Baghdad was in the
nature of a ladder offered to Iraq "to climb down from the precipice".
There was little point for Baghdad to use the ladder without achieving
the minimum political objective of gaining an implicit, if not explicit,
deadline for the end of sanctions and demonstrating that United
Nations actions in Iraq were largely an American show. (The US
secretary of state, Madeleine Albright, has abandoned diplomatic
convention by describing President Saddam Hussein as "just a
congenital liar".) After trying unsuccessfully to resume UN inspections
with American inspectors for form's sake, the UN said the teams were
taking a day off while the US made a point of resuming U-2 spy plane
flights despite Iraqi threats to shoot them down, Baghdad conveniently
deciding that the plane was outside the range of the anti-aircraft
batteries. The political fiction was that the US was flying the spy planes
at the request of the United Nations.

The Iraq crisis was being played out at two different levels. One
was the immediate outcome in terms of the concessions Iraq was able
to extract by bringing issues to a head. American forbearance was due
to its realisation that Washington's policy of continuing sanctions
against Iraq into the twenty-first century had few takers even among
its Western allies, bar Britrain. The other, more important, aspect was
the future of the Western alliance and how the work of the United
Nations was to be defined in a more equitable fashion. To an extent,
the crisis could represent a benchmark in putting an end to the
unchallenged American domination of the world organisation.

American Empire

The truth was that while preaching the virtues of democracy at home
and abroad, the United States kept the concepts outside the field of
international affairs. As the sole surviving superpower, Washington

was quite clear about exercising its prerogatives as the modern Roman empire in having its way and ensuring its dominance as far into the future as possible. History tells us that empires have risen and fallen, and the US was rearranging the world by sequestering Russia in Europe and engaging and containing China in Asia in order to prepare for a time when other power galaxies emerged. The isolationist streak that was an essential component of the American make-up, and employed on occasion to bully the world, would not help because the whole world was wired and no one could be an island unto himself.

The David and Goliath struggle had moved to New York where the battle-scarred veteran Tareq Aziz pursued his diplomacy to achieve a shortening of the crippling sanctions. The Iraqi point was that the world could not be an accomplice to one nation putting a hammerlock on an entire country and forgetting about it. Palliatives such as the oil-for-food deal had not worked. Must all the people of Iraq be made to starve and suffer and die as the world entered the new millennium for the unforgivable act of their leader in invading and annexing a neighbour, a position that was reversed under American command?

Albright Comes Calling

Although Madeleine Albright ended her first visit to West Asia as US secretary of state on a quizzical note, to the echoes of praise from her Jordanian and Saudi interlocutors, she had little to show for her pains. The fault was not entirely hers. She had little new to offer and since the Clinton administration had publicly forsworn putting pressure on the Netanyahu government, there was no incentive for the hardline Israeli prime minister to change course, and he had in his armoury powerful weapons to use against President Clinton were he to alter his pro-Israeli policy.

Saudi praise for Albright surprised her as much as the rest of the world, but it was perhaps meant to encourage her to stay engaged, after she had taken eight months to come. The crumbs of concessions offered by Netanyahu amounted to trifles and the most radical statement to come out of the secretary of state was to ask Israel not to take "unilateral steps" which, in the Palestinian perception, were provocative. This distancing of the Clinton administration from the "Palestinian perception" on such burning issues as blatant new Jewish settlements on occupied land was an interesting demonstration of how Washington continued to coddle Netanyahu.

It would appear that so many of her predecessors had conducted incessant rounds of shuttle diplomacy in West Asia to so little purpose that Albright wanted to distance her watch from the region as much as she could. The Oslo accords, weighted against the Palestinians as they were, at one time seemed to offer a way out of the conundrum, but with Netanyahu's assumption of office, they unravelled, showing how far Palestinians had been short-changed in Oslo. Those (including this writer) who had believed that Oslo did provide the beginnings of an independent Palestinian state were to be disillusioned.

To any impartial outside observer who had visited the so-called Palestinian autonomous area, the manner in which the Israelis police controlled Palestinian lives and movements was a throwback to the days of nineteenth century colonialism. How were Palestinians to run even municipal affairs if the areas they administered—a microscopic percentage of the occupied Palestinian land—could become a prison house in an instant? How long could the Palestinian leadership retain its credibility when Palestinians suffered unspeakable indignities every day?

The irony was that while Netanyahu took Arafat to task for not cracking down hard enough on "terrorists", he was creating more suicide bombers. For there was no greater ally of Hamas and its opposition to the hollow peace process than Netanyahu. The marvel was that Arafat had managed to keep his head above water in the Israeli-created hostile environment. But his virtuosity and exceptional qualities of coping with adversity could not endure forever. And as the Israelis beat the drum of "security" to be instantly joined by the trumpet of President Clinton, more suicide bombers were born to get even with a state that not merely swallowed up Palestinian land but also humiliated them each day.

How could such palliatives as new Israeli–Palestinian meetings in the United States help bring about peace to a region in which a people sought to right historical wrongs suffered in Europe by colonising another people and expropriating their land? How could the fractured Oslo accords be put together again when their hidden ugliness had been revealed by Netanyahu? We should thank Netanyahu for his brutal honesty in telling Palestinians and the world how the state of Israel would function and rule while Palestinians would serve as serfs.

Who would now believe that there was any profit left in the Oslo framework? It might be the only game in town and the United States the only military superpower, and peace-loving governments and leaders in the Arabian Gulf and the larger Arab world might still hope against hope that some good would come out of agreements that had once fired the world's imagination. But did the United States administration really believe that it could still tinker with Oslo and lead the region to peace? Could there be genuine peace in the region with the continuing enslavement of Palestinians?

US Interests

Admittedly, the US had strategic interests in West Asia served by Israel and, despite the high moral tone often adopted by American politicians, morality and imposing the American will on the world did not mix. But Washington could not insulate itself from the march of time. We were no longer living in a world in which old-style colonialism was a profitable or viable industry. Indeed, the French were wise not be accept the pleas of a rebel island of the Comoros to recolonise it. The US was only inviting trouble by underwriting the new colonisation of the Palestinian people by the state of Israel.

The United States was neither willing nor able to acknowledge publicly that the inequities of the Oslo accords had been laid bare by Netanyahu. The Clinton administration, as many other governments for their own different reasons, believed with varying degrees of pessimism that Oslo could be salvaged. The belief was growing, if it had not already taken hold among Palestinians of all persuasions, that Oslo was not worth salvaging, that it promised nothing more than serfdom in another from. Under the protective wing of the United States, Netanyahu was ensuring that the future belonged to Hamas, not Arafat or the mainstream Fatah movement of the PLO.

Albright is an intelligent woman and she was probably reflecting on the Israeli-Palestinian conundrum. But this problem came with the job of secretary of state. It was the undoubted brilliance of the Jewish people that they should have used the American system of democracy to run the White House, as far as West Asian policy was concerned. Once Irish Americans were thought to have the greatest clout in influencing policies of interest to them, but American Jews had proved that they remained unsurpassed in this game.

End of 'Dual Containment'

Quite apart from the ruffled feathers across the Atlantic over Total's audacious deal with Iran, poking a French finger in Uncle Sam's eye, the political ramifications of this commercial and diplomatic coup were far more important. Because, combined with other developments in West Asia, this could represent the beginning of the end of the United States' "dual containment" policy. By Total's act of defiance, supported by the French government and the European Union, the Europeans were telling the Americans that their unilateral sanctions regime would not work.

The new American in Paris, Ambassador Felix Rohatyn, was consoling himself with the thought that US extra-territorial acts, the justified cause of European anger, was a many-dimensional thing like modern art. But while the Europeans were punching holes in the American sanctions regime, the absurdity of the "dual containment" policy was being highlighted every day. Iraq could not defend large slices of its territory because of the American fiat in imposing no-fly zones policed with the help of France and Britain.

The world would simply sigh and look the other way in this post-Cold War world of American dominance were it not for the fact that Iran and Iraq were sitting on some of the world's largest energy reserves. Since the world's appetite is insatiable and there was little prospect of a viable and acceptable alternative energy source on the horizon, Iran and Iraq were important countries. Although Europeans, together with the rest of the world, had accepted American military and strategic leadership and the political decisions that flowed from these strengths, the mercantilist instinct was simply too strong in the European ethic to surrender its economic interests to Uncle Sam's domestic compulsions or world view.

There was an obvious contradiction involved here because of the military and strategic linkages between Europe and the United States, most dramatically highlighted by Europe going cap in hand to Washington to seek help to tackle the problems of a disintegrating Yugoslavia and the European Union's agreement, with varying degrees of enthusiasm, to expand Nato to the former Soviet Union's very borders in order to strangle Russia's future growth and potential. And France, despite its penchant for defiantly flying its own and the European flag, helped the US to police the no-fly zone over Iraq and was junior partner in the American-led Nato mission in Bosnia. French efforts to secure a symbolic measure of dignity for Europeans in the form of obtaining the Nato Southern Command for a European had been rudely rejected.

Saddam Factor

Apart from American power and the trade-offs individual European countries sought from the United States (not counting the United Kingdom, which was content with its retainer's role to US administrations) the "dual containment" policy was withering away under the weight of its own contradictions. With Iraq, the punishing sanctions regime was in place six years after the end of the Second Gulf War because the US wanted to continue them, although some oil-producing states might have concerns over the flow of Iraqi oil into the international market and its impact on price. Officially, the US said, and Britain repeated, that Iraq had to implement all resolutions of the United Nations, it being understood that Baghdad could never satisfy Washington on this score as long as the Saddam regime was in place.

There was widespread suspicion in the region that the longevity of the Saddam regime suited Washington, which was utilising it to increase its military presence in West Asia and make it more palatable.

But whatever trade-offs individual countries received from the American presence, there was growing Arab anger over the consequences of the interminable sanctions on the people of a fellow Arab country. The vibrant Iraqi middle class had been transformed into paupers and children and their mothers suffered permanent disabilities, if not death. The creaking machinery and constraints of the palliative oil-for-food deal were not working as they should.

The Arab world, therefore, could only applaud moves by the Europeans, whatever their motives, to challenge the American world view of Iraq and Iran. No reasonable Arab would defend what President Saddam did to Kuwait; by the same token, no sane Arab could be indifferent to the sufferings of a people being penalised because of an American-led sanctions regime. In relation to Iran, West Asian countries shared the hope of the world that the installation of a new reformist president signified a change that could lead to the maturing of the Islamic revolution. The United States charged Iran with being a state sponsor of terrorism and a country seeking to possess nuclear weapons and missiles (which, in the American view, should remain the preserve of the few). As for the first charge, one could take a leaf our of the book of the American ambassador in Paris by suggesting that terrorism, like modern art, was a many-dimensional thing, depending upon the view and interests of the beholder.

"Dual containment" could not, of course, exist in a vacuum and had been promoted against the central Palestinian-Israeli confrontation in West Asia. That doleful drama, misdirected by the hands that created the Oslo accords, was being played every day. Washington's policy of looking at its strategic interests in the region through the eyes of its Israeli ally, and the powerful American Jewish lobby that manipulated Congress and the White House, meant that Iran could not have nuclear weapons or missiles. It also meant that, given the special American attachment to Israel, peace was not on the horizon.

What remained to be determined was how soon and in what precise fashion the "dual containment" policy would end. The United States would find the going increasingly difficult as it sought to justify why, through its fiat, the world should ostracise Iran and Iraq and why, in the face of Israeli provocations, there were at best whispers of disapproval that could barely be heard above the din of Washington traffic.

Saddam and the US

The Americans had won the battle against Iraq in the United Nations but might have lost the war. The unanimous UN Security Council resolution, after the US had watered down the text sufficiently to secure support, slapped new sanctions on Iraqi officials, cancelled the bimonthly review of sanctions and promised "further measures as may be required". Since Iraq was challenging the authority of the UN

Security Council, which had appointed the Iraq commission in the most draconian American-inspired sanctions measure in UN history, the members of the council had little option but to stand up for the world organisation.

But the debate on the resolution was only the beginning, not the end, of the story. How it unfolded would be determined by President Saddam's decision on ending his regime's non-cooperation with the UN commission, President Bill Clinton's compulsions to act and the attitudes of France and Russia, among other countries. Most countries and peoples would hope that having made its points against the US and the interminable sanctions imposed on it, Baghdad would move away from the brink.

President Saddam, however, had a limited window of opportunity because a gung-ho mood had overtaken the United States, with commentators in mainstream American newspapers demanding the bombing of Iraq's command and operations facilities or a bombing spree as part of a larger political strategy to remove President Saddam. The fact that the demand to bomb Iraq back into the Stone Age was being made not only by the proverbial man in the street fed on a diet of anti-Iraqi theories but also by analysts who, one would assume, would consider the consequences of such action was revealing. It would appear that the US policy-making establishment had either become more insular or was drunk on power unsurpassed in the history of the universe.

One problem, of course, was that the Clinton administration had not been able to frame a long-term policy for West Asia. The "dual containment" of Iran and Iraq was initially a temporary holding operation which had become a policy through inertia. Its inadequacies were well known and while the United States slapped horrendous sanctions of Iraq after leading a coalition and driving it out of Kuwait, it had been conducting an international campaign against Iran and imposed unilateral sanctions on the rest of the world by warning against investments of significant amounts in the country's energy and military structures under pain of being quartered by the all-powerful American regime.

The American propensity to legislate for the world had met with a robust riposte from the Europeans, but a bigger handicap for the Americans was how the Clinton administration had allowed itself to be held hostage to the American Jewish lobby. Prime Minister Netanyahu had pretty nearly destroyed what remained of the Madrid peace process and all that President Clinton or his secretary of state could do in response was to mutter disappointment under their breath Yet the Arab world's perception of America sacrificing its friends in West Asia and its own interests in the region at the altar of Israel would prove to be a terrible handicap for Washington in dealing with the Iraq crisis.

New Roman Empire

If the Americans were to decide to use force to discipline Iraq—a country whose people had been pauperised and starved through nearly seven years of sanctions—it would spark a chain reaction that was unlikely to benefit the United States. Capitol Hill, the world had discovered, was not merely a law unto itself but was the home of many elements that wanted to deal with other nations strictly on their terms, which were composed of jingoism, self-righteousness and evangelism in almost equal proportions. There will always be people and countries willing to do America's bidding (e.g. Britain and Australia), but the majority would revolt against the new Roman Empire seeking to impose its will on the universe.

Indeed, in the case of an American attack on Iraq, the US would give even opponents of President Saddam no option but to support him for refusing to be cowed down by American might. Netanyahu would celebrate the launching of an American attack on Iraq because it would blow sky high the shreds of the Oslo agreements in a Madrid process increasingly unrelated to peace. Iraq's sovereignty and integrity had been compromised for years by the two "no-fly zones" the US had imposed over northern and southern Iraq, and Turkey had in recent months and years been merrily using northern Iraq to battle Kurds of various descriptions while remaining immune from criticism because of American protection.

If America could bring Iraq to its knees, what would happen to Washington's "dual containment" policy? And would it be in the American scheme of things to install a puppet in Baghdad, a role played with distinction in the past by the US Central Intelligence Agency? And if so, how would Washington justify maintaining a large permanent military presence in the region? In Washington's view, a justification is perhaps no longer required. Americans took every opportunity to snipe at French and Russian approaches to West Asia, particularly Iraq, by suggesting that they were determined by visions of profit. For the Arabs, on the other hand, these two countries' attitude represented a more balanced position.

Perhaps one consequence of an American attack on Iraq would be French withdrawal from policing the US-imposed "no-fly zones" over Iraq. Russia had already made it amply clear, together with China, its opposition to resolving the crisis by force. Life is full of ironies and never more so than in this crisis. The United States was upholding the power of the UN Security Council when it refused to pay its dues and UN-bashing was the favorite game in the corridors of power in Washington. The most pro-Israeli US administration in American history was seeking to win friends and influence people in West Asia by targeting an Arab nation while coddling an Israeli regime that tore up peace agreements arrived at. Compared to what has been imposed on the Iraqi people for seven years, the sanction against Prime Minister Netanyahu was that President Clinton might not find time to meet him during a fund-raising visit he was making to the United States.

The marvel was how insular the American foreign-policy establishment had become in an age of unprecedented access to information. Perhaps the world could take comfort in Lord Action's definition about the corrupting influences of absolute power. It was cold comfort.

The Iraq Syndrome

There were several strands in the US–Iraq stand-off that could serve as a guide to the post-Cold War era. One was the sheer power of the United States and its ability to impose its policies on the world, however wrong-headed they might be. Second, the political mood in America was guided by concerns that were increasingly becoming removed from those of most nations. Third, the future geostrategic map Americans were conjuring up could add up to a rash of conflicts and provoke a backlash that would increasingly be led by extremist forces because legitimate forms of national protests were being stymied.

These points reflected the mainstream policy-making establishment's view. Another stream of opinion, espoused in particular by the radical right, argued either for a form of isolationism or for an extreme self-centred policy that punished or rewarded a country in proportion to how it served American interests. The majority of Americans regretfully had little understanding of, and even less interest in, the world and was guided mostly by television news snippets or their pocket book in melancholy proof of the homily that you can make people literate but cannot educate them.

Policy-making in foreign affairs in America was the province of a small section of people in the administration, in the academic world, in the "think tanks" and in the media. Any American administration had great leeway in making foreign policy as long as it could sell it. It is only rarely, as in the case of the Vietnam war, that sustained failure of a policy and an increasing number of American soldiers' deaths trigger a revolt. A contrary mood could also sometimes take hold, as with the revolt of the young in the sixties.

Unlike Richard Nixon, who was a consummate foreign-policy president whatever his other failings, Bill Clinton's basic interest was in domestic, rather than foreign, policy. His first term in the White House was little short of a disaster in conducting foreign affairs, and it had been a painful apprenticeship for him. He had Bosnia to show for his new awareness of the requirements of foreign policy, but in dealing with the larger picture he was handicapped by his lack of vision or a historical sense of how to use power to build a better world.

Henry Kissinger, who had had many *avatars*, was a practitioner of *realpolitik* and always bemoaned the American streak of an idealistic Wilsonian urge. This could be misleading because even before the emergence of Kissinger, idealism never prevented the United States from running the countries of Latin America as virtual colonies or from colonising the Philippines. A distinguishing mark of American diplomatic history had been a domestic interaction among idealistic urgings, isolationism and unadulterated *realpolitik*. With the fall of the Berlin Wall, the end of the Cold War and the disintegration of the Soviet Union, the United States was ill-equipped to lead the world because of the nature of the country's history and the inexperience of its president, with the more experienced George Bush having lost to Clinton.

The Bogeyman

The stand-off with Iraq illustrated President Clinton's and America's handicaps because it showed the failure of the "dual containment" policy of Iraq and Iran, squandered American goodwill in the Arab world and elevated a problem out of all proportion to its capacity for mischief. In the process, moral and humanitarian principles had been thrown to the winds, an entire people had been pauperised and devastated, and for the second time in less than a decade President Saddam has been set up as the bogeyman with whom the world's sole surviving superpower must do battle.

It was revealing that his foolish American policy had strong support from the policy-making establishment, specially Capitol Hill. For the rest of the world, always barring Britain, there had been more questions than answers. Was the United States rushing its military might to West Asia merely to ferret out Iraq's "weapons of mass destruction"? Did the Clinton administration want Saddam to go, as it stated, or did it want him to stay so that it could better control the region by frightening it? Was the US Iraq policy part of a larger strategy to buttress Israel with its generally accepted possession of weapons of mass destruction?

Arafat has been locked into the Madrid process whose resemblance to peace was becoming more remote each day. The PLO chairman might have become a prisoner of the process but how did the US bring peace to the region by encouraging Israel to swallow most of the occupied territory and reduce Palestinians to the permanent status of serfs living in Bantustans? Even assuming that the new oil countries of Central Asia could reduce the importance of oil-producing West Asia, America's interest in protecting, feeding and arming its protégé Israel would remain paramount because American domestic policy so decreed and American Jewry had firm hold over the levers of power in Washington.

If the United States realised its ambition of pulverising Iraq and reducing it to the pre-industrial age because President Saddam had not cried uncle, what profit would come to it? And in the greatest irony of all, America would fight Iraq for the United Nations Americans loved to hate, punishing it while withholding obligatory dues to the world organisation. Communist double-speak the West took such delight in deriding is gone, only to be replaced by American double-speak. America's self-proclaimed mission, after all, was to save the world—after its fashion.

It took President Clinton some time to learn to treat China as a potential superpower (whatever US State Department human rights reports might say). At the same time, the US was keeping its powder dry by expanding defence links with Japan and Australia in a pincer movement. It would obviously take the US much longer to come to the conclusion that treating Russia as a potential enemy by expanding Nato to the east while keeping it out was a sure way to make an enemy of it and divide the European continent again.

American spokesmen had often declared that their country did not want to be the world's policeman. But by its actions and its increasing tendency to tell each nation of the world what it must do, it was falling into that role. For instance, who but a world policeman made an annual inventory of the human rights records of each country of the world and published it as an official document? If the United States went ahead in attacking Iraq in league with is proxy Britain, it would discover that Iraq would come to haunt future American policies in a manner not dissimilar to the decades characterised by the debilitating Vietnam syndrome.

Sounding the War Bugle

While much of the world waited stoically for the Americans to launch military strikes on Iraq even as Washington continued to collect countries rather like a hunter would trophies, history seemed to be repeating itself as farce. Britain's Tony Blair had taken on the role of President Bill Clinton's master of ceremonies in the bizarre business of justifying bombing Iraq and its people back to the Stone Age and is even helping round up support for friend Bill. And the noise of the gathering arms bazaar in West Asia was punctuated with the president's contest back home with the former White House intern Monica Lewinsky.

One wondered what the famous author of "1984", George Orwell, would have made of 1998. There was double-speak enough to last a generation as the United States of America was itching to launch attacks on Iraq variously projected as significant, not pinpricks, and devastating. American legislators could speak their minds better than their president or the State Department. "Go after Saddam" was the unambiguous message. And thereby hangs a tale.

It was easier to fight wars if you demonised your opponent or enemy. Back in the eighties in Paris, researching a book on Unesco, the United Nations Educational, Scientific and Cultural Organisation, I discovered how the US had supported the re-election of the Senegalese director-general, Amadou Mahtar M'Bow with the most fulsome praise. But he had then been turned into a devil and much energy was expended on painting him in the darkest colours. The American objective, as the world was to learn, was to walk out of Unesco to make the point that Washington wanted control of the budget processes in the parent United Nations and all the UN agencies.

It was, of course, a different world and the stakes were higher this time around. It was the post-Cold War era, with the Americans arrogantly demanding their pound of flesh and bullying countries to follow their lead. The difficulty was in discovering the American objectives. No one believed that Washington was after Iraq's "weapons of mass destruction". If the American-dominated and handpicked teams of "inspectors" could not discover what they were after in seven long years while Iraqis starved and died because of lack of adequate food or medicines under the most draconian economic sanctions in UN history, the office of the Central Intelligence Agency should be abolished. Iraq was punished because it had no business to invade and annex Kuwait and fell in an area of American strategic and economic interests. It paid a heavy prices for it.

American Gains

But seven years is a long time to punish a people of a country and even those who were the foremost in condemning Iraq's indefensible action (as I did from the bunker of Al Rashid hotel in Baghdad during the initial bombing raids in 1991) saw the injustice of collective punishment of a nation at the altar of American strategic objectives. It was ironical that the United States made money out of the Second Gulf War and grasped the opportunity to spread its arms (prepositioning them) and men and ships in the region.

The palliative of the oil-for-food deal was offered, and reluctantly and belatedly accepted by Baghdad, with a substantial portion going to meet UN administrative costs in Iraq. And even as the war drums were sounded, first in Washington and then in West Asia and Europe, a bigger oil-for-food deal was offered, with more conditions and more monitors, as an antidote to the new surgery about to be performed on Iraq. At the end of this exercise, there would doubtless be fewer Iraqis to feed, with the latest in American weaponry doing its job.

We had it on the authority of the US administration that Iraq was continuing to hide weapons of mass destruction, a heinous sin in the

American dictionary as far as countries such as Iraq (but not Israel) were concerned. And judging by the fuss Israel was making of a possible biological attack from Iraq, UN inspectors having taken care of Iraqi nuclear capacity, manufactures of gas masks were making a fortune. After the United States became the sole surviving superpower with the end of the Cold War and the disintegration of the Soviet Union, Israelis could hardly believe their good fortune and set about fashioning a Greater Israeli state. Under the benign eyes of Bill Clinton, they got pretty far, and Netanyahu was having the time of this life swallowing up more occupied Palestinian land while Arafat flew around the world seeking support and sympathy.

The Americans had divided Iraq into three parts, northern Iraq now serving as a target practice area for Turkey. There were calls from Capitol Hill not only to go for Saddam but to put in his place a collection of Iraqi opposition exiles. What about the weapons of mass destruction Iraq was allegedly harbouring?

If they were there, they could be destroyed and they would have served the American propaganda purpose in any event. There was some doubt whether the American objective was, indeed, to remove Saddam Hussein. He had proved so useful in serving Washington's objectives that many in the US State Department and the Pentagon would be loath to see him go. Many in the world were wondering what all this fuss about WMD (weapons of mass destruction) was about. Others believed that if the Americans carried out their threat they would merely succeed in fracturing the world along new fault lines, with the Arab world and Russia and China and the developing world ranged against the United States and Britain, with France uncomfortably in a middle camp. And the scars of the new war against Iraq would remain.

Some American legislators believed that the world was ungrateful for not coming immediately to their side as soon as the war bugle had been sounded. Much of the world believed that the United States was getting too arrogant for its own, or the world's, good and was seeking to reorder peoples and nations to its whims or Machiavellian designs. One must, however, sympathise with the American experts who bemoaned the fact that the newest weapons in the American armoury were not quite ready for the new Gulf war.

Louder War Cries

A curious thing was happening in the United States. Even as the war cries got louder, with a battery of old administration heavies were weighing in for air strikes extending to the demolition of Saddam Hussein and the cabinet line-up was repeating tired old arguments, more and more people were discovering that the emperor had no clothes.

The heckling of the Clinton administration's A team at Ohio University was one indication of a revolt of the young. Interestingly, sober American analysts were asking the question, what would the air strikes achieve? Even those in the gung-ho camp of bringing Saddam down were saying that President Clinton's heart was not in what he was about to do: bomb Iraq. Others said that the US administration had allowed itself to be boxed in; yet others that the White House had no clear idea of the consequences of the impending attacks, despite the amateur efforts afoot to bolster an Iraqi opposition and finance it to replace Saddam.

Some Americans seemed undeterred by their experience in conducting social engineering experiments in such places as Vietnam, Chile and elsewhere in Latin America. One problem was that the United States was stuck with Saddam because of its habit of personalising the fight with "enemy" countries, now magnified many times over by a hungry electronic media. Many more Americans, for instance, would be happy to let their armed forces "go for Saddam" (not the declared American policy) although its requirement of putting ground troops in would not be popular in the country and on Capitol Hill.

In a strange way, the wheel had almost come full circle. It look the United States a long time to come to terms with the misadventure in Vietnam and the Vietnam syndrome had still left scars. "Body bags" became a dirty evocative phrase to denote the number of American soldiers dead in a war which came to have no aims except ultimately to devise an honourable exit formula denied the US. The end of the US military role in Vietnam came in a memorable photograph of the forced and chaotic departure of the last Americans by helicopter from an American diplomatic compound in Saigon, at it was then called. The Vietnam war scarred a whole generation because when the soldiers came home from what had become a dirty war, they were not welcomed as heroes; they had acquired some of the unsavoury aspects of the war they had fought.

Sunny Ride Up

Ronald Reagan did much to restore national confidence during his two terms. He was the sunny and Teflon president reflecting his own and his countrymen's natural optimism. He had simple solutions for the world's problems, the Soviet Union being the "evil empire" although he was later to do business with the last Soviet president, Mikhail Gorbachev. But it was during the watch of George Bush in the White House that the Vietnam syndrome was tackled head on. Saddam Hussein gave him the opportunity by doing the indefensible in 1990, invading and annexing Kuwait.

The surprise was that the United States waited for months until it put together a coalition and brought an impressive array of American and other military power to the region before beginning the attacks on Iraq. A lesson Bush, and his successor, learned from Vietnam was that domestic support for a foreign military venture was directly proportionate to the number and frequency of "body bags". Indeed, the modernisation of American weapons had the major aim of reducing the risks involved for American fighters. In hunting terms, the new American tactic would be the equivalent of getting an army of 100 hunters with high-tech precision guns to corner and shoot one poor tiger.

The 1991 Gulf War was a success because it cost relatively few American lives, and President Clinton was reluctantly but surely led to putting American soldiers on the ground in Bosnia, a problem West Europeans and Russia failed to resolve. But this was the post-Cold War era of a sole surviving superpower and American soldiers were to stay on in Bosnia for another extended time because, despite grumbling, it had been a practically cost-free exercise, in terms of American lives. However, as the young demonstrators in Ohio and elsewhere in the US were beginning to suggest, President Clinton's planned military offensive against Iraq, with the old Gulf coalition in tatters and much of the non-Western world ranged against it, was acquiring an ominous ring.

American power gathered in the region was even more high-tech than it had been the last time around as many countries had been dragooned into a new shaky coalition. Outside of Kuwait, the Arab world was against a new war whose biggest sufferers would be the Iraqi people. And such a war would pose the threat of breaking up Iraq, cause a new confrontation between Israel and the Palestinians and set off a new refugee exodus.

American Gallup polls indicated that the great majority was for the bombing of Iraq. Saddam had been demonised and his potential in threatening the world with chemical and biological weapons had been so exaggerated that most were frightened about what he would or would not do. Thanks to a rather small band of Americans who had kept cool heads, an unease about the impending war was beginning to grow. But sane reasoning was drowned by the war cries. In the popular imagination, the "bad" Saddam had to be punished and the gleaming American war-fighting machine was tantalisingly close to its guarry.

A Parable

A parable reportedly told by Saudi Arabia's Crown Prince Abdullah bin Abdulaziz to US Secretary of State Madeleine Albright in February 1998 had a resonance in West Asia. According to the London

Times account, he had told her the story of a shepherd who was angry that a wolf was killing one of his lambs every week. He bought himself two guard dogs, only to find he then had to kill a lamb every day to feed the dogs. "He decided to live with the wolf," Abdullah explained.

The parable formed the backdrop to regional reaction to the whirlwind six-nation trip to the Arabian Gulf of US Defence Secretary William Cohen. Because although his mission was an omnibus one, including setting in place a mechanism for inducting US troops in an emergency, "to buck up morale" of US troops in the area and sift the winds of Arab opinion on Iraq and Iran, the centrepiece was to sell the concept of a future missile-defence system.

Before setting out for the trip from Washington, Pentagon figures for the American military presence in the region were put at 24,050 troops, 24 navy ships and 170 warplanes and helicopters. Further, it was claimed that the US troop strength could be increased up to 40,000 in 96 hours and we had it on the authority of Cohen that the number of cruise missles available had been doubled since "tensions (over Iraq) started to increase" in October 1997.

The traditional American scenario was to broadcast the twin threats posed by Iraq and Iran, but the urgency of Cohen's mission was determined by US Congressional pressure on protecting US troops in the region after the bombings of two US embassies following the Saudi Arabian tragedy. The "Theatre High Altitude Area Defence" Programme had already cost the Pentagon $3.2 billion and although the experiments had proved to be a failure, Cohen wanted them to be continued.

US Sales Pitch

It was in this context that the US defence secretary made his pitch for a theatre missile protection system to replace the ageing Patriot missiles used in the 1991 Gulf War, eventually found to be not as great as they were billed to be. The message to the Gulf sates was simple. The US was looking at several systems for the long term, the one finally decided upon would be both expensive and sophisticated and the states of the Arabian Gulf should chip in with contributions to fund the research or at least agree eventually to buy the new system. The sales pitch was that the missiles would protect both US troops and the countries of the region.

Cohen was realistic enough to declare that the regional states' involvement in the futuristic project would be limited in view of the prevailing low oil prices, but the impression he left as he hopped from one country to another was that this was only the beginning of a proposal that would be buttressed from time to time. The US defence secretary did not set out for the trip to finalise or sign any new arms deals in what his officials had described as "a lucrative arms market".

Few American defence secretaries had been given a tougher assignment. Prince Abdullah's parable—apocryphal as it may be—expressed a widespread feeling in the Arabian Gulf. The Second Gulf War depeted the treasuries of many of the states and the price of American protection was growing. Second, the American "dual containment" policy had been largely abandoned, and although Washington's process of reconciliation with Teheran would take time, both sides were making tentative moves towards it. Third, since the declared aim of US policy was to give Israel a qualitative edge in weapons, the Arab states would presumably be given an inferior version.

The obvious question that presented itself was: Must the Arabian Gulf states fund a missile system on a hypothesis that might change by the time the programme was ready? Granted we lived in a dangerous area in a dangerous world, but should random threats in the future determine immediate expensive plans beyond the AGCC states' own road map for the integration of the air defence system?

America's fascination with anti-missile air defence reached its climax during President Ronald Reagan's Star Wars extravaganza. The grand plan lost some of its shine after he left the White House and after the costs and visionary nature of the scheme were added up. Anti-American feelings fuelled by US support of Israel in the latter's confrontation with Palestinians resulting, most recently, in the bombings of two American embasies had built up a momentum for dusting the cobwebs off Reagan's Star Wars. Cohen's parting words before leaving the region were that the Arabian Gulf countries were "quite receptive" to his missile plan, an assumption that remained to be determined.

The Simmering Pot

No one doubts the capacity of the United States to wreak greater havoc in Iraq, but the dogfights between American and Iraqi warplanes over the unilaterally declared no-fly zones over Iraq, after the four-day Anglo-American bombing spree in December 1998, highlighted the larger political consequences of Washington's approach. At the end of the day, the US, with satellite Britain, was playing a losing game.

This was so quite apart from the West Asian leaders' views on President Saddam. Despite the American obsession with Saddam, the core issue related to the American and Western approach to the region. Thanks to eight years of cruel sanctions against Iraq, the American coddling of Israel's Netanyahu and his predecessors had come into sharp focus as was the subjugation of the United Nations to American interests.

The United States, as the pre-eminent superpower, had its national interests in West Asia and was pursuing them, but if the pattern of its policies went against the people and countries of the region, Washington would have to pay a high price. Every one knew that the US had its geostrategic interests, greatly reinforced by the powerful American Jewish lobby, in backing Israel. But no previous American administration had allowed itself to be blackmailed by Israel to the extent the Clinton administration had.

Few Arab leaders held a brief for President Saddam. But no Arab leader could dismiss the suffering of the Iraqi people for eight long years nor the contrast between the kind of punishment meted out to the Iraqis for non-compliance with draconian UN resolutions while the red carpet was rolled out for Netanyahu for treating the UN and the resolutions it had passed as scraps of paper and responding to a public call by US Secretary of State Madeleine Albright for "a time-out" on settlements with building new illegal settlements and ex-panding existing entities.

The Clinton administration had given ample evidence that the United Nations was a dispensable commodity, brought into the picture only when it suited Washington's interests. The UN Security Council was ignored before America decided to bomb Iraq, but the operation of the UN inspections regime in Iraq had been dear to the US admini-stration, with a credible report in the *Washington Post* suggesting that UN Secretary-General Kofi Annan was disturbed by the use Washington had made of the snooping by UN inspectors of Iraqi communications with a view to overthrowing President Saddam.

Ironical Behaviour

It is an indication of the state of mind of US policy-makers that they did not see the irony in their waxing eloquent over the impermissibility, under UN rules, of Iraq seeking the ouster of US and British aid personnel. To the world, Richard Butler's claims to impartiality sounded strange, given his behaviour and the report he handed out, giving Washington the justification, however tenuous, for carrying out the December bombing. Nor did it strike President Clinton as strange that his selective enthusiasm for the United Nations should co-exist with his country's refusal to pay its dues.

The American approach to West Asia was creating new and more acute problems in the region because of the failure of the Clinton administration to realise that the more frequent use of greater force against Iraq was becoming increasingly counter-productive. If the Clinton administration was happy counting the region's leaders who did not love President Saddam, it would get him nowhere.

The nub of the problem was simple. The sanctions against Iraq should be lifted to allow the Iraqi people to breathe and live. Toppling

President Saddam should not be the policy of one member state towards the leader of another, now that we were supposedly past the colonial era of gunboat diplomacy or America's own traditional approach to South America. There could be no regional stability if, in pursuit of its national interests, one country was willing to sacrifice the lives and prosperity of 22 million Arab people.

President Clinton had proved to be inept and wrong-headed in the pursuit of his foreign policy goals. When domestic issues determined a country's foreign policy, it could only appear jaundiced. And if this was laced with visions of grandeur in making the rest of the world a mirror image of the United States, and strangulating such former enemies as Russia who could not be remoulded, the world sat uneasily on the brink of a precipice.

There was little ground for optimism that the Clinton administration would change course on Iraq or Israel before its term was up. There would, therefore, be more sweat and tears for the Iraqi people, further humiliation for the Palestinians, and the West Asian pot will be kept simmering, if not on the boil. And we had it on the authority of BBC Television that it was a "provocation" for Iraqis of fly in their own air space because the United States had unilaterally decided that it would enforce "no fly" zones over Iraq!

Spies in UN Hats

Some Americans were calling their countrymen to arms to do battle with UN Secretary-General Kofi Annan and Iraq's President Saddam. It was a fall-out from the charges that were multiplying each day about the chief UN arms inspector, Richard Butler, letting the United States misuse the UN mandate to spy on Iraq and its president. And American officials had been quoted in the *Washington Post* as being ready to fight for Butler to the end.

Poor Butler! In his efforts to be helpful to the United States to the disregard of his UN duties and loyalty to his boss Kofi Annan, he had realised too late that he was a mere pawn in the bigger game. The Pentagon was boasting about the senior Iraqis killed and the damage caused by the strikes it undertook in December 1998, courtesy the information gathered under the garb on UN inspections.

The disturbing aspect was not so much the spying—a charge Iraq had been making for years—but the climate of opinion at the policy-making level in Washington. It was not merely an expression of arrogance as the sole surviving superpower but also one of reckless disregard of the perils of an unthinking Rambo-like policy on the United Nations and the world in the new millenium. It was as if the United States had divorced itself from the world and was living on another planet and could not care less about what others thought of its irrational actions on Iraq—or trying its own president, for that matter.

Indeed, the United States was busy refining a policy that would not only crown its unilateral right to take military action anywhere in the world without reference to the UN but also bring in the Cold War organisation Nato to do the same thing under American leadership. This issue was slated for the Nato summit in the US in April 1999 and one would hope that the Europeans, their spirits boosted by the launch of the euro, would have the good sense to turn down the gratuitous offer. But for Europe as well as the world, American policies and actions portend a bleak beginning to the last year of the twentieth century.

Take the American approach to the United Nations. That the world organisation had become something of a dirty word on Capitol Hill was not a secret. The US Senate had appropriated to itself the right to determine how much its contribution to the UN should be and a succession of American presidents had used the payment of obligatory dues as a lever to force their views on the organisation. The Congress had now imposed a set of conditions before partial payment of the old dues could be made; the arrears remained unpaid.

Yet the United States had been a major beneficiary of the United Nations—in conducting the Korea war under the garb of the UN in the 1950s as in continuing a savage eight-year embargo against Iraq under the UN umbrella. And Washington decided that it did not need the sanction of the UN Security Council to bomb Iraq. It had been irked by Annan's diplomacy in warding off earlier air strikes as in averting strikes again when US bombers were up in the air.

Alarm Bells

The United States single-handedly refused a second term to the previous secretary-general Boutros Boutros-Ghali because he was not sufficiently subservient. However, the fortunes of individuals were less important than the crisis the American attitude created for the future of the world organisation. The United States had it in its power to destroy the United Nations, as it destroyed the League of Nations in other circumstances, but it was time for others to ring the alarm bells for what its actions added up to for the new millennium.

The Iraq crisis would be resolved one day but the world could not live without a United Nations; interestingly, the American conservative Heritage Foundation had suggested at one stage that it could. Must the world continue to witness the unravelling of the United Nations by one member state? Were there no sanctions for not paying dues, for decreeing how much less the US should pay, for using UN-mandated sanctions to spy on a country, to shut the UN out of the world's most potentially explosive Israeli–Palestinian confrontation?

To cap it, American commentators professed to be scandalised that the rest of the world did not salute and follow the great words of wisdom emerging out of Washington. After gathering awesome power, the United States had become disoriented. There was a time when it was said that for Americans a country was either for it or against it; there were no greys perceived or permitted.

That was in the bad old days of the Cold War. The new game was called the US versus the United Nations. If the world organisation was not with the US in the policies it chose to follow in the pursuit of its national interests, it was against the US and should be punished for its temerity. If the UN persisted in looking after the interests of all members, rather than one member, its days were numbered.

One could only hope that before the US buried the UN with full military honours, some Americans would speak up. Or were we destined to repeat the follies of the past?

A Pantomime Show

A century hence, students of history reading about developments in the last year of the twentieth century would marvel at the pantomime show over Iraq. US Secretary of State Madeline Albright had said in so many words before launching bombing and missile raids on Iraq in December 1989, with Britain in tow, that she knew UN arms inspectors might not be able to go back, but it did not really matter.

Yet the Australian Richard Butler, after giving Washington the pretext for launching raids, presented a 250-page report to the UN Security Council saying why it was so necessary to continue to ferret out weapons of mass destruction in Iraq. And the work of the UN commission was totally compromised by a multitude of credible reports showing that the United States was using the inspections as a cover for spying and pinpointing targets it bombed last December. Sending back UN inspectors of the Butler variety would be worse than a farce. It would be a tragedy.

And Richard Butler was presumably being paid out of the rationed money Iraq was allowed to earn by exporting oil to try to feed its people and give them some of the urgent medicines the sick needed.

Albright, meanwhile, hopped from Moscow to Cairo, to Saudi Arabia while pronouncing that one of her goals was to coordinate the toppling of Saddam. In between, of course, there was the little problem of threatening Yugoslavia's Slobodan Milosevic with bombs and missiles if he did not give the Kosovars their independence under the guise of "self-government".

The UN Security Council, ignored by the US with a scarcely-veiled contempt while bombing Iraq, was now deadlocked. France and Russia had made proposals, eminently sensible ones, in moving the process forward, essentially by lifting sanctions on Iraq in exchange for future long-term monitoring and maintaining curbs on arms. Such proposals were anathema to the US, which did not have any of its own proposals to offer. It did not need to. The UN Security Council that Washington refused to acknowledge when it suited it purposes could be a useful vehicle on occasion because America had a veto that permitted it to make the Iraqis suffer for eight long years—and far into the future as long as Saddam was in place.

A Catalyst

President Saddam himself, was of course part of the pantomime show. He was the essential catalyst for America's ability to rampage through international agreements and obligations to the United Nations, to tear up the sovereignty of a nation and tell the world that it was embarked on such tasks as the toppling of a leader of another country by giving money to his opponents, cutting up the country into three parts to maintain two 'no-fly zones' (the modern equivalent of gunboat diplomacy) and nurturing a spy network in the North.

At least one Iraqi Kurdish group and the Shi'ite opposition to Saddam have had the courage to refuse American largesse. One could imagine the credibility among Iraqis of the other opposition groups that were apparently accepting CIA money to get rid of the legal ruler of their country through subterfuge and armed revolt.

If Saddam was not helping his own or his country's cause by the rhetoric emanating from Baghdad, would the Arab cause or that of the wider world be enhanced by American policies? There would be a world after Saddam to nurture and protect. Should we lose all the fruits of post-World War II progress because one country was drunk on power and sought to rule the world?

Yet the consequences of American policies would stay with us. The UN Security Council, the most vital peace-keeping and peace-making organ of the only world organisation, lay wounded and panting. It used to be said that the UN never had a chance to function as it was intended to because of the advent of the Cold War shortly after its formation; vetoes then ruled the sessions.

The end of the Cold War was hailed as a new era, the golden moment for the United Nations, with the so-called peace dividend on the horizon. The golden moment had turned into a dark night because the US was choosing the option of avoiding the Security Council altogether and was moulding Nato, the Cold War organisation, into a new world policeman under its command, with no vetoes to frustrate its wishes.

The peace dividend had vanished into thin air. Americans had informed us that it was a wicked world we lived in. There were new threats, new 'rogue states', new and hidden dangers and therefore the US national defence budget should be increased, with the Republican opponent of President Clinton suggesting that the increase was not big enough.

One wonders how long it would take the UN Security Council to retain its dignity, if the world organisation was not to be thrown into the proverbial dustbin of history, the destiny of the old League of Nations. There could not be one nation, however powerful, above the law the rest of the world had to obey. And one nation, even with satellites, could not rule the world.

As the world watched the pantomime, with Butler performing his act, Saddam Hussein his own and Madeleine Albright her double-take, we would, all of us, suffer.

Clinton's Goal

It was typical of the manner in which President Bill Clinton had pursued his foreign policy goals insofar as he had identified them that in unveiling his agenda for the remaining two years of his second term in San Francisco, he remained tentative, unfocused and without a reliable compass to guide him. He had won his election the first time on promising to focus on domestic economy and had all but made foreign policy an adjunct of trade and commerce.

As President Clinton began to learn on the job, he relished striding the world stage, as all politicians did as a relief from domestic chores, but he had little to show for his pains. In world terms, the American contribution to Haiti's fragile peace counted for little. The President's role in Northern Ireland was commendable and apparently driven by domestic dividends, but Bosnia remained a questionable success.

An American president's job was not an easy one and his responsibilities as the leader of the sole surviving superpower were immense. It was equally true, however, that President Clinton had been surprisingly profligate in frittering away George Bush's legacy. President Bush had contained the disintegration of the Soviet Union and the fundamental change in Europe with Germany's unification, built a coalition to defeat Iraq and reverse its invasion of Kuwait, and finally begun the West Asian peace process in Madrid in 1991.

Looking at the Clinton record, the obsession with duplicating the American market system helped in the near-implosion of the Russian state, with all its consequences for the suffering Russians and for Europe and the world. Russia followed South-east and East Asia as the economic meltdown in Thailand set off a contagion. Further, in a singularly irrational attempt at containing Russia in the post-Cold war world and dividing the European continent again, America forced an eastward expansion of the North Atlantic Treaty Organisation, despite the promises made to the last Soviet president Mikhail Gorbachev at the time of Germany's unification.

In West Asia, the flexibility American presidents had was very limited, guided as Washington's relations with Israel were by geostrategic considerations and the great power of the American Jewish lobby. President Clinton made his options even more limited by identifying himself completely with Israel, and when a difficult customer in the shape of Prime Minister Netanyahu appeared on the scene, the White House was left defenceless.

Netanyahu's Victory

In cameos that would not be duplicated, Netanyahu stared down at President Clinton and won on at least two memorable occasions. There was US Secretary of State Madeleine Albright publicly declaring that Israel should take "time-out" on building illegal settlements on occupied Palestinian land, only to receive a slap in the face by Tel Aviv initiating more settlements. And after President Clinton had invested days in personally taking charge of negotiations on getting Israel to accept withdrawal from a measly 13 per cent of occupied land (an American proposal), Netanyahu went home and tore up the Wye River Memorandum, the President quietly pocketing his pride.

West Asia sat precariously perched on a Palestinian house left half-built and remaining unfurnished as Israel went about grabbing more occupied land as and when Tel Aviv was ready to talk seriously to Palestinians. And on Iraq, President Clinton had chosen the worst of all options by prolonging the suffering of Iraqis for eight years while periodically bombing that luckless country and peppering the so-called "no-fly" zones with lethal bird shots nearly every day. Overthrowing President Saddam had been elevated to state policy in Washington.

By contrast, President Clinton seemed to have undergone a total conversion on China. The wheel had come full circle, from candidate Bill Clinton attacking President Bush for coddling China to defending Beijing against the report of his own administration released the day of his foreign policy speech in San Francisco condemning China's human rights record. The most favoured nation status for China had been de-linked from human rights earlier. Outside of Israel, China seemed to be the only country that inspired fear and deference in the White House. The difference, of course, was there was no China lobby to compare with the Jewish lobby to dictate to US presidents and administrations.

America's dubious distinction as the only remaining ideological state in the world required that goals, however discursive and ad hoc they might be, should be tabulated and set out as principles or "challenges", as President Clinton chose to call them in San Francisco. The five challenges he listed were: building a more peaceful twenty-first century world; bringing Russia and China into the international system as "open, prosperous, stable nations"; protecting against dangers of weapons proliferation, terrorism, drugs and climate change; making a world trading and financial system that benefited ordinary people; and maintaining freedom as "a top goal".

The list recited by President Clinton in his virtual State of Foreign Policy address tellingly revealed the chinks in his armour. He was, above all, an amateur in foreign policy without possessing a conceptual framework or the ability to marshal his country's immense power for achieving goals. Choosing soft—and exceeding cruel—options like penalising an entire population for eight years through sanctions could not be described as wise policy. Nor could the Clinton trademark "comply or we bomb you" make for coherence in determining foreign policy goals.

President Clinton's grandiose themes, on the other hand, were taking him to dangerous paths. After the April summit in Washington, Nato was to be the world's policeman surpassing the UN Security Council. And what was the point of threatening Belgrade with bombing Serbia to pulp for misbehaviour in Kosovo or refusal to let 30,000 Nato troops police a Serbian province to oversee the virtual independence it had been promised?

Henry Kissinger, the *éminence grise* of America's foreign policy establishment, had raised the question of defining where the US should intervene in dousing the flames of ethnic conflict since it could not extend its reach everywhere. But President Clinton had been unmindful of other percepts of the former secretary of state and national security adviser as well. He had decreed that the president himself should not conduct negotiations, except when agreement has been reached or was within grasp. Second, a major power should not threaten to use force unless it was prepared to do so and ensure its victory.

American World Order

It was Warren Christopher, the former US secretary of state, who had made what then seemed the preposterous proposal that the United Nations should persuade American legislators to pay up arrears. What the United Nations Organisation had to do with different feuding branches of the US establishment was not explained.

This belief in US exceptionalism had been taken to its logical conclusion by the new US ambassador, Richard Holbrooke, aided and abetted by UN Secretary-General Kofi Annan, inviting the chairman of the US Senate Foreign Relations Committee to the Security Council. This unprecedented invitation provided the setting for Jesse Helms to lecture the UN on how American laws had precedence over what the UN might legislate, and, in good measure, he asked the world organisations to keep its hand off American citizens.

Encouraged by the exceptional world stage he was able to command, Helms invited the Security Council to come to Washington to talk to his committee. In other words, the key organ of the United Nations should now be willing to be grilled by the legislative arm of a member state on its attitudes and decisions.

Ostensibly, the Helms exercise was to sell the American diktat to the United Nations. If the UN wanted part of the money the US was obliged to pay in full on time, it should reform itself, agree to reducing the US peace-keeping share from 31 per cent to 25 per cent and its regular budget share from 25 per cent to 22, then 20 per cent. America was too powerful to be bound by rules and obligations, and, among other sins, Helms had not forgiven the UN for probing *American* human rights abuses. And he ended his discourse with a veiled threat that the US could leave the UNO, pointedly bringing up the American rejection of the League of Nations which doomed it.

And what was Annan's response to this challenge to the authority and very *raison d'être* of the world organisation? According to his spokesman, "He feels it's a positive step to open the dialogue. He feels we've turned the corner in the relationship between the US and UN". If anyone doubted where the secretary-general's loyalties lay, here was unambiguous proof that he was repaying the US for getting him the job by espousing American positions, however detrimental they might be to the world organisation and its future.

Above the UN

The simmering crisis precipitated by the American approach to the United Nations had come to the boil, and since the secretary-general's attitude could only harm, rather than help, the organisation, the burden of saving the only universal institution fell on the shoulders of three of the five permanent members of the Security Council—Russia, France and China—and the wider membership. If the United Nation were to accept the American logic, that they were above the United Nations and were not bound by its laws other than those they chose, it would be the beginning of the end of the end of a second attempt at making a universal organisation work.

Helms believed that not only did the United States have the right to intervene in a crisis across national borders (he was maladroit in singling out Ronald Reagan's exercise of power in Grenada), but that the UN Security Council had no business to put a damper on such exercises. Annan, of course, agreed with the American thesis on humanitarian interventions disregarding the boundaries of nation states and could add little to further the debate.

President Bill Clinton had a problem with Capitol Hill and, in his second term, he sought to resolve it by wooing Helms, first through

Secretary of State Madeleine Albright and latterly through Holbrooke whose own nomination was held up by the Senate for close to a year. Why President Clinton should inflict his domestic problems on the world organisation was for member states to rebel against. And in a remarkable display of sycophancy, Holbrooke told the Senate Foreign Relations Committee meeting in New York after Helms' oration in the Security Council that Japan was considering legislation similar to America's on lowering its own contribution to the UN budget standing at 19 per cent, capping it with, "They're watching you, Mr. Chairman. You're their hero".

How President Clinton chose to deal with his Congress was his business, but Helms had put the world on notice that in the American vocabulary, the United Nations counted only to the extent it agreed with US aims and priorities. The UN had lasted longer than the League of Nations but its middle-age crisis following America's superpower supremacy after the end of the Cold War could prove fatal. The US had tested the waters in the eighties by withdrawing from Unesco, and remained outside it until 2002. With its veiled threat to leave the parent United Nations, the stage was set for a more portentous battle.

The UN should be saved—from Helms, the American impresario Holbrooke and Annan.

A Father's Legacy

Back in January 1991, as we were herded in pyjamas into the basement of Al Mansour hotel in Baghdad early one morning after American and British aircraft had painted the sky in pyrotechnical colours, few of us could have imagined that a son of President George Bush would be wrestling with President Saddam a decade later. The decision of the younger Bush, now a President in his own right, to order American and British planes to strike at targets close to Baghdad for the first time in two years was only the opening gambit. (Britain's agreement with Washington's policies on Iraq was taken for granted.)

Even before assuming charge, Secretary of State Colin Powell had given an indication of the new Bush administration's Iraq obsession. Later, it was suggested that Washington was groping towards a sanctions regime that was more effective and targeted the ruling elite, rather than the people. With the air strikes at targets outside the northern and southern no-fly zones, W, as he is called after his middle initial, had appropriated the baggage of the previous Clinton administration in relation to Iraq even as he fashioned a new policy.

Judging by the opprobrium he had invited from the better part of the world for ordering the strikes, W was in a hurry to make his point: a tough posture on Iraq. In the process, he had saddled himself with a no-win situation, whatever the future held for President Saddam. The most draconian sanctions regime engineered by the United States against any country in United Nations history had impoverished a people, destroyed a generation and decimated the middle class. After a decade, the sanctions regime was frayed, with Egypt and Syria having signed free trade agreements with Iraq and more countries' airlines flying into Baghdad.

The senior Bush and Clinton legacy on Iraq was daunting enough. A no-fly zone over northern Iraq was set up in 1991 to protect the Kurds; in August 1992, a southern no-fly zone was declared and later expanded, to protect Shi'as. Neither of the zones had UN sanction. The saga of United Nations inspections, ostensibly to ferret out and destroy weapons of mass destruction, was too well known to need elaboration. The weapons inspectors were withdrawn in December 1998 before American and British planes unleashed days of bombing of Iraq as punishment for its refusal to cooperate fully with the inspection regime.

The US had thus appropriated the right to be the world's policeman in places it wanted to police, untrammelled by what the UN Security Council might or might not desire. The open-ended sanctions regime had been brought into disrepute and, together with the erosion of the UN's political authority, its moral authority was sapped as the world witnessed Iraq's continuing tragedy with dismay.

How the new Bush administration would be tougher than its predecessor remained to be determined. A decision to give the anti-Saddam opposition grouping $ 29 million in assistance impressed no one, given the contentious nature of the opportunist combine and its acceptance of American bounty to fight domestic foes. Whatever views the Iraqi people held about their president, they could not look kindly on fellow countrymen seeking the help of those who had brought devastation to their land long after Baghdad was punished for invading and annexing Kuwait.

Bush's Message

Powell was to embark on his first West Asian tour soon and might pick up a few useful tips in evolving a new regional approach. But the pitch had already been queered by the message the new President was keen to send on Iraq. It would seem that W's obsession with Saddam was clouding his administration's judgement in framing a new foreign policy. The Arab world was asking itself whether the son's desire to answer his father's critics for not taking Desert Storm to its logical conclusion 10 years earlier would lead the region to new troubles and travails.

The crux of George W. Bush's foreign policy as it had been elaborated was that the US would choose its areas of intervention selectively and strike hard to make its power prevail when it decided to move. The administration's initial unfolding of the National Missile Defence plan would indicate an even stronger streak of unilateralism than was displayed by the Clinton dispensation. Significantly, neither France nor Canada was informed, much less consulted, before the new strikes near Baghdad. And there was dismay in UN corridors that the strikes came barely 10 days before scheduled talks between UN and Iraqi officials on breaking the stalemate over new inspections.

The ostensible reason for retaining sanctions against Iraq was that UN inspectors had not cleared Baghdad on a full accounting of weapons of mass destruction. The real reason, it was almost universally acknowledged, was that the US would ensure that sanctions remained in place as long as the Saddam regime was in power. There were palliatives such as the oil-for-food programme and after UN inspectors were withdrawn before the intense bombing spree of December 1998 by American and British warplanes, the Security Council went through a convoluted series of meetings. The result was the setting up of another inspection regime with a bigger carrot offered to Baghdad, but President Saddam was not biting.

Given the stalemate in the Israeli–Palestinian process and the level of unrest on the West Bank and in the Gaza Strip, it made sense to look at the broader regional picture. The new administration was swearing by its adherence to discipline and strategy, but its fixation on Iraq was in danger of distorting its perspective. The Israeli–Palestinian confrontation was causing unease in many Arab capitals and this central issue would continue to cast a long shadow.

A more belligerent American posture on Iraq would serve to feed forces inimical to American interests while making the lives of regional rulers more uncomfortable. If Powell followed the new US Defence Secretary, Donald Rumsfeld, in his style of consultation in the form of the lecture the latter gave Nato allies on the merits of the National Missile Defence plan, a combustion in West Asia would not be long in the making.

A New Fork

It was ironical that it should require the labours of the Mitchell Commission to pinpoint a transparent fact, that the entire Oslo process between Israelis and Palestinians could be little more than a charade if the occupying power set about changing the contours of the occupied territories while it talked peace. Yet that was precisely what had been happening for the past eight years and more under both Labour and Likud dispensations.

The question to ask as relations between Israelis and Palestinians reached a new fork was whether there was the proverbial light at the end of the tunnel. As the second intefada raged in the occupied territories and the hardline Israeli Prime Minister Ariel Sharon used warplanes and invaded the supposedly autonomous Palestinian territories, had we reached the bottom?

The detached stance of the Bush administration was unsustainable because the cards were stacked against Palestinians, thanks to American geopolitical interests and the clout of the American Jewry. Once these interests were threatened by the level of violence and the outrage in the Arab world, Washington had perforce to intervene. President George W. Bush was coming to recognise this even as his negotiating tactic would be different from his predecessor's.

For all his sins, Ehud Barak made a valiant attempt at belling the cat but failed and a divided Israeli nation that could have inched towards facing reality reacted by swinging to the other extreme. Oslo, flawed as it was, was built on the principle of land for peace. In the end, there was little land transferred to the Palestinians and peace remained elusive. As Sharon was discovering yet again, answering stone-throwers with warplanes and live ammunition was not the answer. Nor was the Sharon proposal of shelving the difficult issues the answer because it would translate into consolidation and expansion of the occupation, with Palestinians perennially living under the threat of curfews and blockades, their livelihood gone and their lives in tatters. Oslo had left the difficult issues till the end and what happened? The final issues were never genuinely discussed under the Oslo framework, deadlines of Israeli withdrawals slipped and more occupied land was colonised.

Former president Bill Clinton's high profile interventions highlighted the nature of the problem. While Oslo could serve as an umbrella, only Washington had the power to resolve the problem. His successor's arm's length approach was, in effect, a gift to Israel. Tel Aviv received all the protection and benefits of the American connection while it was free to deal with the Palestinians as it wished.

The Impasse

If peace proved a mirage for the Israelis under Barak, security was proving a mirage under Sharon. A divided nation had yet to find the answers even as it switched leaders and its American mentor and protector took a measure of the problem. Palestinians were at the receiving end of much of this because occupation begot violence and as curfews and prohibitions blighted their lives and livelihood, the young in particular rebelled at their lot while partisans with other agendas promoted their causes.

The way out of the impasse was shown by Barak's failed attempt, and the US had to be intensively involved to get the parties back to the drawing board. There was no option but to tackle the basic issues of occupation, settlements, Jerusalem's status and the right of refugees' return. But Israel was flirting with the seducers who promised security even as the situation had been muddied by the decision of Peres to lend his support to the Sharon experiment.

The Israelis were mortgaging their future the longer they shied away from facing reality and the more they relied on their edge in weapons and technology to keep Palestinians in check. Some of the Israeli conservatives' scenarios were so fanciful that their implementation would bring disaster. There would be many more years of blood and tears for Palestinians and Israelis alike if the Sharon way of doing things was allowed to proceed unhindered.

Yet the contours of a fair settlement were now well known and recognised. There had to be a contiguous, viable Palestinian state. East Jerusalem, particularly areas covering the Muslim holy sites, had to return to Palestinians. Settlements on occupied land had to go because a future Palestinian state could not allow another state to exercise sovereignty over pockets on its land. Settlements clubbed around Jerusalem could be given to Israel in exchange for Israeli land elsewhere. Israel should concede the principle of the refugees' right of return while seeking to limit and regulate their flow.

As previous colonial powers had discovered on leaving their colonies, reconciliation began when colonised peoples were treated with dignity. The Israeli twist was that it was not a distant metro-politan power that could go away. Israelis were not merely occupying Palestinian land but coveted it and in the end had to co-exist with the colonised. Although tilted against Palestinians, Oslo was a recognition of this fact. In retrospect, Israelis found it easy to use individualist terrorist acts directed by Palestinians opposed to Oslo to deny and ultimately frustrate the basis of the accords.

The Bush administration was learning the hard way that its own options were limited. It sounded good to declare that Americans could not be keener to resolve the Israeli-Palestinian problem than the parties concerned. But the problem in its present form was created and defined by US geopolitical interests and affinity with Jews. For the Palestinians, it had never been a level playing field and their problems had merely been accentuated by the end of the Cold War and the emergence of Israeli's protector as the sole superpower. This geopolitical reality and the Arab states' own divisions were responsible for the impasse. There could not be a resolution of the problem on Sharon's terms.

Tail Wags the Dog

The Bush administration was learning the hard way that it did not have the luxury of disengaging from West Asia. Nor could it impose its will on a problem that had major domestic ramifications and strategic implications for America. If former President Bill Clinton was a hands-on man in seeking a way out, his successor had graduated from a hands-off policy to a band-aid method of coping with a problem that would not go away.

A succession of US officials who headed to the region—from the CIA chief George Tenet to Secretary of State Colin Powell—had been tinkering with the periphery. The American assumption was that since Sharon would not begin to talk to the Palestinians unless there was calm, a formula had to be devised to bring it about.

Periods of calm were part of the formula, latterly of one week followed by six weeks of cooling-off period. But it was plain for all to see that unless the definition of 'calm' was fudged, there could not be calm for any such length of time. It was not in Arafat's power to rein in all the anti-Israeli groups. And as Palestinian stone-throwers became the recipients of Israeli rubber bullets or worse and more funerals were held, they provided the impetus for fresh attacks on Israeli settlers who lived behind fortifications on occupied land.

The Bush administration's therefore was, at best, a holding operation —until such time that the wheel turned full circle and Israel reverted to a leader and party that could make peace with Palestinians on anything approaching a fair settlement. Sharon's rise to power was the proverbial swing of the pendulum because his predecessor Ehud Barak made peace his slogan but brought insecurity to Israelis instead. The Israeli electorate then threw away the baby with the bath water.

The Israeli–Palestinian problem was unique in the conduct of American foreign policy because the tail wags the dog. An American president's freedom of action was circumscribed not merely by his country's strategic interests in keeping Israel afloat in a hostile region but in Tel Aviv's ability to discipline the White House through the powerful American Jewish lobby and the threat of using Capitol Hill against a president thought to be going against core Israeli interests. This ultimate weapon had been unleashed on occasion.

One piece of fiction perpetrated by both Israelis and Arabs, for different reasons, was that the United States can be an 'even-handed' mediator. Washington made no secret of being Israel's main strategic ally in the region. Nor was it a secret that the US State Department's West Asian division was traditionally dominated by officials of Jewish faith, in addition to American Jewry exercising a veto over Washington's West Asian policy. True, US administrations had to make gestures to allies in the Arab world, but Arab disunity and the need for an American military umbrella blunted the edge of Arab states' protests.

The Israeli tragedy was that Peres, a leader of sensibility, should have compromised himself by agreeing to serve as foreign minister in Sharon's national unity government to further his political career. Traditional political folklore has it after Richard Nixon's successful overtures to China that only hardliners could resolve longstanding contentious problems. If Sharon was to transform himself into a new *avatar* of peace, he had given little indication of his intentions.

Barak's Role

Even more than Rabin, it was Barak who confronted the difficult problems of bringing about real peace. The significance of his final proposals was not that he failed but how close he was to succeeding. Barak could not surmount the last hurdle because his peace constituency ran out of patience and the dying days of the Clinton presidency did not give Arafat sufficient time to present a realistic counter-proposal. It was wrong of Clinton to blame Arafat for his failure.

Under Sharon and the presidency of George W. Bush, we had a Catch-22 situation. There could not be political talks between Israelis and Palestinians while blockades of Palestinian areas, deaths of Palestinian youth killed by Israeli bullets and the daily humiliation of Palestinians proceeded apace. And the Mitchell commission report, which was the new guiding star, was often invoked but remained implemented. One would have imagined that the simple contradiction between negotiations on the future and Israel's continuing expansion of Jewish settlements on occupied land would have been plain. Yet the freeze on settlements, if it took place, had been made dependent upon the observance of 'calm' and other conditions.

Nobody underestimated the difficulties of bringing about peace between Israelis and Palestinians, but a beginning towards a solution could only be made if the Palestinians received justice and fairness. The contours of a fair settlement were clear enough. The crucial question that remained to be answered was how much more bloodshed and turmoil it would take before the larger Israeli public and its American ally realised it.

A Deadly Combination

Orient House in occupied East Jerusalem is a villa that would be indistinguishable in a suburban European setting. The morning I drove past it, it stood serene, its gates firmly shut, a Palestinian flag fluttering in the lazy breeze. Yet this house had served as a potent symbol of Palestinian nationalism and foreign dignitaries had traditionally wended their way there, against Israeli wishes, to pay their symbolic tribute to the incipient Palestinian state.

Israel had occupied Orient House in response to a suicide bombing in Jerusalem to try to snuff out Palestinian nationalism. In practice, Israel had ended up gaining another bargaining chip against

Palestinians. By now, Israel had a graveyard of bargaining chips and one more or less had ceased to matter in the game of escalation the world had been witnessing.

What was new about an old confrontation was that the combination of the new Bush administration and Ariel Sharon was, in the short term, proving deadly for Palestinians. President George W. Bush seemed to be following a policy suggesting that the power of the United States was so great that the anger of the Arab street and the hand-wringing of the so-called moderate Arab governments would not harm its interests in the region.

Sharon is an intelligent man and could read the signs and he had taken full advantage of the not-so-benign neglect by the US administration. First, the so-called autonomous Palestinian areas were invaded and homes demolished. Then the American supplied F–16 fighter jets were used to flatten Palestinian buildings. Helicopter gunships were employed to assassinate individual Palestinians.

There were, of course, the continuing refinements of using the old colonial methods of the previous century to deal with Palestinian dissent. Palestinians were often bottled up in their restricted areas, unable to earn a living, often unable to meet one another from one Bantustan to another. Whether it was Sharon or his Labour predecessor Ehud Barak, settlement expansion went on merrily encroaching more occupied land, with more roads built to secure inter-settlement traffic.

The US administration made pro forma noises about Israeli provocations, took Arafat to task for not exerting himself sufficiently to rein in violence, the suicide bombers and the terror attacks. US Secretary of State Colin Powell listed the time he had spent telephoning regional and other leaders on the Israeli–Palestinian problem. It was as if, after giving Israel all the trump cards, the US had taken a holiday from West Asia.

Arafat, for his part, flew around the world, had innumerable meetings with Arab and other leaders, issued appeals and promised action. For the better part, he received tea and sympathy from the outside world. Europeans were more sympathetic to Palestinians and less in thrall to Israel. But apart from paying the better part of the aid bill for Palestine, they seemed to be able to do little because the Israeli–Palestinian problem was an American preserve, with even the United Nations being allowed in under strict guidelines. UN Secretary-General Kofi Annan's last visit to the region was at the behest of the Bush administration.

Sharon's Penchant

The world knew Sharon's penchant for using force in resolving problems. One had only to look at his record as defence minister and the massacres that took place in the refugees camps in Lebanon in the

1980s. Even assuming that the spiral of violence would continue, with stones being met by bullets, suicide bombers by F-16s flattening the poor Palestinian infrastructure, something would have to give. A limitless escalation of violence, like Mao Zedong's permanent revolution, was a rhetorical argument not rooted in reality.

What then was the solution? There could be none as long as the Bush administration pursued a policy which, in effect, encouraged Sharon to pursue his policy of maximum force and killings of Palestinians. But there would come a time when even the unilateralist W would have to bend, as he had in relation to China, because his deliberate neglect of the Israeli–Palestinian confrontation would simply prove to be too expensive.

Proponents of the separate development of Israel and Palestine were gathering steam and suggested that Israel should wall itself in. The rub lay in the need for defining its borders, the fundamentalists believing that the whole of the occupied West Bank belonged to Israel. The only working model Israelis and Palestinians could go back to was the last round of the meeting Barak had with Arafat under President Bill Clinton's auspices. Under it, 95 per cent of the occupied West Bank was to go to a new Palestinian state. The right of the refugees' return to Israel proved a sticking point and the question of Palestinian sovereignty over the holy sites in occupied East Jerusalem in particular was not quite resolved. Settlements around Jerusalem would be clubbed together with the city, with Palestinians being compensated by receiving land in Israel proper.

In immediate terms, the rise to power of Sharon and the ugly Israeli mood in the wake of a succession of suicide bombings had given a fillip to the hardliners in Israel even as Hamas in the Palestinian areas was gaining more supporters as funerals of Palestinians become a daily occurrence.

The trouble with an ideological state is that it becomes difficult to give large minorities their dues. There were more than a million Arabs in Israel proper. How would they feel as their cousins were treated even as they themselves were discriminated against?

A Catastrophe

It was the enormity of it that never ceased to surprise as the world sat glued to television sets to watch real life science fiction unfold in all its horror. The terrorist acts that demolished the twin towers of the World Trade Centre in New York and damaged a section of the Pentagon outside Washington had transformed America and the world in some ways. They had also set in train a chain of events that would have a ripple effect for a long time.

The United States had lost its sense of invulnerability for the first time since the MAD (mutual assured destruction) regime of the Cold War made the country reasonably safe from a nuclear attack. America's love affair with high-tech served little purpose because the plotters took civilian aeroplanes of everyday use to employ them as deadly missiles to slam into the twin towers and the Pentagon. Even as President George W. Bush had been single-mindedly promoting his National Missile Defence plan ostensibly to cope with threats from 'rogue' states, it would have proved irrelevant to the attack on the symbols of American financial and military power.

Initially, the US paused to establish leads to the perpetrators of the crime even as it sought to gather a 'coalition' for what President Bush had termed the first war of the twenty-first century. That in itself was a revolutionary concept for W with his penchant for unilateralism. Second, for the first time since the end of the Cold War, the American administration was using a familiar yardstick to measure friendship and loyalty: either you were for us or against us.

The Bush administration understood that fighting terrorism was for the long haul. Unlike state actors, the enemy was shadowy and finding terrorist networks to destroy him was a painstaking task. Terrorist training camps were easier to destroy than more obscure facilities and the tightly knit ideological groups were almost impossible to infiltrate. W had stated that the Saudi dissident in Afghanistan, Osama bin Laden, was the prime suspect, a finding that would come as no surprise.

On the military plane, no one doubted the American capability and will to inflict heavy damage on terrorists and terrorist networks. How far the United States would go in punishing states it saw as accomplices of the outlaws remained to be seen. But a military response to tackle terrorism could not achieve all that the US might wish. A state actor could be defeated and suppressed for a time but eradicating terrorism required a broader political approach that addressed the root causes of large-scale disaffection of peoples and countries.

In the short run, things would get worse in West Asia because the terrorist acts in New York and Washington gave Sharon a freer hand in tackling Palestinians even as he employed to his advantage President George W. Bush's hands-off approach to the region. Using F-16s helicopter gunships and missiles to settle scores with Palestinians would, however, exacerbate, rather than help resolve, the Israeli–Palestinian problem.

Low-Tech Havoc

It was too much to hope that the Bush administration, baptised by fire, would take a fresh look at West Asia once it had set in motion its military response? The horror of the terrorist acts on mainland America had given rise to many emotions: sadness, anger, calls for revenge and even a willingness to sacrifice American lives in fighting terrorism. Time would temper some of these emotions but the sense of hurt would remain, particularly because the world's sole surviving superpower had proved to be vulnerable to a diabolical low-tech plot.

No one doubted the role of the unresolved Israeli–Palestinian confrontation in the terrorist bombings in the US. If there was one issue destabilising a region and other parts of the world, it was the central problem of reconciling Israelis with Palestinians. The tragedy was that Palestinians had not received justice or their state and the only effective mediator, the United States, had amply proved its partisanship. Bill Clinton came closet to offering Palestinians—through Ehud Barak—something approaching a Palestinian state. Sharon had all but repudiated the land-for-peace principle that was the basis of the flawed Oslo accords.

America was Israel's protector and benefactor. But it did not have to follow that Palestinians had to languish without a viable state for all time. This is a hurt—a hurt greater than that of Americans after the terrorist bombings—Palestinians carried. This hurt became desperation on occasion.

The better part of the world supported the US in its fight against terrorism. Senseless acts of terror against innocent civilians are particularly loathsome. But as the American experience in Vietnam and the Soviet experience in Afghanistan revealed, force alone did not succeed in winning wars. And wars against non-state actors were particularly difficult to win.

Military, economic and other coercive methods had their place in fighting terrorism but they should have a moral dimension to succeed. That dimension is provided by the willingness of the strong to give justice to the weaker party in a complex historical problem that straddles a sensitive area. Would the Bush administration have the foresight to listen to Palestinian voices crying for justice even as it sought to get after terrorists and their dens?

World, Post-September 11

The September 11 terrorist attacks in New York and Washington are destined to take their place alongside the fall of the Berlin Wall and the disintegration of the Soviet Union. For like those epochal events, the attacks on the symbols of America's financial and military might were redefining Washington's relations with the better part of the world.

As far as Afghanistan is concerned, the American accent was on a post-Taleban dispensation. But in the process of achieving this goal by going after Osama bin Laden and his network, the US would also transform its interaction with the nations of Central Asia, Pakistan and Russia. The strategic aspect of the new configuration would come into greater prominence once immediate American goals receded.

The Bush administration had left no one in doubt that it would be a US-imposed New Order, admittedly with the help of sets of coalitions. The United Nations was being encouraged to bless America's efforts but would not be in the driver's seat. The contours of a new geopolitical relationship between the United States and the former Soviet Central Asian states bordering on Afghanistan were beginning to emerge. Once Russia decided to make a virtue of necessity by acquiescing in the American foray into its 'near abroad', Washington moved quickly into Uzbekistan to employ the significant military base for logistical and rescue and reconnaissance purposes. Uzbekistan was keen on a more permanent military relationship with the US.

Russia's President Vladimir Putin himself had taken a number of steps to express his support for the US anti-terrorist campaign and took the unprecedented decision of visiting the headquarters of Nato. It would, however, be a mistake for the West to interpret these moves as a Russian suspension of disbelief in Nato's capacity for mischief. Rather, President Putin's stance was more in the nature of hedging his bets in uncertain times.

Despite the obvious problems Pakistan faced in the wake of an American resolve to punish and dethrone the Taleban, President Pervez Musharraf had also been offered the opportunity to put his country's affairs in order. Thanks to his support for the US effort, he had been given a new economic lifeline and could be better placed in tackling domestic extremists and the consequences of the ferment in the North.

Two American characteristics that had again come into play were their penchant for focussing on one problem at a time, to the exclusion of much else, and their limited attention span. The new strains between Sharon and the Bush administration were an indication of the first characteristic as was the short shrift being given to Indian concerns falling outside the Osama bin Laden-defined terrorism. And Pakistanis were only too aware of Americans saying good bye once their immediate mission was accomplished, leaving the horrendous consequences of actions they encouraged and financed in the lap of their erstwhile host. In other words, nations, like individuals, are selfish. Such selfishness is often described as national interest.

Intriguing Possibility

The new developments, however, had thrown up an intriguing possibility. The anti-Iraq coalition put together by the United States to drive Iraq out of Kuwait highlighted an embarrassing anomaly in the American position effectively exploited by Baghdad. While a succession of US administrations had been supporting Israel to the hilt despite its continuing occupation of Palestinian land, George Bush Senior was quick to start building a coalition to chase Iraq out of Kuwait.

Out of the Gulf War was born the Madrid peace process, which led to the promise of the Oslo accords—a promise that had been buried by a succession of Israeli governments presiding over a divided nation afraid to exchange land for peace. If the new anti-terrorist campaign promised to be a long one, as Bush Junior never tired of repeating, Washington's aims could not be achieved without beginning a new process to bring a fair settlement to the Israeli–Palestinian confrontation. Perhaps it was this realisation that led Sharon to his extraordinary outburst warning America not to emulate Britain's surrender to Hitler in 1938 by "appeasing" the Arabs.

These were early days but an important relationship that was likely to be affected by the post-September 11 American world view was the transatlantic one. Leaving aside Britain, which served as a Jeeves to America's Bertie Wooster, the European allies were generous in their support of the US. The invocation of Nato's Article five, saying that an attack on one member was tantamount to an attack on all, was speedy. But it did not take long for Europeans to realise that Washington did not wish to seek Nato's military help. Rather, it would deal with members bilaterally for military or other help in order to maintain full autonomy in decision-making.

Europeans had been seeking to strike out an independent path in translating their economic clout into political and military muscle. The concept of building a Rapid Reaction Force was the boldest expression of the European wish to cut themselves loose from American apron-strings in the post-Cold War world. The fight against terrorism had galvanised much of the world, but if the US were to interpret the widespread support it had received as a licence to build a New World Order unilaterally, it would face European and other opposition.

The tragedy was that the United Nations was led by a man who conceived his duties as being mindful of American interests and concerns. Kofi Annan was installed as secretary-general by an American veto, but after he had obtained a final second term, he could perhaps be more attentive to the interests and concerns of all the members of the world organisation. There was a distinction between a secretary-general being on the right side of the world's sole surviving superpower in order to be able to function effectively and one who was subservient to one member state.

A Path of Disaster

Against the backdrop of the American campaign against terrorism, the Israeli–Palestinian confrontation was reminding President George W. Bush that after US forces would have left Afghanistan the unresolved problem in West Asia would mock the sole surviving superpower. Americans had always titled towards Israel for a variety of well-known reasons, but never more so than under the present US administration.

The debate in Washington was how further to isolate and humiliate Arafat, already under virtual house arrest, surrounded by Israeli tanks, his helicopters destroyed as were the Gaza airport runway and the sea port. If the world had doubts about how the Israelis conceived of a Palestinian Authority and a Palestinian state, here was a vivid demonstration of Tel Aviv's wish list. And the Bush administration had weighed in on Israel's side, condoning its policy of assassinating individual Palestinians and Israeli invasion of Palestinian-administered territory to destroy houses and kill and arrest people. F-16 fighter planes targeted Palestinian areas. Cease-fires came and went as the cycles of violence fed on the actions of either side. Israel—and now increasingly the US—held Yasser Arafat responsible for any and every terrorist attack against Israelis.

A boatload of arms intercepted early in January 2000, apparently bound for the Gaza Strip provoked new American anger, with President George W. Bush suggesting that he was "very disappointed" with Arafat and accused him of "enhancing" terrorism. And the US administration had been debating further steps to express its displeasure with the Palestinian Authority even as it prepared to welcome Sharon to the White House. Neither the Americans nor the Israelis seemed to know where they were going. The Palestinians and the wider Arab world had been at the receiving end of American policies. Even as the governments of the Arab world lined up with the US in the coalition against terrorism, the new twist to the Israeli–Palestinian confrontation was taking shape. Sharon had assumed power in Israel with a proclaimed lack of faith in the Oslo peace process, his hardline policies a sure recipe for Palestinian retaliation in the shape of terrorist acts by extremist factions. Sharon was greatly helped by the new US administration's initial hands-off policy.

A central objective of Sharon's policy had been to demonise Arafat, in one instance comparing him to Osama bin Laden. Every act of terror committed by a Palestinian faction was laid at the door of the Palestinian leader while the ferocity and disproportionate nature of the Israeli response invited further Palestinian retaliation. And with the capture of the boatload of 50 tonnes of munition, Sharon had swung President Bush entirely to his side, reinforcing W's posture of keeping Arafat at arm's length.

It seemed likely that Sharon had finally succeeded in burying the Oslo peace process. There had been precious little peace since Sharon assumed office and a succession of his predecessors had done their bit to repudiate Oslo by reneging on the land-for-peace formula and piling on more Jewish settlements on occupied land. Ehud Barak, identified with the doves, saw the greatest colonisation of occupied land. The new high-stake game in West Asia came at a difficult time in Washington's relations with the Arab world. Sharp differences had emerged on two aspects: America's military presence in Saudi Arabia and US plans to target Iraq in its continuing war against terrorism. The Americans were suddenly discovering flaws in Saudi mores and restrictions placed on the use of the military facilities in the kingdom. And on the Iraq issue, Arab states had made it amply clear that military action against Baghdad would be little short of disastrous.

Saudi Warning

Unusually, a senior member of the Saudi ruling family had thought it fit to warn America in an interview to the *New York Times* of the dangers of weakening Arafat. Washington was reported to have given Arab governments evidence of the links between the boatload of seized arms and the Palestinian Authority. Israel had already declared Arafat "irrelevant" and W seemed inclined to follow that path. But the question posed by Prince Nawwaf bin Abdul Aziz, director of the Saudi military intelligence, was pertinent: Who will then come forward to make peace on the Palestinians' behalf?

The Palestinians knew they were in a weak position and even as they had taken out a demonstration in support of their leader, Arafat had called for American engagement again. Ironically, former president Bill Clinton was shouting from the housetops that Arafat spurned his marathon attempts at giving Palestinians most of what they wanted in terms of a viable state and divided sovereignty over Jerusalem. The truth was somewhat different, as one of the participants in the Camp David summit revealed in the *New York Review of Books* on August 9, 2001, but the formula proposed would remain a benchmark.

Sharon was doubtless patting himself on the back for folding his own agenda seamlessly into W's war against terrorism. But anyone with an even cursory knowledge of the Israeli–Palestinian confrontation would realise that the Israelis and Americans were setting out on a road to disaster. The answer was surely not in finding pliant Palestinians to do the Israeli bidding. Indeed, it would become increasingly counter-productive for the Israelis to continue to rule over a resentful Palestinian population in occupied land. The situation had never been as hopeless since the Oslo accords were announced on the lawn of the White House. The peace camp in Israel lay dormant as the killing of Israeli civilians strengthened the war lobby each day.

Target Iraq

America had a problem, a big problem. President Saddam remained in power in Baghdad after having lost the mother of battles led by a coalition headed by Bush Senior a decade earlier. He was thus an affront to President George W. Bush and to the unparalleled status of the United States as the seat of the Second Roman empire. The problem was how to topple President Saddam.

Even before the September 11 events brought Afghanistan into focus, the new administration of Bush the son had fixed its gaze on undertaking the unfinished business Bush Senior had neglected to accomplish. After a decade of the most severe sanctions regime imposed on any country in the world, the privations of the Iraqi people, the oil-for-food programme and the biased clearance mechanism for approving imports into Iraq had combined to tilt the world's sympathy towards the Iraqis.

The US had been unsuccessfully trying to refine the sanctions, with few immediate takers. America's perspective on the world changed after September 11 and it was immediately made clear that the Afghan operations were only the first phase of the anti-terrorism operations. The next phase, as amplified, would take in Baghdad, only to draw a blank. Americans had been half-heartedly trying to support a disparate Iraqi opposition, and this support had been firmed up.

President Bush, meanwhile, had been building an ideological framework for toppling President Saddam by describing Iraq as being a member of "an axis of evil", juxtaposing it improbably with Iran and North Korea. At the same time, the American attempt was to make the brief of new United Nations weapons inspectors so onerous that Baghdad would refuse to have them. Baghdad, for its part, seemed to be playing a waiting game.

Iraq's refusal would then be a cause for the United States to launch a military strike on Baghdad, presumably followed by ground action with American troops and a ragtag army of Iraqi exiles and factions of Kurds. The planned justification would be that Iraq was building weapons of mass destruction and represented a danger to the region and the world. Such an act would send a fearful message to peoples and countries.

Shorn of the rhetoric and propaganda offensive that would precede a likely US military offensive, the message would amount to a declaration of a unilateral right to intervene any time anywhere. Were such action to be clothed in the garb of the "war on terror", in the American idiom, it would discredit the laudable cause of actually fighting terrorism. The United Nations had been effectively marginalised except when Washington wanted to use it, principally in feeding the refugees of war. The European Union's offer of help in fighting the war against terrorism in Afghanistan was, for the better part, spurned. The EU's role, in American eyes, was largely to finance the Palestinians and others and keeping the peace, leaving America to fight the wars it wanted to.

Terror under Beds

Was this then the emerging shape of the New World Order? Signs were multiplying that Americans were working themselves into a frenzy, with the "war on terror" having replaced the old Commie-bashing exercises. Instead of Reds, Americans were looking for terrorists under their beds and an impervious shadow seat of governance has been set up to take into account the hazards of nuclear or biological attacks.

Two questions should be asked. Did the new anti-terrorism offensive satisfy an American need for an enemy to keep the military–industrial complex of President Eisenhower's description moving? Second, the world was, for the first since the September 11 tragedy, examining the motives of American actions. In other words, was the anti-terrorism campaign being used merely as a cover for achieving American foreign policy goals that would otherwise have been difficult to accomplish?

The Iraq issue had alerted the world to the latter danger because while people everywhere sympathised with the loss of American and other lives in the September 11 attacks, there was a growing suspicion of a hidden American agenda in meeting the terrorist threat.

It was the American-dominated air war on Yugoslavia that first set alarm bells ringing in Europe. The European Union quickly agreed to form a Rapid Reaction Force to meet emergencies without the United States. But the American air war on Afghanistan had administered an even ruder shock; America did not need Nato to fight its wars, the argument now being reduced to discussing the possible obsolescence of Nato in the New World Order.

But America had still to face the problem of riding roughshod over the world to achieve essentially selfish objectives. Could one country, however powerful, set itself as the arbitrary emperor in an incredibly inter-connected world? Fighting terrorism, to begin with, should be an international endeavour to be effective. Besides, the prosperity of the United States was partly dependent upon its ability to trade with and do business in other countries. Could the haughty airs of a new imperial power serve these American interests?

India and West Asia

Tilt Towards Iran

Two aspects of the Shah of Iran's talks in Delhi in December 1974 deserved attention. It was a symbolic visit and it was successful in what it set out to achieve by underlining the increasing commitment by the two countries to building a new kind of relationship.

No dramatic initiatives were taken during the visit, nor were any expected. But the joint communiqué gave an indication of how far India was prepared to go in accommodating Iranian views. India's need to fashion special relations with a new oil-rich nation was obvious. For the Iranians, there were advantages in having closer ties in the east to balance their none-too-happy relations with the Arab world.

During his talks with Indira Gandhi, the Shah was believed to have made no secret of his disenchantment with the Pakistani leadership. In any event, Pakistan's relations with some of the Arab countries were too close for Iranian comfort. India fell into a different category as far as Iran was concerned.

India had no hesitation in endorsing the Shah's proposal for the "formation of an economic inter-relationship in the northern part of the Indian Ocean region". In fact, Indira Gandhi would have gone further in supporting Iranian views had the Shah spelled out the concept of the economic organisation he had in mind.

India had its own ideas of a South Asian Common Market although efforts to implement them had made show progress. Talks were in progress with Sri Lanka. The Indian proposal envisaged taking in Burma, Sikkim, Bhutan, Bangladesh, Pakistan, Nepal and Afghanistan. The attempt was first to suggest tariff cuts by a certain percentage in a traditional Common Market arrangement. The model was the tripartite arrangement between India, Egypt and Yugoslavia.

There would be obvious advantages in an oil-rich country like Iran making a similar proposal, although New Delhi would have to decide whether to abandon the initiative to Teheran and how wide the new economic relationship should be. South-east Asian countries had their own ASEAN arrangement and the broader concept implied by the Shah was on the face of it a long-term project. There were also obvious problems in bringing Pakistan into an economic arrangement, particularly in view of a new hardening of Pakistan's attitude towards India.

Revealing Communiqué

Unlike most such documents, the joint communiqué was revealing because it recorded the Indian tilt towards Iran on a number of issues. There were reportedly difficult sessions in arriving at an agreed formulation, but the Indian side finally agreed to make the necessary concessions to Iran.

Thus the importance to the security and stability of the Persian Gulf was specifically recorded and the Straits of Hormoz were given special attention. Further, there was agreement on maintaining peace and tranquillity in that region by "cooperation among the littoral States". On Cyprus, India had for the first time given the minority Turkish community almost equal rights in working out future political arrangements. Again, Indira Gandhi agreed to support Iran's proposal for a nuclear weapons-free zone in West Asia.

Even in relation to the Indian Ocean, it could be argued that references in the communiqué—for example, when it called on the Great Powers to cooperate in establishing the ocean as a zone of peace—were less pro-Soviet. The economic concessions obtained by India were not spelled out, although the terms of Indo-Iranian cooperation had been softened in New Delhi's favour.

One implication of the Indian tilt towards Iran was that Indira Gandhi had decided to seek a new equilibrium in West Asia. India's relations with Iraq were not as cordial as could have been expected. But although the Iranians might have extracted more political concessions than New Delhi could have thought wise, there was no mistaking the search for a new basis of relations with the countries of West Asia.

India could not cash in on the basis of religion, a choice open to Pakistan and Bangladesh. Besides, in view of the new tensions building up between Iran and Pakistan, India was a natural complementary factor in the former's need to promote good relations on its eastern flank.

There were few regrets in South Block over the concessions given to Iran. The speed with which agreed Indo-Iranian projects were being processed was an indication of the Indian resolve to buttress economic relations between the two countries. Indo-Iranian projects had a wider connotation in foreshadowing a new phase in Indian economic policy. For instance, the Kudremukh iron ore project was something of a foreign undertaking that would operate on Indian soil virtually free of foreign exchange regulations, the first time a project of this nature was being attempted since 1953. The joint shipping line project, on the other hand, would be financed by Iran. It would tap Indian expertise and cater to the growing volume of trade between the two countries. The desire to implement the major trade and commercial arrangements with Iran had induced the government to free one sector from the constraints operating on the bulk of Indian industries.

Given the growing amity and bilateral trade and commercial arrangements with Iran, how would India reorder its relations with the Arab world? One choice before India was to seek cordial relations with countries like Oman and Saudi Arabia, without unduly neglecting Iraq and Egypt.

On the political plane, it was remarkable that Indian official spokesman have had nothing to say about the channelling of US equipment to Pakistan through Iran. The supply of US helicopters by Iran to Pakistan excited Indian misgivings over US policy towards India and there was no criticism of the Iranian action.

Since the new relations were being built on the benefits each hoped to receive from the other, they had a chance of survival. For Iran, the political implications were as important as its desire to use Indian manpower and technical competence to the maximum extent. In India's case, the economic advantages outweighed other benefits.

A Plaything

Foreign policy was not destined to determine the outcome of the January 1980 election. But in a campaign in which there were few real issues except those relating to the politicians' capacity to govern the country at an acceptable price, it was inevitable that the pro-tagonists' speeches should be laced with matters relating to foreign affairs.

An interesting outcome of the campaign was that all the major parties had thought it fit to move left—to swing away from the West and to adopt a more pro-Arab stance, at Egypt's expense. More predic-tably, jingoism had been given some play.

Indira Gandhi set the ball rolling by using foreign policy as an integral part of her omnibus attack on the Janata government's record. Her attempt had been to paint the Janata regime as a pusillanimous one, giving away too much to neighbours, and titling towards the West. She chose the example of tiny Bhutan making eyes at India (a reference to its vote in Havana) to drive home her point that the nation's interests were not safe in Janata's hands.

The Charan Singh government she had sought to demolish by recalling the Lusaka fiasco and spreading the fanciful story of a deal with Pakistan to create a border diversion in order to postpone the elections. Perhaps her objective was to deny Charan Singh any kind of excuse to delay elections, rather than make people believe such a cock-and-bull story.

The US, at any rate, had been Indira Gandhi's favourite whipping boy, and if it served her purpose by painting the Janata government as an American stooge, it could hardly do her much harm. The anti-West stance could always be moderated were she to return to power; meanwhile, it was politically profitable to strike a nationalistic posture to suggest that she was the only one capable of keeping India's flag flying.

Henry Kissinger had unwittingly helped Indira Gandhi in her objective. Excerpts of his memoirs in *India Today* had done her a world of good by his presentation of her as a consummate practitioner of the international power game. The contrast this presented with S. N. Mishra's performance at Lusaka was too telling to need further comment.

Indira Gandhi had no hesitation in bringing into her fold H. N. Bahuguna whose name had been bandied about as a KGB agent by no other than the caretaker Prime Minister, despite Charan Singh's later ambiguous retraction. And when she had in her ranks an alleged KGB agent, she must perforce introduce a CIA one, alleged to have passed on her government's secrets to the Americans. She was only being non-aligned in her fashion.

Charan Singh had not been found wanting in steering his party to a more leftist position, whatever his own views on world affairs by hastily dropping "genuine" from non-alignment, but he scored by paying Indira Gandhi back in her own coin. In a brilliant transfer of imagery, he painted her next government, should she come to power, as one which would conduct public floggings à la General Zia-ul-Haq of Pakistan. This was the kind of language everyone understood and was worth a mountain of theses on the evils of dictatorship.

Perhaps, Charan Singh also realised that trailing behind the other two major groupings in the race for power, he had greater freedom in striking up a populist posture on the nuclear question. In his August 15 speech, he had said India might be forced to review its nuclear option if Pakistan exploded a bomb, and his Defence Minister, caretaker though he be, had been giving further airing to this view, despite Y. B. Chavan's public disapproval.

Jagjivan Ram had been forced to reiterate India's traditional policy on the nuclear question; a man who expected to be Prime Minister could not play with an issue which bristled with international implications. And Indira Gandhi, who would have loved to become a pro-bomb protagonist, probably felt she was too near the Prime Minister's chair to start throwing foreign chancelleries, including the Russians, into panic.

Pakistan was not an issue in the Indian election and there was a consensus on having good relations with it. But India was too close to events in the neighbouring country for developments there not to have an impact. Indira Gandhi's promise of a strong government had to be sufficiently tempered not only because of the Emergency excesses but also because General Zia was a constant example of what could happen to a country when it was run by a dictator. And, of course, an "Islamic bomb" would have an immediate reaction in India.

Approach to Arabs

For his part, Jagjivan Ram had thought it wise to mend the Janata Party's fences with the Arabs, perhaps with an eye on Muslim votes in UP in particular. He held an extraordinary meeting with a number of Arab envoys to push his party closer to their prevailing views on that part of the world. He·suggested that the Janata government's attitude to the Arab question should have been different in Havana. Poor S. N. Mishra, who was merely following the Janata policy as best he could!

The pleas of A. B. Vajpayee, who did a creditable job as Foreign Minister, that foreign policy was not an issue in the election, were going unheeded in his own party. Even Indira Gandhi privately agreed that it was not an issue, but some of its aspects were too tempting to ignore in a free-for-all election. Nobody in Janata talked of "genuine" non-alignment; it had become a dirty word for all political parties.

The Russians had not directly figured much in the election campaign, except for the controversy over H. N. Bahuguna's Russian credentials. But party strategists were putting their heads together to try to discover the persons and parties other than the CPI they were backing. It was taken for granted that Russian money flowed in every election. If the version making the rounds in Delhi — that the Russians were backing Y. B. Chavan and his Congress and the Communists aligned with him — was correct, Soviet understanding of Indian election politics left much to be desired.

In any event, the Russians could only be pleased with the policy stance the major parties had adopted. There was in Jagjivan Ram's talk with the Arab envoys the suggestion that India would take a more pro-Soviet line in the Non-aligned Movement. Indira Gandhi, temporarily in league with Bahuguna, continued to berate the Americans. And Charan Singh was so anxious to appear "with it" that he had turned a radical.

Mercifully, China had not figured in the election campaign. There was no prospect of a dramatic breakthrough in relations between the two countries and no party, except the CPI and other pro-Moscow elements, could have much quarrel with keeping the lines to Beijing open.

Was there a national consensus on foreign policy, as suggested by Vajpayee, and how genuine was the swing to the left that had taken place? Every political party, except those on the extreme fringes, swore by non-alignment, and even Janata, which tried to steer the country towards a more even-handed relationship with the two superpowers and inserted the word "genuine" before non-alignment, was professedly following Nehru's foreign policy.

There was admittedly a national consensus on India professing non-alignment but since the concept was elastic, it could be interpreted in various ways. Governments in India had found it easier to side with the Soviet Union than with the West for national and psychological reasons. For non-alignment was often a convenient cover for pursuit of national goals and the Western colonial legacy still haunted many.

One of the problems facing the non-aligned was that in view of the increasing rivalry between the Soviet Union and China, the Russians had been attempting to tilt the movement to their side. It was not merely a question of choosing between the West and the East but between the Soviet Union and China. Only those beholden to the Soviet Union, financially or otherwise, could plead that India should support the Russians on every issue.

While in power, Indira Gandhi had found it profitable to operate her foreign policy on a populist, vaguely left base, buttressed by her own anti-Americanism. Her election campaign gambits had been in keeping with this approach. But Jagjivan Ram had felt it necessary to take Janata's foreign policy away from Morarji Desai's genuine non-alignment to a more leftist and pro-Soviet orientation. Presumably, he had done this for hard-headed electoral reasons.

For many parties, adopting a left posture in foreign policy was merely to play safe in a confusing election. Indeed, should the left parties improve their position in the Lok Sabha, they would have more bargaining power in demanding their pound of flesh, particularly in the field of foreign policy.

Testing Syrian Waters

Rajiv Gandhi's foray into West Asia in December 1988 raised an important question. Was his visit to Syria a tactical exercise in relation to the PLO, Afghanistan and Pakistan? Or did it portend a new linkage India was seeking to create in the context of a policy framework in West Asia?

In Jawaharlal Nehru's days, India's dealings with the Arab world were through Egypt. This was inevitable in view of President Nasser's pre-eminence in the Arab world and the Non-aligned Movement. The latter buttressed the close rapport Nehru had with Nasser, although the economic benefits from this relationship proved illusory for both countries.

Nasser's era was the romantic age in the Arab world, and Nasser himself made several mistakes because he was susceptible to the Arab myth of its omnipotence. Egypt, together with the rest of the Arab world, learnt the hard way, through defeats on the battlefield, that it had to put its own house in order before taking on Israel.

The post-Nasser era was necessarily a period of confusion and a scaling down of Egypt's ambitions. And then President Sadat came along to change the face of Egypt and West Asia through a separate peace agreement with Israel under American auspices. Sadat's reasoning was simple. Egypt could not hope to defeat Israel in view of US assistance and commitment to it.

A continued Arab–Israeli confrontation, Sadat felt, was largely at Egypt's expense, in view of its important strategic position in the Arab world. Therefore, it was prudent to get back Sinai through a separate peace arrangement and suffer rebukes and isolation from the Arab world for a period. Such suffering was mitigated by a massive and continuing American economic and military aid package, second only to that offered to Israel.

From India's point of view, Egypt was no longer a credible interlocutor in the Arab world. In any event, Indira Gandhi had made an astute move to seek a linkage with Iran with two objectives: to weaken the Teheran–Islamabad link and to sell the Shah the idea that in the economic and technical fields, the two countries were ideal complementary partners. Against the background of the Shah's ambitions, his money, combined with Indian manpower and expertise, could provide an ideal partnership of mutual benefit.

The fact that the Shah grasped the Indian invitation enthusiastically was apparent from such projects as Kudremukh. And there were growing indications of an effort by the two countries to project the burgeoning relationship into the strategic field. Where such efforts would have led India became an academic question with the fall of the Shah and the birth of the Iranian revolution.

The result was that India was left with no real interlocutor in West Asia. India's own domestic problems merely tended to accentuate the trend towards a less activist role in the region. Rajiv Gandhi's personal rapport with King Hussein of Jordan was not a real policy option, and India's main symbolic ally remained the Palestine Liberation Organisation and its leader Yasser Arafat.

Indeed, India had been consistent in its support to the main Fatah faction of the PLO. But the PLO remained a movement, not a government, and could not, from India's point of view, serve as one. And the PLO itself was beset with a number of problems: exclusion from Lebanon and the Syrian-backed efforts of the Abu Musa faction to dislodge Arafat from the organisation's leadership.

The six-month-long uprising in the Israeli-occupied territories of the West Bank and the Gaza Strip had two consequences. It brought to the fore the PLO—the organisation and its leader won the ringing endorsement of the Arab summit in Algiers, from which Egypt was necessarily excluded, and it forced the Arab states to pay attention to a problem they had swept away under the carpet. The fact that Washington had recognised the untenability of continued Israeli occupation of the territories was clear from the Shultz Plan and the incessant journeys the US secretary of state had made in the region.

Divided Arabs

The Arab world remained divided, despite the endorsement of the PLO at Algiers. The one thread that united the member nations was a healthy respect for Israeli power, in addition to the undoubted emotional appeal that forced the Arab states to appear to hasten the process of Palestinian emancipation. The truth was that many countries of the region are beset with their own problems. Gradually, Egypt was emerging out of its isolation but it could not join the Arab League because its treaty commitments with Israel conflicted with the League's charter.

Jordan knew that it was sitting on a powder keg, with a majority of its population being Palestinian and the West Bank's future still undetermined. King Hussein wisely went along in supporting an independent Palestinian state although everyone felt that a likely solution to the problem of the West Bank, at least in the first stage, would lie in a confederation with Jordan. The Arab world was also suitably wary of the shock waves of the Iranian revolution of Ayatollah Khomeini although each state in the region was forced to make compromises to denote its religiosity.

Syria occupied an interesting position in the Arab world. It had, of course, its own problems, chiefly in Lebanon, which it viewed as falling in its sphere of influence. But Lebanon was proving to be a difficult problem, with religious and ethnic groups and the factions of the PLO tearing it apart. Besides, the Syrian Golan Heights still remained under Israeli occupation.

Syria was secular in its official orientation and traditionally took a radical stance. After a succession of coups, President Assad had provided his country with a long period of stability although this has come at the price of an oppressive state structure and the propagation of a personality cult which was remarkable. Interestingly, Syria alone among the major Arab states maintained a linkage with Khomeini's Iran for which it was rewarded in the form of economic assistance.

President Assad had shown a great measure of flexibility in dealing with his problems. Following the uprising in the occupied territories, Syria and Jordan were working in tandem. The Palestinian uprising and Abu Jihad's murder by suspected Israeli agents in Tunis also helped bring Assad and Arafat together for a face-to-face meeting. Syrian reservations had not been allayed because Arafat had proved far too shrewd and independent for Assad's linking.

Syria had sought to buy American goodwill by helping the process of the release of Western hostages in Lebanon. President Assad was seeking American understanding, if not help, in resolving the Lebanon problem, particularly in relation to the Moronite Christians. Syria had, of course, close relations with the Soviet Union.

For India, Syria provided as good a window on the Arab world as was available. In immediate terms, there was a measure of similarity in the view of the two countries in relation to Afghanistan. Outside Iran, few countries in the region would want an Iranian-style regime in Afghanistan but they chose to be guided by Pakistani perceptions and interests in this respect. There was also some sympathy in Syria for India in the context of its problems with Pakistan. Pakistan's close relationship with Saudi Arabia and alignment with the United States would also seem to militate against Syrian interests.

There was, therefore, some basis for a closer Indo-Syrian relationship, but it would be foolhardy to exaggerate the similarities. While giving Rajiv Gandhi head of state treatment during his stay, the Syrians underlined the long Indian neglect of this relationship. In the short term, the very fact of the Prime Ministerial visit served to the balance the Indian relationship with the PLO.

The Syrians are inheritors of a long and distinguished history and although officially they forswear any ambition for building a Greater Syria, except in the cultural sense, they believe in a more glorious future destiny.

Missing the Boat

In just over a decade, a major world development had caught India totally unprepared for the second time. When Soviet troops marched into Afghanistan, the caretaker Prime Minister, Charan Singh, was in office and, understandably, was without a clue on how to react to the Soviet ambassador informing him of a dangerous twist to events in India's immediate neighbourhood—after the event.

Again, with events moving at an unbelievable speed, with the Berlin Wall breached, the External Affairs Ministry remained unmanned at the political level. Both the minister, P. V. Narasimha Rao, and his minister of state, Natwar Singh, left the store unattended for some two weeks to put all they had into their election campaigns. Their thoughts were far removed from the Berlin Wall.

Yet the happenings in East Europe, particularly in East Germany, were set to transform Europe and the world. They would inevitably have a major impact on India's relations with the East and the West as the post-war structure decreed at Yalta was in the process of a transformation.

Not even Mikhail Gorbachev could have anticipated the speed with which his revolutionary concepts of *glasnost* and *perestroika* would take East Europe by storm. Solidarity rode to power in the first partially free elections in Poland in 40 years. The Hungarian Communist Party decided to transform itself into a West European-style social democratic party, with free multi-party elections slated.

Even more remarkably, the German Democratic Republic's *éminence grise*, Erich Honecker, was swept out of office and power in a hurricane.

The youngest politburo member, Egon Krenz, took charge as hundreds of thousands demonstrated for freedom and thousands made their way to the West through Hungary and other East European countries.

And lo and behold, Krenz decided to punch holes in the Berlin Wall and give his countrymen unhindered exit in a desperate bid to stem the tide. Krenz held on to the two tenets: the communist system should remain and so should the country's commitment to the Warsaw Pact. At the same time, he promised free elections and a package of reforms to correct what were described as distortions in the socialist system. Demonstrators, in their tens of thousands, continued to demand more; they remained to be convinced of their leaders' good faith.

In an instant, as it were, the East German events transformed the comfortable assumptions of the post-war world. Gorbachev, having helped put an end to the Cold War era though his "new thinking" on foreign policy predicated upon *glasnost* and *perestroika* at home, unveiled his concept of the "Common European Home". But East European events had overtaken Gorbachev because they called into question the sanctity of the present borders between East and West Germany.

The reunification of the two Germanies was now firmly on the world agenda as the two superpowers and West Germany and its European allies scrambled to man the barricades. Henry Kissinger believed that the reunification would come about in 10 years, if not five. What was worrying the two superpower capitals and many in West Europe were the consequences of a possible reunification.

President George Bush had welcomed the breach in the Berlin Wall and changes in East Germany, but the underlying mood in Washington was cautious. In a sense, recent developments called into question the future military role of the United States in Europe and with it the role of the North Atlantic Treaty Organisation. West Germany was the frontline state in the East–West confrontation, with massive allied military equipment on its soil and large numbers of American and other allied troops.

Soviet Dilemma

While welcoming the changes in East Europe, partly influenced by Gorbachev, Moscow had been careful to underline the warning that the post-war borders in Europe were inviolable. In other words, the fact that East Germans could now freely visit the other Germany did not imply that the borders between the two states did not exist. However, given the continuing ferment in East Germany and the groundswell of opinion in West Germany, Moscow might be in no position to enforce its writ, except at an unacceptable cost.

West Germany's European allies' anxieties related to the economic might of a reunified Germany and its temptation to impose its dominance on Europe. President François Mitterrand called an emergency summit of the European Economic Community to come up with a collective response. The most notable outcome of the summit was a public assurance given by West Germany's Helmut Kohl of his country's continuing enthusiasm for the EEC and the Western alliance.

President Bush and Gorbachev would have much to talk about in their informal summit off Malta. The two Germanies would provide the central focus of their political discussions and they were, ironically, one in wanting to arrest the speed of future developments. But the question that would remain to be answered was how far they could moderate the hurricane.

German Reunification

President Mitterrand's attempt was to speed up the economic integration further to tie West Germany to the West's mast. Opinion in West Germany was divided over reunification, with the Christian Demacrats being more enthusiastic about it than the Social Democrats. But given the choice, no West German politician could survive by refusing to countenance the reunion of the "Fatherland".

The conventional wisdom was that the Soviet price for the reunification of the two Germanies would be the neutralisation of the two. But Nato and the Warsaw Pact would lose much of their relevance if events in the two Germanies would push them into a reunion.

What consequences would the dramatic developments in East Germany have on India? For one thing, a possible change in the timetable of the EEC's integration would inevitably affect India's trade strategy. Second, India would need to accord Germany a far higher priority in trade and political consultations. Third, the political consequences of a reunified Germany on the world would be many-sided.

If the US military commitment to West Europe was reduced dramatically, would Washington wish to increase its forces in other regions such as the Persian Gulf and the Indian Ocean? Besides, since Gorbachev could hardly have foreseen the time-frame for the "Common European Home" as it was finally likely to emerge, would Moscow speed up the bridge-building exercise with Japan and focus more on East Asia?

If a reunited Germany were to impose its dominance on Europe, in particular in dealings with the East, what corrective action would other West European nations take? Unlike today, France and Britain would discover that they had a common language, and perhaps the smaller West European nations would coalesce around them.

The irony was that events often stood conventional wisdom on its head. Washington had feared for long that one of the Soviet objectives was to de-couple it from Europe. A reunion of the two Germanies could achieve that purpose, irrespective of Soviet wishes. Gorbachev's hypothesis on the "Common European Home" was that it would be a gradual gentlemanly exercise which would respect accepted European frontiers, with the reunification of the two Germanies not in the intermediate agenda.

At Sea

The cut and thrust of the first debates in the new Parliament had demonstrated the emergence of the Congress strategy in seeking to pull down the Vishwanath Pratap Singh government. It was a two-pronged attack: to paint the National Front government as being subservient to the United States and the West in general, and to bring to the surface the underlying contradictions of the communists' "unconditional" support to it.

The first opportunity was provided by the American invasion of Panama and the mild New Delhi reaction to it. But the Congress had subsequently expanded the charges against the government by bringing in the trade disputes with the US, symbolised by "Super 301" and the continuing negotiations in the General Agreement on Tariffs and Trade forum on such issues as intellectual property rights and services. The former American ambassador's newspaper interview suggesting that the V. P. Singh government would be more amenable to seeing the virtues of the American position was grist to the Congress mill.

The message the Congress was seeking to send out was that ideologically the new government tilted to the United States and would be unable to protect vital Indian interests. Thereby, it was taunting the communists to stand up and be counted while trying to refurbish its own leftist credentials.

The communists, who had chosen to support the National Front government for their own opportunistic reasons, were unlikely to be easily provoked, but the Congress tactic would make life more difficult for them. Above all, it struck at a vulnerable chink in the National Front armour: its almost total immersion in the domestic agenda without any great interest in or understanding of the world.

The first weeks of the National Front government had, indeed, highlighted the inward-looking nature of the government. Its initial dealings with Sri Lanka and Nepal represented more a change of stance than policy. While a friendly posture was useful in dealing with sensitive neighbours, it could not be confused with policy or national interests. For perfectly understandable reasons, our neighbours, as others, were happy to deal with a government in New Delhi that was perceived to be weak.

The bloody events in Romania, culminating in the success of the revolution and the downfall and execution of the hated Ceausescu, underlined the limitations of the new government in the field of foreign policy. Days after the event, there was silence in New Delhi, the government initially remaining content with letting a Janata Dal spokesman welcome the end of the reign of terror.

The epoch-making developments in Romania came at the end of a breathtaking series of events in Eastern Europe as one country after another repudiated its communist masters, with the envisaged reunion of the two Germanies foreshadowing the end of 40 years of the post-War dispensation. First, India was too wrapped up in the election and campaign fever to pay much attention to Europe. And, with the accession of the National Front to power, foreign affairs had been considerably downgraded.

As the Janata Dal's performance in the parliamentary elections dramatically demonstrated, foreign policy issues did not win or lose elections. Foreign affairs were on the periphery of the Dal's manifesto, with the little attention span the party had for events abroad devoted almost entirely to neighbours. But the consequences of a national government paying little heed to dramatic changes in the world were a different matter.

The Janata Dal had successfully merged the corruption issue represented by the Bofors scandal with the nation's security, unfairly denigrating the gun in the process. The Congress was attempting to elevate the issue of foreign policy to a matter of national prestige and the lack of the new government's interest in it as being tantamount to a betrayal of national interest.

Congress Contradictions

There were obvious contradictions in the Congress stand. It was the Rajiv Gandhi government that took Indo-US relations a considerable stage further in coaxing high technology items out of the United States and in the increased interaction between officials and politicians of the two sides in the defence and other fields. Its greatest contribution in this field was perhaps to take Indo-US relations out of the evocative national agenda. Few paid much heed to the standard communist rhetoric on the alleged American perfidy.

The previous government's policy made obvious sense because in an increasingly non-ideological world, with the superpowers seeking to bury the Cold War, normal and civil relations with the United States were to India's advantage. With the Soviet Union's new domestic agenda and the ferment in Eastern Europe, Indo-Soviet relations were bound to be less exclusive in nature.

Such contradictions were hardly likely to deter the Congress from painting the new government as being pro-American to show up the nature of the communists' support for it and to cash in on the arrested political development in India in terms of the country's failure to surmount the confines of clichés in the new world. In view of the poverty prevailing in India, it was still fashionable to be left and pro-left after communist countries were abandoning their outdated and unworkable ideological prescriptions.

In a larger sense, the Congress had a point in bringing to the fore issues of foreign policy, albeit for its partisan advantage. India was too large a country to shut itself off from the world. The danger, in that case, would be that the new and old power centres would reorder the world to their advantage, and to India's disadvantage.

The new external affairs minister, I. K. Gujral, is a capable man with some experience of diplomacy. But he had to operate within the confines of an insular party and government. Besides, with his services frequently required for firefighting operations in Punjab and Kashmir, he could not devote his full attention to his primary charge.

It was already clear that the orientation of the new leaders and the minority nature of the government would add up to the country taking a low-profile posture in world affairs. This would give the Congress more opportunities to show up the National Front weakness. The greater the contrast between the Rajiv Gandhi government's basically successful and often high-profile foreign policy, the greater would be the Congress onslaught on the National Front for demoting India to the status of a third rate power.

From the country's point of view, it would be a great pity if Congress partisan welfare were to combine with the new government's insularity to make a plaything of foreign policy. The country needed to pay more, rather than less, attention to foreign affairs in an era of dramatic changes even as it should seek to resolve major national issues.

As parliamentary debates showed, the National Front would seek to meet the Congress challenge by pitting domestic issues against the pursuit of India's foreign policy goals. This was not an adequate answer, and the National Front might discover that a foreign policy disaster, through a wrong decision or neglect, could rub off on to its domestic standing.

Taking Fright

Few tears were being shed for India in the world as the V. P. Singh government picked up the pieces of its policy—or non-policy—in relation to Iraq's invasion of Kuwait and the Gulf crisis it had caused. Having followed a weak-kneed policy in bending over backwards in not displeasing President Saddam Hussein, India had met with a swift retribution at Iraq's hands.

For despite Iraq's rhetoric, the real hostages of the Gulf crisis were not the few thousand Western men remaining in Iraq and Kuwait, the women and children being helpfully ferried home by chartered Iraqi planes, but the hundreds of thousands of Indians and other Asians. The Iraqis had told India that it should break the United Nations sanctions to send food or let its people starve. Or they should make the painful desert journey to Jordan, live in hell holes of camps until they were ferried out.

Not only did India make the gentlest of statements asking for the withdrawal of Iraqi troops from Kuwait but the External Affairs Minister, I. K. Gujral, went to Baghdad and Kuwait to fraternise with Saddam—the bear hug of the two men was repeatedly shown on Iraqi and Kuwaiti television. On Iraq's orders, India promptly closed down the Indian embassy in Kuwait.

The *quid pro quo* of this journey was that Iraq would help get the sizable Indian population out. Iraqi planes, it was suggested, would directly fly out the Indians. Indian ships could dock in Kuwait to take more Indians out. Then came the riders even as Doordarshan was showing clips of interviews, or how well Iraqi soldiers were treating Indians in Kuwait. Iraqi planes taking Indians out should be stocked with food and medical supplies on their return journey. Ships should come laden with food to evacuate Indians. Finally, Iraq washed its hands of feeding Indians in Kuwait and Iraq.

While Indian officials were quick to point to the West's double standards in paying the Iraqis for chartered planes to get its women and children out, despite United Nations sanctions, they were reticent in discussing Iraq's behaviour. Yet Saddam's message was clear: no one respected a coward or a weak-kneed nation. Having sized up the Indian government, Saddam knew that he could use it to his own purposes—get India to raise hell to break the United Nations embargo.

Why did the V. P. Singh government behave as it did? From the beginning, it was clear that India had two immediate compulsions: the safety of its nationals in Kuwait and Iraq and ensuring supplies of oil. The latter was more a question of price than of availability because the other oil producing countries were only too willing to raise production quotas.

There were other compulsions: the close relations with Iraq and its relatively secular approach to such questions as those of Kashmir and the considerable trade potential. Second, the building of a large Western armada on India's doorstep was an unwelcome development for the risks it presented and the opportunity it gave Pakistan to serve American strategic purposes and claim its reward in military assistance. Third, the threat of choking off India's trade lifeline to the West involved obvious risks. Fourth, instead of the "peace dividend" the end of the

Cold War promised—a greater economic interaction with Europe and West Asia—the Gulf crisis posed the threat of war.

It spoke of the nature of the V. P. Singh government that it concentrated on the first two immediate compulsions without paying any attention to the wider ramifications. What was even worse was the manner in which it chose to seek its first objective, oblivious of the exhibition the country was making of itself. And in the process, India gave a handle to Saddam to extract the last drop of propaganda by forcing New Delhi to fight Iraq's battle against UN sanctions. Saddam had shown little respect for the welfare of the large Indian community in Iraq or Kuwait.

What would India have done, given the brazen nature of the Iraqi invasion and annexation of Kuwait? First, India should have activated its diplomacy in the major non-aligned capitals, if non-alignment had any relevance left.

A Failed Test

Yugoslavia, the then chairman of the Non-alignment Movement, was preoccupied with domestic events and two of its republics even questioned the need for non-alignment for their country. It was, therefore, for India to take the initiative in testing the non-aligned capitals in the crisis. It should have implied Gujral going to Cairo, Algiers and Tunis, rather than Baghdad and Kuwait, for attempting to evolve a common position.

The Arab world was split down the middle and it was important for India to consult Arab leaders on both sides of the fence to play its non-aligned card. Instead, Gujral gave the impression of studiously avoiding any Arab capital ranged against Iraq's action. And it proved disastrous for India because it became a partisan in an essentially Arab quarrel, giving a handle to Saddam to treat New Delhi as of no consequence.

India's belated efforts to retrieve the situation came too late in the day. Writing letters to the permanent members of the UN Security Council or to the two foreign ministers of the superpowers carried little conviction. Nor did the ultimate stance adopted by India about the need for a peaceful resolution of the crisis on the lines of the Soviet stand have much meaning. And no one was impressed by the fact that a group of three non-aligned foreign ministers, including that of India, met at Belgrade some five weeks after the Iraqi invasion of Kuwait.

Having lost sight of the wider implications of the Gulf crisis and having hesitated in calling a spade a spade, India's foreign policy had become hostage to the Indian hostages in Kuwait and Iraq—the Indians who could not get out of these countries remained hostages. Reaching food to the Indians in Kuwait and Iraq while Saddam kept the

Westerners he reviled in great comfort had become the sum total of Indian ambitions.

The answer to India's sorry plight in the world lay in the nature of the Janata Dal. The main constituent of the National Front government remained parochial, with little interest in or understanding of the wider world. Its ken had been limited to the neighbourhood and of the three visits V. P. Singh made outside the area, one had been the obligatory trip to Moscow, a ceremonial visit to Namibia and a journey to Kuala Lumpur for a non-aligned group meeting.

There was no attempt among the political leadership in Delhi to comprehend the amazing changes taking place in the world and to reassess India's role. While the Non-aligned Movement suffered from atrophy and the end of the Cold War gave a new twist to the past half century's alignments and increased, rather than reduced, the potential for regional conflicts, India could not remain mired in its old attitudes.

It was fashionable among the Janata Dal leaders to decry the Rajiv Gandhi regime's interest in the world and his frequent travels abroad. But the anti-foreign policy postures of the government were a luxury India simply could not afford. The world might not have become a global village, but as the events in the Gulf proved, developments in one part of the world could have immediate and debilitating consequences for the country.

By its hesitancy and pro-Saddam attitude, the National Front first ruled itself out of playing any meaningful role in the Gulf crisis. And after Saddam had shown India the door, the country was left simpering and grasping at straws in getting its hostages out of Kuwait and Iraq.

Out of Depth

India had, not for the first time, found itself totally out of depth in coping with the world and the country's place in it. Charan Singh was the caretaker Prime Minister when Soviet troops marched into Afghanistan. But even that sorry display by India paled into insignificance in the face of the momentous events in the Soviet Union or what would become of it — events that were changing the face of the world and future power equations.

Quite apart from the kind of reaction India mustered, the Congress, which had been constantly berating the two previous minority governments for neglect, and worse, in the field of foreign policy, was displaying a strange lack of will in pursuing Indian interests. It was as if, having returned to office albeit as a minority government, it was suffering a case of nerves. Self-confidence was a quality totally lacking in an area that dwarfed all others in the consequences it would have.

The surprise appointment of Madhavsinh Solanki as Foreign Minister, one had assumed, had been made because P. V. Narasimha Rao, who had two spells as Foreign Minister, wanted to be in the driver's seat in making foreign policy. This would have been a perfectly legitimate arrangement had the Prime Minister been in reality the Foreign Minister as well. In any event, the executive head of the government had become the most important foreign policy-maker.

But Narasimha Rao had shown little interest in assuming the reins of foreign policy-making and Solanki's modesty in understanding the vast complexities of his new office, though praiseworthy in itself, had failed to measure up to the demands of the situation. It was patently unfair to put a new minister through a crash course in a field which required a level of understanding that was taxing the veterans.

To make matters worse, India had been witnessing guerrilla action within the Narasimha Rao cabinet in the field of foreign policy. The Home Minister, S. B. Chavan, was seeking to fill the vacuum that existed in the making and articulation of foreign policy with a passion that immediately raised questions.

Was he articulating a new policy different from that being pursued, insofar as it was, by the government? If so, was he building his own constituency on the assumption that in a bewildering world of vanishing myths and what were until recently verities, enough people in India would want to remain locked up in a bygone era of the two power blocs and America-bashing to cheer Chavan's vision of the future of India rooted in the make-believe world of the past?

A Loose Cannon

First, we had the astounding statement from Chavan all but accusing the United States of possible complicity in the assassination of Rajiv Gandhi. Then, we were treated to a full-scale attack on the United Nations at the unlikely forum of the All India Small and Medium Newspapers Federation in New Delhi.

Chavan's attack on the United Nations was, it seems, a thin veneer to train his guns on the United States again. A Press Trust of India report on the event said the minister cautioned small and medium newspapers against "an attempt by international organisations to project only one kind of thinking".

On the United Nations, the Home Minister suggested that the international organisation had lost its importance "the day it took upon itself the role of policing in the Gulf War". In his view, the UN should have used persuasive powers to attain its objectives, and the sending of the US army into Iraq would have "consequences and results" for the international community.

In the past, during the rather brief and varying tenures of non-Congress governments at the Centre, ministers blithely made pronouncements on all subjects under the sun, without regard to accepted policy formulations of the government and without consulting the minister concerned. One of the merits of a Congress government, one had assumed, was that such anarchy in the articulation of policy did not exist.

Parliamentary government functions on the basis of collective responsibility. A minister who disagrees with the Prime Minister's, or a joint, decision has the freedom to tender his resignation. And when he publicly chooses to question government policy in an area outside his responsibilities, he puts himself outside the pale.

Narasimha Rao needed the support of every section of the Congress, in addition to elements of the opposition, to survive in office. If Chavan was seizing upon this weakness of the government to pursue his own political agenda, he was weakening Narasimha Rao's position and jeopardising Indian interests.

That there might be other foreign elements, in addition to the Sri Lanka Liberation Tigers, in the assassination of Rajiv Gandhi was a perfectly legitimate field of investigation. But for the Home Minister of the country publicly to cast aspersions on the United States without a shred of evidence could be ascribed only to deep-seated anti-Americanism and a desire to pander to a constituency, in addition to hampering Indian efforts further to improve relations with the United States.

The United Nations' role in Iraq was bound to remain a controversial question for a long time. The enormity of Iraq's crime is marching into another sovereign country and annexing it was unparalleled in post-World War II history. President Saddam misjudged the era and the phase of a new Soviet foreign policy following the virtual end of the Cold War to an extent that seemed incomprehensible to an outsider.

The United States used its advantage of being the only functioning superpower and the Soviet need for assistance from the West to build up an alliance with other Western nations and Arab states even as it began ferrying vast masses of men and fighting machines to the region for a military showdown, if necessary. At the same time, Soviet cooperation meant that the UN Security Council became a handy instrument for pursuing American strategic and political interests.

The five permanent members of the Security Council, with the US in the driver's seat, took the war to Iraq in the face of continuing defiance by Saddam Hussein. And out of this operation, hopes were raised that the original purpose of the UN Security Council as the world's policing agency could now be fulfilled. Such a role was, in fact, envisaged by Mikhail Gorbachev in his book *Perestroika* before events overwhelmed him and his country.

Sad Days

Those were sad days for India—sad not only because of the muddle we were witnessing in a period of political transition from a single dominant party rule to a new dispensation whose precise contours were not quite clear. They were sad because we had chosen to advertise our domestic weaknesses to the world.

The view of the Gulf War from India was so jaundiced and partisan that it bore little relation to the conflict or to the country's abiding interests. It was one thing for the government to give the impression of stirring itself on the issue through the perambulations of the External Affairs Minister, V. C. Shukla, or to try to activate the UN Security Council. It was quite another for the other political parties to see the conflict through the prism of the Muslim vote banks with an eye on the next elections.

Vishwanath Pratap Singh, who displayed a singular lack of interest in the world beyond the country's immediate neighbourhood during his stint as Prime Minister, now waxed eloquent over the Chandra Shekhar government's alleged misdemeanours in relation to the Gulf conflict. The Communist parties had the virtue of consistency in condemning the United States on the conflict as on everything else, but the Congress of Rajiv Gandhi was also getting into the act in the hope of garnering Muslim votes.

Rajiv Gandhi's missive to Chandra Shekhar could only serve the purpose of distancing himself from the government's policy, or lack of it, on the Gulf. To suggest that more time should have been given to peace initiatives before launching the attacks after the United Nations deadline of January 15 was saying nothing new. And to try to call a session of the UN Security Council was a barren road.

The Bharatiya Janata Party had at least the merit of refraining from offering a grand formula for the resolution of the crisis. But for most parties, the refuelling of American planes in India on their way to and from the Gulf region had given a godsend opportunity to berate the government on something more substantial than airy formulae.

What India needed was a man of the vision of Jawaharlal Nehru who could examine the concept of non-alignment in the light of a changed world and had the courage to scrap it. Until such a leader emerged on the scene, it was well to recognise reality about the Gulf conflict. India had largely become irrelevant to resolving the conflict because of its domestic problems and because of its failure to build a new nucleus which would have a greater impact on world affairs than a moribund Non-aligned Movement.

The Gulf conflict as it had developed against the background of a fast-changing world proved that President Saddam Hussein over-estimated his power and underestimated world reaction in invading and annexing Kuwait. The United States' response was almost immediate and it chose to go through the United Nations machinery, instead of acting unilaterally, in a successful effort to carry the Soviet Union and China with it. In the meantime, it built up a coalition against Iraq's Saddam regime.

Although it is arguable whether the United Nations should have imposed a deadline, there had been opportunities enough for Iraq to withdraw from the brink through a whole range of intermediaries. Saddam, for his own reasons, chose not to do so and sought to link his indefensible action in relation to Kuwait to the wider Palestinian issue and gave it a religious colour to gather support.

Before the January 15 deadline, the position of the US-led anti-Saddam coalition was clear to Iraq as it was to the world. If Iraq withdrew from Kuwait, no harm would come to it. But if it chose not to, not only would Kuwait be freed but Iraq's military potential would be sought to be destroyed.

The offensive of the US and its allies came sooner than expected, but having placed its superpower reputation on the line by inducting an armada into the region, by sending more than 400,000 troops and by deploying an awesome panoply of air power, President Bush had to work to fulfil his maximalist aims. In other words, Iraq itself had to be punished in addition to Kuwait being liberated.

The US and its allies were relying so heavily on air power to pulverise Kuwait, Basra and other targets in Iraq for two reasons. They wanted to reduce casualties on their side in the ground fighting. But a second important reason was that once Kuwait was liberated, the Americans would have no justification for destroying Iraq's military and economic potential.

Iraq's Folly

One of the many miscalculations made by President Saddam was to overlook the cardinal fact that with the domestic convulsions and changes in the Soviet Union, Mikhail Gorbachev's priorities had changed. The Soviet Union became not only inward-looking but was seeking crucial help from the US and the West in reordering its domestic order. It had, therefore, given up its balancing role vis-à-vis the United States in international crises.

It must at the same time be conceded that President Saddam made it extremely difficult for the Soviet Union or many of Iraq's other well-wishers to help him get out of a crisis he created. His obduracy in refusing to leave Kuwait, his intemperate rhetoric and the crude propaganda efforts made by his regime defeated the most zealous of the peace-makers, including the UN secretary-general, Javier Perez de Cuellar.

Although the outcome of the conflict could lead to only one conclusion, Saddam had raised the political stakes for the United States. His effort to combine Arab nationalism with Islam while linking them to the Palestinian issue had been a marked success. At the terrible cost of largescale destruction of his country, he was creating conditions for new convulsions in the region, which would turn increasingly hostile to the American military presence.

Given this background, the Americans and their principal Western allies would not stop short of achieving their immediate military aims. In any event, the Non-aligned Movement was moribund and India, in its prevailing state, could voice little more than platitudes.

While waiting out events in the Gulf, it was incumbent on India to assess the consequences of the Gulf conflict on the geopolitical map of the region and how it would affect the country in the wake of the collapse of the bipolar world. A new era of instability in the region was likely, and such instability would snowball if a serious attempt was not made to resolve the Palestinian issue. Israel and the United States would need to summon the political will to end a festering sore that made even men like Saddam Hussein credible to a large part of the world.

Belated Decision

India's decision to grant full-scale diplomatic recognition to Israel in 1992, surprising only in its timing, posed two interesting questions. What did it mean for India's relations with West Asia? Second, to what extent did it signify a rethinking of the country's traditional assumptions of its foreign policy?

India's earlier vote at the United Nations for rescinding the "zionism is racism" resolution was a trial balloon launched to test the country's reaction and its impact further afield. There was satisfaction on both scores for New Delhi's policy-makers, and it increasingly became clear that after China's recognition of Israel, apart from the earlier Russian decision, there was little to be gained by a step-by-step approach and if India had to make residual capital from the move, it had better go the whole hog.

One need not tarry over the criticism of the Indian decision dictated by a dated ideology or a mind-set formed in concrete in the early years of independence. But, having missed the bus in the early fifties by recognising Israel without agreeing to full-scale diplomatic relations, Indian policy was inhibited by two factors. They were the sensitivities of the country's Muslim population against the shadow of the sub-continent's partition and India's vigorous economic and other relations with West Asia.

Thanks to the dramatic changes in the world and American success in getting Israel and the Arabs to the historic peace conference in Madrid, forging full diplomatic ties with Israel presented itself in a new light. The danger of adverse Arab reaction was minimal and the scope of Pakistani mischief-making potential in the region was further reduced by the recognition accorded to Israel by Pakistan's traditional friend and ally, China.

The more interesting point was that, after months of fumbling, the Indian foreign-policy making establishment had decided to review its old policy in the light of a starkly changed world. It took months of agonising and some hard knocks for New Delhi to acknowledge the fact that the old Soviet Union had indeed vanished and that the technical successor state, Russia, had a very different way of doing business with countries such as India.

Beset with domestic problems, particularly in the field of economy, and the minority nature of the government, P. V. Narasimha Rao gave low priority to foreign policy. He was content to let the establishment chant the old slogans, hopelessly dated as they were, and sought to change the focus indirectly by emphasising the economic and trade interests in the pursuit of foreign policy goals.

That the government's effort was totally inadequate to the demands of the changing world was apparent in many ways. There was the embarrassment of India hugging a 20-year extension of the friendship treaty, complete with its security clauses, with a Soviet Union that was no more. The country's formulations of non-alignment sounded quaint against the backdrop of a new world where the countervailing Soviet presence was no more, with the United States remaining as the only superpower in the military field while competing power centres were emerging in Europe and Japan.

India's journey in redefining its national interests in the foreign policy field in the new world—there was no order on the horizon, of President George Bush's description or other countours—had just begun. The full recognition of Israel meant that New Delhi was at least prepared to take a second look at some of the hoary postulates of its foreign policy.

The decision to recognise Israel gave New Delhi some elbow room in the pursuit of its policy, but the major hurdles remained to be crossed. It could of course be argued that India's new economic policy projections by themselves indicated a change in political direction. And since original thinking is not the forte of Indian politicians, the old rhetoric held sway.

But the urgent need was to take the problem of redefining Indian foreign policy head on. The two areas crying out for attention were our adherence to non-alignment and the placing of India in the new world.

Shared Problems

It is axiomatic that India, belonging as it does to the South, had many interests in common with the developing world. Therefore, it needed a forum to consult other similarly-placed countries to frame a joint strategy as also to negotiate with the North. The real point was whether the Non-aligned Movement, which played a notable role in the world that was, remained the best vehicle for achieving these objectives.

The Group of 77 developing countries—the actual number was far higher—was an even more amorphous outfit than the Non-aligned Movement. Indeed, the Egyptian proposal to change the name of NAM had great merit because it would signify that the developing world was moving with the times in jettisoning its old ideological baggage.

To argue about the virtues of non-alignment on the philosophical plane took us nowhere. India had to deal with a real world and that world had changed beyond recognition. If it had to preserve the name, redefining the characteristics of NAM to bring it in tune with 1992 was necessary. With Yugoslavia having surrendered its privileges as NAM's chairman long before the movement's next summit, there was something comical about India swearing undying loyalty to it.

The fact that the Cold War mind-set was no longer operative opened up immense possibilities in placing India in the new world. There was an intensification of Indo-US relations in the diplomatic, economic and defence fields. New Delhi needed to do some homework on how far this relationship could grow without detriment to the country's interests.

The US triumph in the Gulf War came with the rider that it could no longer be the world's sole policeman. In other words, in protecting American interests, the United States needed friendly regional powers to mind the store. Such a regional power status for India could be compatible with the country's own interests, as long as the convergent and divergent interests were made clear.

India's traditional psychological propensity to invest all its political capital in a relationship with one major country was a handicap. A supreme effort was needed to get out of this trap in the emerging multi-polar world. There were several competing forces in the world and India would be foolish to limit its options to one power centre.

This problem brought to the fore the domestic limitations in the pursuit of a sane foreign policy. Apart from India's communists who, by and large, wanted to live in the past, there were any number of cold warriors who refused to leave the world of the two-power equation. In the face of a challenge to Nehru's nationalism by the Bharatiya Janata Party, the old loyalists drew comfort from living in a time warp.

But the world was no respecter of national fallings and foibles. And the ideological lodestar was no longer a reliable guide to chart the country's future course. Rather, India's political establishment needed to move away from many of the old postulates—valid as they might have been in another era—to an assessment of the real world.

Indian Interests

It is a truism, repeated times without number, that a country does not have permanent friends, only permanent interests. It is then all the more amazing how often this piece of conventional wisdom is disregarded. Independent India's history is replete with instances of our forgetfulness in respecting the old adage, the *Hindi-Chini Bhai Bhai* phase being only the most glaring example.

Indeed, India as a nation and people suffered from an excess of emotionalism in relations with the outside world. India's web of relations with China, Bangladesh and Nepal would have followed a steadier course had we been less emotional. And in seeking to tackle the riddle of Pakistan, our emotionalism had stood in the way of understanding the limits of mutuality of interests.

Was India then about to commit itself to another assault on national interests by displaying its brand of emotionalism in relation to Israel? There was a new warming of relations with Israel and our television presenters blithely announced that the two countries faced similar problems of terrorism and India sought Israeli advice on how to counter it.

There was no reason why India should not have close and beneficial relations with Israel. India could share their agricultural expertise, import their high-tech weapon systems and indulge in profitable trade in other areas. By any yardstick, Israelis are a remarkable people and, together with Palestinians, represent the brightest men and women in West Asia.

At the same time, India had to consider its national interests in relation to the Arab world. There were some three million Indians in the Gulf states, with about a million in the United Arab Emirates alone. Their remittances home were a useful source of foreign exchange and their earnings abroad had helped to lift countless numbers of people into the middle class on their return home.

Dynamic and modern as it is, Israel is a small territory in an Arab sea. Most disturbingly, it has been locked in a bloody battle with the Palestinians. It was sitting on occupied land, was loath to give it up and had distorted the Oslo peace process by repudiating agreed deadlines while building and expanding Jewish settlements. Israel's ability to dictate terms to the Palestinians was a direct result of the bountiful American support it enjoyed in military and economic assistance and in Washington's guarantee of its security. Thanks to the clout of the American Jewish lobby, Israel exercised much influence on US West Asia policy.

American efforts to mediate reached a climax towards the end of the Clinton presidency when a proposal for the return of some 95 per cent of occupied land on the West Bank and 100 per cent in the Gaza Strip to Palestinians was mooted. The Palestinians would have some kind of sovereignty over holy Muslim sites in Jerusalem. The right of the refugees to return home was left unresolved. The Palestinian leader Arafat was under virtual siege, or felt he was, and did not obtain the assurances he sought. What Bill Clinton and Israeli spokesman later described as Arafat throwing away the best settlement he could have had was plainly untrue. He could not have walked away without satisfying in a measure two cardinal Palestinian demands: the right of refugees' return and unqualified Palestinian sovereignty over East Jerusalem.

Facile Parallel

Television presenters in India who facilely drew an analogy between troubled Kashmir and what was happening in the occupied territories controlled by Israel did the country grievous harm. In Kashmir, India was fighting terrorists trained, armed and financed abroad for the express purpose of fuelling an insurgency. In the Israeli-controlled territories, Palestinians have been fighting a colonial ruler to seek independence. To overlook or erase this vital difference was asking for trouble. Both Israel and India might be fighting militant Muslims, but India could not base its policy on this coincidence.

The whole basis of the Oslo process was the recognition by the Palestinian Authority of the existence of Israel, and India's role should be to use its good relations with Tel Aviv to encourage a reconciliation predicated upon fair play and justice. Washington was zealous about its exclusive role as a mediator and had rebuffed United Nations and European Union mediation, except on the margins and in extending economic assistance to Palestinians.

The new levels of violence and Palestinian suffering flowed from the assumption of office of Ariel Sharon, Washington's toleration of harsh Israeli reprisals and the activities of the Palestinian factions indulging in terrorist acts. India could be a mere sympathetic spectator in the impasse until the situation improved. The hardliner that Sharon is, he won support from the Bush administration whose initial hands-off policy gave the Likud leader all room he needed for pursuing aggressive policies.

The moral of the story is that India should curb its emotionalism to pursue good relations with Israel without forgetting the wider national interests it should promote in the Arab world. These are difficult times for the Arabs because the context in which their relations with the principal West Asian power, the US, were taking shape was changing. For one thing, terrorism had assumed forms detrimental to the Arabs themselves. It refused to be bottled up in one country, as the multi-national terrorist network revealed. Second, the social and political pressures on the Arab regimes had become more pressing.

Once Israelis saw their way to giving Palestinians their birthright, a viable and free state, they would be integrated into their neighbourhood, to everyone's benefit. First, Sharon would have to make way for a more pragmatic leader. It could not be in America's interest to have permanent strife in an area which provided the world with much of its oil. But the Bush administration's policies would have to change as well.

India's role, meanwhile, should be to look after its own interests while seeking the friendship of Israel and the Arab world.

Epilogue

Epilogue

Everything, it seems, runs in cycles in the Israeli–Palestinian confrontation. Hopes alternate with despair, peace talks with violence, and, not unsurprisingly, Israeli hardliners embrace Palestinian suicide bombers to frustrate a settlement because they oppose the land-for-peace deal, despite the Oslo accords, despite the efforts of countless men and women on the two sides.

The injustice of the continuing Israeli occupation of Palestinian land captured in the 1967 war remains, buttressed by a level of unparalleled American support for the nation state of Israel in money, weapons and export of ideologically-inclined Jews. While Palestinians waited for the Oslo process to bring benefits and Israelis constantly delayed meeting obligations, both the Likud and Labour parties in Israel went about diligently building new illegal settlements on occupied land. Settlements particularly proliferated during the term of the supposedly dovish Ehud Barak.

The closest Israelis and Palestinians came to a settlement was in the dying days of the Clinton presidency, at Camp David and at Taba. Americans and Israelis are now unfairly blaming Yasser Arafat for his failure to grasp a rare opportunity. Those who know the twists and turns of these negotiations know that Arafat alone was not to be blamed. There were enough snags in the outline on offer to trip up any leader and the unfortunate tactics of the loner Ehud Barak who had lost parliamentary support, combined with President Clinton's frenzy in achieving a result before his time ran out, were sufficient reasons for the talks' failure.

What Israelis and Palestinians came close to agreeing was the return of the Gaza Strip and some 95 per cent of the West Bank to Palestinians to form a contiguous independent state. There was a less than satisfactory proposal for Palestinians to exercise authority over the holy Muslim sites in East Jerusalem and the right of Palestinian refugees' return was left hanging in the air.

Palestinians would achieve a contiguous independent state, without the right to maintain a standing regular army, and they would be compensated for the land they would lose, chiefly the illegal settlements around Jerusalem to be absorbed by Israel, by equivalent land in Israel proper.

The right of return, an evocative demand for Palestinians, would be finessed by Israel granting a symbolic number permission to return to their original homes while the others would be compensated and settled in the new Palestinian state or elsewhere.

Gloomy Picture

Whatever the finer points of these discussions, such ideas seem far from Israeli thoughts as I write these lines. Ariel Sharon is, for the present, firmly in power, and thanks to the unprecedented support he has won from President George W. Bush, he has been given the licence to do pretty much as he pleases. Not only has Sharon successfully folded his own agenda in the American "war on terror" after the horrific events of September 11, 2001 but he has successfully sold his animosity towards Arafat to the White House, with disastrous results for Palestinians and peace.

Indeed, Sharon has spectacularly exploited the rash of Palestinian suicide bombings to reoccupy Palestinian cities for shorter or longer periods, answered Palestinians with F-16s, helicopter gunships and battle tanks and exercised the self-appropriated right to murder individual Palestinians. Beyond these acts of war, there has been a determined Israeli objective of seeking to destroy the Palestinian will to fight by bombing all the symbols and infrastructure of the Palestinian Authority, and grounding Arafat before declaring him irrelevant and an enemy.

Judging by President Bush's June 24, 2002 speech, he has put America right behind Sharon, to the extent of seeking Arafat's ouster and placing impossible conditions before Palestinians could be given an undefined state in three years without specifying when the clock would start ticking. American attitudes can change but the burden W has placed on what was at best a dying peace process became insupportable.

There are understandable geopolitical and other reasons for America's support of Israel. The zionist pioneers' burning desire for a Jewish state, their ruthless guerrilla war and the support of the West, in particular Britain as the then authority, harbouring a guilty conscience over the holocaust—a European phenomenon—brought Israel into being in a non-European setting. But increasingly, the United States took over the role of chaperoning Israel through the hostile choppy Arabian sea.

The Arab states collectively aided Israel's statehood and expansion as they sought to right a historical wrong through an exaggerated view of their strength and belief in their own overblown rhetoric. It was after the disastrous 1967 war that lost the Arab world the West Bank and Gaza Strip that Egypt's Anwar Sadat decided to act.

Egypt came to the conclusion that discretion was the better part of valour and Sadat successfully sought to sue for peace, realising that the United States would never let Israel go down. The separate peace Sadat made under American auspices got it back the Sinai and massive American assistance at the cost of earning it pariah status in the Arab world. Sadat's successor Hosni Mubarak led his country back into the Arab fold.

It has, indeed, been a recurring theme in the Israeli–Palestinian conflict that Arab states have been divided, each with its own interests and defence arrangements with the very Western powers they sought to vilify, a phenomenon that gathered greater strength after the defeat of Iraq by the American-led coalition. The Nasser phase of pan-Arabism did not last long. And as Ayatollah Khomeini led Iran to a Revolution, he became something of a role model, with Arab masses embracing different versions of Islam, including a radical variety, after their secular God had failed them.

Israeli Ambitions

The fall of the Berlin Wall and the demise of the Soviet Union were further blows for Palestinians who lost the countervailing power to the United States. The Second Gulf War led to the calling of the Madrid peace conference, spawning in turn the Oslo accords. Israeli sabotage stemmed from Tel Aviv's ambivalence towards making peace with Palestinians and security became the watchword after the rash of suicide bombings by desperate Palestinians. Finally ended an Oslo process, observed more in the breach. Since the coming to power of Sharon and the beginning of the Bush presidency, Israeli ambitions have broadened. Left to themselves and with implicit American support, even the last Camp David version of peace is no longer on offer.

When the pendulum in Israel will swing again remains to be seen. Suicide bombings, in more recent times, played into hardline Israeli hands, but before the world condemns them, as it must, it should understand their rationale. Of the two phases of intefada, the first was more productive in placing the Palestinian problem centrestage. Besides, how do a people boxed in by an occupying power using disproportionate force protest against injustice? With the Arab states preoccupied with their own affairs and beholden to the very power that underwrites Israeli actions, where are they to turn? Admittedly, organisations like Hamas have their own agendas and a section of Palestinians, though in a minority, do not accept the legitimacy of a Western-imposed Jewish state in their heartland.

Sharon and his supporters are banking on their ability to turn the clock back in the hope that their free ride on the American "war on terror" will be a long one. Yet it is clear to any rational person that increasing doses of repression are counter-productive and the very objective Israelis seek, peace and security, will prove elusive. More than Palestinians, Israelis are a tortured people because the only way they can legitimise their presence in the eyes of their neighbours and the better part of the world is to give Palestinians a state and justice.

Calamitous Time

During my two visits to Israel I gained the distinct impression that young Israelis want nothing more avidly than to live in a normal nation state. Yet in recent years, the prospect of such a denouement has been receding. In political terms, the end of the Cold War and the September 11 events have been calamitous for Palestinians. At the same time, they have done a great disservice to Israel for giving many Israelis the illusion that they can trick history and justice by retaining Palestinians as vassals.

For its part, the United States administration, increasingly conscious of its unparalleled power in the world, is in an arrogant mood. As history reveals, no post-World War II American administration, with the exception of Eisenhower's, has been able to take on Israelis on a major issue. The hold of Israel on Washington's West Asian policy is phenomenal through the working of the American Jewish lobby. Few American legislators can challenge Israeli interests and remain in the Senate or the House of Representatives. In the wake of September 11, such support from Capitol Hill and the White House has never been more full-throated.

The Saudi origins of Osama bin Laden, the man painted as the evil genius of September 11, and the Saudi nationality of the bulk of those who commandeered civilian American planes to such destructive effect have brought Muslims in general and Arabs in particular under a cloud of suspicion in the popular American imagination, if not in the corridors of power. The prevailing climate in the US has naturally delighted Sharon and his loyalists because it makes it so much easier to paint Palestinians in the same corner.

This interpretation would suggest that only a change in the dominant Israeli mood could induce a US administration to change its attitude to Palestinians having a state of their own. One would hope that the law of cycles will apply to the future as well and more and more Israelis will realise that men of the ilk of Sharon offer no hope for the future. Logically, the Israeli hardliners can only take their country to the status of a perpetual garrison state at the cost of sacrificing the very system they are proud of—democracy. Already, the substantial minority of Israeli Arabs are treated as second class citizens and are distrusted by their Jewish neighbours and the state.

It is sad to see yesterday's persecuted become today's persecutors of a people who have had little to do with the tragic Jewish history in the modern age.